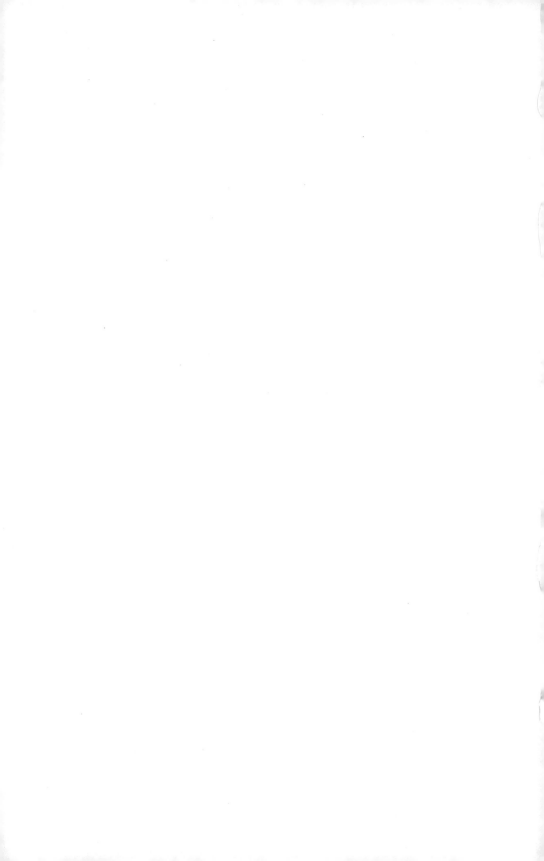

Malignancies of the Upper Gastrointestinal Tract

Editor

DAVID H. ILSON

HEMATOLOGY/ONCOLOGY CLINICS OF NORTH AMERICA

www.hemonc.theclinics.com

Consulting Editors
GEORGE P. CANELLOS
EDWARD J. BENZ JR

June 2024 • Volume 38 • Number 3

ELSEVIER

1600 John F. Kennedy Boulevard • Suite 1800 • Philadelphia, Pennsylvania, 19103-2899

http://www.theclinics.com

HEMATOLOGY/ONCOLOGY CLINICS OF NORTH AMERICA Volume 38, Number 3
June 2024 ISSN 0889-8588, ISBN 13: 978-0-443-29596-6

Editor: Stacy Eastman
Developmental Editor: Shivank Joshi

Hematology/Oncology Clinics (ISSN 0889-8588) is published bimonthly by Elsevier Inc., 360 Park Avenue South, New York, NY 10010-1710. Months of issue are February, April, June, August, October, and December. Business and Editorial Offices: 1600 John F. Kennedy Blvd., Ste. 1800, Philadelphia, PA 19103–2899. Customer Service Office: 3251 Riverport Lane, Maryland Heights, MO 63043. Periodicals postage paid at New York, NY and at additional mailing offices. Subscription prices are $498.00 per year (domestic individuals), $100.00 per year (domestic students/residents), $525.00 per year (Canadian individuals), $100.00 per year (Canadian students/residents), $597.00 per year (international individuals), and $255.00 per year (international students/residents). For institutional access pricing please contact Customer Service via the contact information below. International air speed delivery is included in all *Clinics* subscription prices. All prices are subject to change without notice. **POSTMASTER:** Send address changes to *Hematology/Oncology Clinics of North America*, Elsevier Health Sciences Division, Subscription Customer Service, 3251 Riverport Lane, Maryland Heights, MO 63043. Customer Service (orders, claims, online, change of address): Elsevier Health Sciences Division, Subscription **Customer Service, 3251 Riverport Lane, Maryland Heights, MO 63043. Tel: 1-800-654-2452 (U.S. and Canada); 314-447-8871 (outside U.S. and Canada). Fax: 314-447-8029. E-mail: journalscustomerservice-usa@elsevier.com (for print support)**; **journalsonlinesupport-usa@elsevier.com (for online support)**.

Reprints. For copies of 100 or more, of articles in this publication, please contact the Commercial Reprints Department, Elsevier Inc., 360 Park Avenue South, New York, New York 10010-1710; Tel.: 212-633-3874, Fax: 212-633-3820, E-mail: reprints@elsevier.com.

Hematology/Oncology Clinics of North America is covered in *MEDLINE/PubMed (Index Medicus), EMBASE/ Excerpta Medica, and BIOSIS*.

Printed in the United States of America.

Contributors

CONSULTING EDITORS

GEORGE P. CANELLOS, MD
William Rosenberg Professor of Medicine, Department of Medical Oncology, Dana-Farber Cancer Institute, Boston, Massachusetts, USA

EDWARD J. BENZ Jr, MD
Professor, Pediatrics, Richard and Susan Smith Professor, Medicine, Professor, Genetics, Harvard Medical School, President and CEO Emeritus, Office of the President, Dana-Farber Cancer Institute, Boston, Massachusetts, USA

EDITOR

DAVID H. ILSON, MD, PhD, FASCO, FACP
Attending Physician, Member, Professor or Medicine, Memorial Sloan Kettering Cancer Center, New York, New York, USA

AUTHORS

GHASSAN ABOU-ALFA, MD, MBA
Attending Physician, Department of Medicine, Memorial Sloan Kettering Cancer Center, Professor, Department of Medicine, Weill Medical College, Cornell University, New York, New York, USA; Trinity College Dublin, Dublin, Ireland

LAYAL AL MAHMASANI, MD
Senior Fellow, Department of Medicine, Memorial Sloan Kettering Cancer Center, New York, New York, USA

OLEKSII DOBRZHANSKYI, MD
Surgical Oncologist, Upper Gastrointestinal Tumors Department, National Cancer Institute, Kyiv, Ukraine

JOHNATHAN D. EBBEN, MD, PhD
Fellow, Division of Hematology, Medical Oncology and Palliative Care, Department of Medicine, University of Wisconsin School of Medicine and Public Health, University of Wisconsin, Madison, Wisconsin, USA

MARIA CLARA FERNANDES, MD, MSc
Assistant Attending, Department of Radiology, Memorial Sloan Kettering Cancer Center, New York, New York, USA

KARYN A. GOODMAN, MD
Professor and Vice Chair for Research and Quality, Department of Radiation Oncology, Icahn School of Medicine at Mount Sinai, New York, New York, USA

JAMES J. HARDING, MD
Assistant Attending, Department of Medicine, Memorial Sloan Kettering Cancer Center, Instructor, Department of Medicine, Weill Medical College at Cornell University, New York, New York, USA

EMILY C. HARROLD, MB BCh, BAO, MRCPI
Visiting Investigator, Department of Medicine, Memorial Sloan Kettering Cancer Center, New York, New York, USA; Department of Medical Oncology, Mater Misericordiae University Hospital, Dublin, Ireland

VETRI SUDAR JAYAPRAKASAM, MBBS, FRCR
Assistant Attending, Department of Radiology, Memorial Sloan Kettering Cancer Center, New York, New York, USA

KHALID JAZIEH, MBBS
Physician, Division of Medical Oncology, Mayo Clinic, Rochester, Minnesota, USA

GEOFFREY KU, MD
Associate Attending Physician, Gastrointestinal Oncology Service, Department of Medicine, Memorial Sloan Kettering Cancer Center, New York, New York, USA

MONIKA LASZKOWSKA, MD, MS
Gastroenterologist, Gastroenterology, Hepatology and Nutrition Service, Department of Medicine, Memorial Sloan Kettering Cancer Center, New York, New York, USA

JAEYOP LEE, MD, PhD
Medical Oncology Fellow, Department of Medicine, Memorial Sloan Kettering Cancer Center, New York, New York, USA

MENGYUAN LIU, MD
Fellow, Department of Surgery, Memorial Sloan Kettering Cancer Center, New York, New York, USA

ERIC MEHLHAFF, MD
Fellow, Division of Hematology, Medical Oncology and Palliative Care, Department of Medicine, University of Wisconsin School of Medicine and Public Health, University of Wisconsin, Madison, Wisconsin, USA

ROBIN B. MENDELSOHN, MD
Associate Attending, Gastroenterology, Hepatology and Nutrition Service, Department of Medicine, Memorial Sloan Kettering Cancer Center, New York, New York, USA

DEVON MILLER, MD
Fellow, Division of Hematology, Medical Oncology and Palliative Care, Department of Medicine, University of Wisconsin School of Medicine and Public Health, University of Wisconsin, Madison, Wisconsin, USA

VIKTORIYA PARODER, MD, PhD
Associate Attending, Department of Radiology, Memorial Sloan Kettering Cancer Center, New York, New York, USA

LISA RUBY, MD
Fellow, Department of Radiology, Memorial Sloan Kettering Cancer Center, New York, New York, USA

SMITA SIHAG, MD, MPH
Assistant Professor of Thoracic Surgery, Thoracic Service, Department of Surgery, Memorial Sloan Kettering Cancer Center, New York, New York, USA

ZSOFIA K. STADLER, MD
Assistant Attending Physician, Department of Medicine, Memorial Sloan Kettering Cancer Center, New York, New York, USA

VIVIAN E. STRONG, MD, FACS
Iris Cantor Chair and Attending Surgeon, Vice Chair, Department of Surgery, Surgical Innovations and Outcomes, Gastric and Mixed Tumor Service, Memorial Sloan Kettering Cancer Center, Professor of Surgery and Associate Dean, Weill Cornell Medical College of Cornell University, New York, New York, USA

EMILY E. STROOBANT, MD
Surgical Research Fellow, Gastric and Mixed Tumor Service, Department of Surgery, Memorial Sloan Kettering Cancer Center, New York, New York, USA

LEILA T. TCHELEBI, MD
Associate Professor, Department of Radiation Medicine, Northern Westchester Hospital, Mount Kisco, New York, USA; Donald and Barbara Zucker School of Medicine at Hofstra/Northwell, Hempstead, New York, USA

NATALIYA V. UBOHA, MD, PhD
Associate Professor, Division of Hematology, Medical Oncology and Palliative Care, Department of Medicine, University of Wisconsin School of Medicine and Public Health, University of Wisconsin, University of Wisconsin Carbone Cancer Center, Madison, Wisconsin, USA

ALICE C. WEI, MD, MSc
Attending Surgeon, Department of Surgery, Memorial Sloan Kettering Cancer Center, New York, New York, USA

JIN WOO YOO, MD
Clinical Fellow, Gastroenterology, Hepatology and Nutrition Service, Department of Medicine, Memorial Sloan Kettering Cancer Center, New York, New York, USA

HARRY YOON, MD
Assistant Professor, Division of Medical Oncology, Mayo Clinic, Rochester, Minnesota, USA

KENNETH H. YU, MD, MSc
Associate Attending, Gastrointestinal Oncology Service, Cell Therapy Service, Memorial Sloan Kettering Cancer Center, New York, New York, USA

MOJUN ZHU, MD
Medical Oncologist, Division of Medical Oncology, Mayo Clinic, Rochester, Minnesota, USA

Contents

The goal of a gastric cancer operation is a microscopically negative resection margin and D2 lymphadenectomy. Minimally invasive techniques (laparoscopic and robotic) have been proven to be equivalent for oncologic care, yet with faster recovery. Endoscopic mucosal resection can be used for T1a N0 tumor resection. Better understanding of hereditary gastric cancer and molecular subtypes has led to specialized recommendations for MSI-high tumors and patients with pathogenic CDH1 mutations. In the future, surgical management will support minimally invasive approaches and personalized cancer care based on subtype.

Radical esophagectomy with two or three-field lymphadenectomy remains the mainstay of curative treatment for localized esophageal cancer, often in combination with systemic chemotherapy and/or radiotherapy. In this article, we describe notable advances in the surgical management of esophageal cancer over the past decade that have led to an improvement in both surgical and oncologic outcomes. In addition, we discuss new approaches to surgical management currently under investigation that have the potential to offer further benefits to appropriately selected patients. These incremental breakthroughs primarily include advances in endoscopic and minimally invasive techniques, perioperative management protocols, as well as the application of local therapies, including surgery, to oligometastatic disease.

Radiation therapy is an effective treatment modality in the management of patients with esophageal cancer regardless of tumor location (proximal, middle, or distal esophagus) or histology (squamous cell vs adenocarcinoma). The addition of neoadjuvant CRT to surgery in patients who are surgical candidates has consistently shown a benefit in terms of locoregional recurrence, pathologic downstaging, and overall survival. For patients who are not surgical candidates, CRT has a role as definitive treatment.

The Trastuzumab for Gastric Cancer (ToGA) trial marked a pivotal moment in the adoption of trastuzumab for treating advanced human epidermal growth factor receptor 2 (HER2)-positive esophagogastric (EG) cancer. The KEYNOTE-811 trial brought to light the synergistic effect of immune modulation and HER2 targeting. Additionally, the emergence of trastuzumab deruxtecan (T-DXd) highlighted the potential of new pharmaceutical technologies to extend response, particularly for patients who have advanced beyond initial HER2-targeted therapies. This review aims to navigate through both the successes and challenges encountered historically, as well as promising current trials on innovative and transformative therapeutic strategies, including promising first-in-class and novel first-in-human agents.

Immune checkpoint inhibitors are rapidly transforming the care of patients with esophagogastric cancer. Particularly, anti-PD-1 therapy has demonstrated promising efficacy in metastatic and resectable disease. In this review, the authors discuss landmark clinical trials, highlight challenges and opportunities in this field, and propose potential directions for future work.

Substantial progress has been made toward understanding biology and developing new therapies for pancreatic ductal adenocarcinoma (PDAC). In this review, new insights from genomic profiling, as well as implications for treatment and prognosis, are discussed. New standards of care approaches with a focus on drug therapies are discussed for the treatment of resectable and advanced PDAC. The role of targeted and immune therapies remains limited; cohorts likely to benefit from these approaches are discussed. Promising, preliminary results regarding experimental therapies are reviewed.

A multimodality approach, which usually includes chemotherapy, surgery, and/or radiotherapy, is optimal for patients with localized pancreatic cancer. The timing and sequence of these interventions depend on anatomic resectability and the biological suitability of the tumor and the patient. Tumors with vascular involvement (ie, borderline resectable/locally advanced) require surgical reassessments after therapy and participation of surgeons familiar with advanced techniques. When indicated, venous reconstruction should be offered as standard of care because it has acceptable morbidity. Morbidity and mortality of pancreas surgery may be mitigated when surgery is performed at high-volume centers.

Biliary tract cancers continue to increase in incidence and have a high mortality rate. Most of the patients present with advanced-stage disease. The discovery of targetable genomic alterations addressing IDH, FGFR, HER2, BRAFV600 E, and others has led to the identification and validation of novel therapies in biliary cancer. Recent advances demonstrating an improved outcome with the addition of immune checkpoint inhibitors to chemotherapy have established a new first-line care standard. In case of contraindications to the use of checkpoint inhibitors and the absence of targetable alterations, chemotherapy remains to be the standard of care.

Gastroesophageal cancers are highly diverse tumors in terms of their anatomic and molecular characteristics, making drug development challenging. Recent advancements in understanding the molecular profiles of these cancers have led to the identification of several new biomarkers. Ongoing clinical trials are investigating new targeted agents with promising results. CLDN18.2 has emerged as a biomarker with established activity of associated targeted therapies. Other targeted agents, such as bemarituzumab and DKN-01, are under active investigation. As new agents are incorporated into the treatment continuum, the questions of biomarker overlap, tumor heterogeneity, and toxicity management will need to be addressed.

Beyond the few established hereditary cancer syndromes with an upper gastrointestinal cancer component, there is increasing recognition of the contribution of novel pathogenic germline variants (gPVs) to upper gastrointestinal carcinogenesis. The detection of gPVs has potential implications for novel treatment approaches of the index cancer patient as well as long-term implications for surveillance and risk-reducing measures for cancer survivors and far-reaching implications for the patients' family. With widespread availability of multigene panel testing, new associations may be identified with germline-somatic integration being critical to determining true causality of novel gPVs. Comprehensive cancer care should incorporate both somatic and germline testing.

Upper gastrointestinal cancers are among the leading causes of cancer deaths worldwide with exceptionally poor prognosis, which is largely attributable to frequently delayed diagnosis. Although effective screening is critical for early detection, the highly variable incidence of upper gastrointestinal cancers presents challenges, rendering universal screening programs suboptimal in most populations globally. Optimal strategies in regions of modest incidence, such as the United States, require a targeted approach, focused on high-risk individuals based on demographic, familial, and clinicopathologic risk factors. Assessment of underlying precancerous lesions has key implications for risk stratification and informing clinical decisions to improve patient outcomes.

Advances in the Imaging of Esophageal and Gastroesophageal Junction Malignancies   711

Lisa Ruby, Vetri Sudar Jayaprakasam, Maria Clara Fernandes, and Viktoriya Paroder

Accurate imaging is key for the diagnosis and treatment of esophageal and gastroesophageal junction cancers . Current imaging modalities, such as computed tomography (CT) and 18F-FDG (2-deoxy-2-[18F]fluoro-D-glucose) positron emission tomography (PET)/CT, have limitations in accurately staging these cancers. MRI shows promise for T staging and residual disease assessment. Novel PET tracers, like FAPI, FLT, and hypoxia markers, offer potential improvements in diagnostic accuracy. ^{18}F-FDG PET/MRI combines metabolic and anatomic information, enhancing disease evaluation. Radiomics and artificial intelligence hold promise for early detection, treatment planning, and response assessment. Theranostic nanoparticles and personalized medicine approaches offer new avenues for cancer therapy.

HEMATOLOGY/ONCOLOGY CLINICS OF NORTH AMERICA

SERIES OF RELATED INTEREST

Surgical Oncology Clinics
https://www.surgonc.theclinics.com
Advances in Oncology
https://www.advances-oncology.com

THE CLINICS ARE AVAILABLE ONLINE!
Access your subscription at:
www.theclinics.com

Preface

Malignancies of the Upper Gastrointestinal Tract

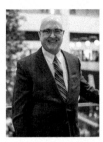

David H. Ilson, MD, PhD, FASCO, FACP
Editor

Treatment of upper gastrointestinal (GI) cancers has undergone a significant transformation over the past decade. The move to minimally invasive surgical approaches has led to potential better surgical therapy tolerance, lessening of surgical complications and enhanced recovery times, and potential enhancement of delivery of adjuvant therapies. Adjuvant treatment has advanced across the spectrum of GI cancers with improved survival with more contemporary chemotherapy regimens. Increasingly neoadjuvant strategies are being employed across the spectrum of upper GI malignancies, and participation in multidisciplinary discussions and treatment planning is the new care standard. The role of radiotherapy is being more clearly defined with more selective application of radiotherapy in treatment management. In advanced disease, immune checkpoint inhibitors have moved to first-line treatment in gastroesophageal and biliary cancers. The potential usage of immunotherapy in the adjuvant setting continues to be under investigation and has already achieved success in esophageal cancer. The subset of patients whose cancers have mismatch repair protein deficiency, manifested as positive testing for microsatellite instability (MSI), has emerged as a patient category highly responsive to immune checkpoint inhibitor therapy, with study of these agents in both locally advanced and metastatic MSI high cancers. Agents targeting HER2-positive cancers also have emerged as therapy options in first- and later-line treatment. Other novel targets are emerging with implications across upper GI cancers, including claudin 18.2, the fibroblast growth factor receptor, and other pathways. Molecular profiling has identified specific molecular targets, which have been successfully exploited with specific agents, leading to gene-specific approval of novel agents in advanced disease. The knowledge base of potential hereditary cancer syndromes will continue to expand with the broader application of genomic and germline testing in

Hematol Oncol Clin N Am 38 (2024) xiii–xiv
https://doi.org/10.1016/j.hoc.2024.02.004
0889-8588/24/© 2024 Elsevier Inc. All rights reserved.

upper GI cancers. Significant advances in imaging will have an effect on tumor staging and response assessment as new technologies continue to evolve.

David H. Ilson, MD, PhD, FASCO, FACP
Memorial Sloan Kettering Cancer Center
300 East 66th Street
New York, NY 10065, USA

E-mail address:
ilsond@mskcc.org

Advances in Gastric Cancer Surgical Management

Emily E. Stroobant, MD[a], Vivian E. Strong, MD[b,c],*

KEYWORDS

- Minimally invasive gastrectomy • Robotic gastrectomy • Laparoscopic gastrectomy
- Gastric cancer surgery • Gastric cancer • Stomach cancer • Total gastrectomy

KEY POINTS

- Gastric cancer should be resected with a negative microscopic margin.
- D2 lymph node dissection has been proven superior but should be done by experienced surgeons.
- Minimally invasive techniques for appropriately selected patients have equivalent oncologic outcomes with reduced hospital stay, less pain, less blood loss, faster return to work/life activities, and fewer adhesions. This approach also may facilitate sooner adjuvant systemic treatment.
- Endoscopic resection is supported for properly selected T1a N0 cancers due to lower risk of nodal metastasis.
- We are moving toward individualized treatments based on molecular/genetic features.

INTRODUCTION

Gastric cancer has been declared a public health concern by the World Health Organization and is the fifth most common cancer worldwide and the third most common cause of mortality.[1] Although not as prevalent as in the East, the United States has an estimated 26,380 new cases each year with 11,090 deaths,[2] and incidence in the West is rising in younger populations (ages 25–39 years).[3] Surgery remains the mainstay of treatment. In the past 30 years, the surgical approach has evolved with the advent of laparoscopic and robotic surgery. The debate regarding the extent of lymphadenectomy has been settled with the acceptance of D2 lymph node (LN) dissection as superior. However, reconstructive methods are still being investigated with no single

[a] Gastric and Mixed Tumor Service, Department of Surgery - H1216, Memorial Sloan Kettering Cancer Center, 1275 York Avenue, New York, NY 10065, USA; [b] Gastric and Mixed Tumor Service, Department of Surgery, Memorial Sloan Kettering Cancer Center, 1275 York Avenue, New York, NY 10065, USA; [c] Weill Cornell Medical College of Cornell University, 1300 York Avenue, New York, NY, 10065, USA
* Corresponding author. Department of Surgery - H1217, 1275 York Avenue, New York, NY 10065.
E-mail address: strongv@mskcc.org

Hematol Oncol Clin N Am 38 (2024) 547–557
https://doi.org/10.1016/j.hoc.2024.01.003
0889-8588/24/© 2024 Elsevier Inc. All rights reserved.
hemonc.theclinics.com

preferred method. As we look toward the future, tailoring treatment to genetic and molecular subtypes will further guide our approach to surgery.

FUNDAMENTALS IN TECHNIQUE

As with other forms of oncologic surgery, negative resection margin and lymphadenectomy are fundamentally important to surgical technique. Negative resection margins constitute a critical factor in gastric resection, as positive resection margin is an independent predictor of poor survival.[4,5] Therefore, the goal of surgery is successful R0 resection (microscopically negative surgical margin) to reduce chances of local recurrence, which has been observed in 16% of patients with a positive surgical margin.[4] Owing to the importance of R0 resection, intraoperative frozen sections can be used to verify a negative resection margin and reduce the risk of local recurrence.[6] The diagnostic accuracy of frozen sections in esophagogastric adenocarcinoma ranges from 93% to 98%, though caution should be used in cases of signet ring cell (SRC) cancer due to a higher prevalence of false negatives in this subtype.[7,8] Previously the National Comprehensive Cancer Network (NCCN) guidelines recommended a 4 cm gross surgical margin; however, the 2023 guidelines have been updated to recommend a negative microscopic margin only.[9,10] Of course, as previously stated caution should be taken with diffuse or SRC cancers due to their propensity to spread within the submucosa and cause false-negative margins.[7,8] Therefore, resections should be planned with either subtotal or total gastrectomy as needed to obtain negative margins.

Although the extent of lymphatic dissection has been extensively debated, the importance of positive and total number of resected LNs after pathologic review has been established as one of the most important prognostic factors for gastric cancer.[11] It improves the accuracy of staging[11] and is associated with increased survival.[12] The ideal number of LN to be retrieved during lymphadenectomy has also been debated, with literature ranging from 15[11] to 29,[12] and the current NCCN guidelines recommend at least 16 for localized resectable gastric cancer.[9,10]

To inform the extent of lymphadenectomy, LN stations have been grouped into 3 levels: D1, D2, and D3. D1 dissection consists of the perigastric LNs only (stations 1–7).[13] A D2 dissection includes stations 1 to 12a and adds the hepatic, left gastric, celiac, and splenic nodes.[13] D3 dissection includes stations 1 to 16 and adds the porta hepatis and periaortic nodes to D2 dissection.[13] The appropriate method of LN dissection has been debated, and incongruence remains between approaches in the East and West. However, after years of randomized controlled trials (RCTs) D2 dissection has emerged as superior. Although initial studies indicated increased morbidity and mortality,[14,15] Western studies (Dutch and Italian) with 15 year follow-up have confirmed that D2 LN dissection has been found to have a significantly improved disease-specific survival, a lower risk of gastric cancer-related death, and lower locoregional recurrence versus D1 without significant increase in rate of complications.[16,17] It has also been shown that there is no benefit to D3 dissection, given no evidence of survival benefit with possible increased morbidity especially with pancreatectomy and splenectomy, which is no longer recommended except in cases of direct tumor extension/vascular encasement.[18–20] The NCCN guidelines currently recommend D1 or modified D2 dissection for localized resectable gastric cancer, again with the goal of ≥16 LN.[9] They recommend D2 dissection be completed by experienced surgeons in high-volume centers.[9]

TRANSITION TO MINIMALLY INVASIVE SURGERY

Surgical treatment of gastric cancer has now evolved beyond open gastrectomy, although it still may remain necessary in cases with considerable adhesions, patients with significant comorbidities, or with inaccessible tumor location. Regarding gastric conservation, studies established that subtotal gastrectomy, when feasible to achieve R0 resection, had identical long-term survival to total gastrectomy with possible lower morbidity and mortality rates.[21,22]

After the advancement of laparoscopic surgical techniques in the 1980s, the first laparoscopic gastrectomy was performed in Japan in 1994,[23] proving the feasibility of laparoscopic resection for gastric cancer. Several RCTs followed from 2005 to 2010 showing the oncological safety of laparoscopic resection, as well as suggesting that minimally invasive surgery (MIS) techniques lead to reduced blood loss, reduced time to oral intake, and earlier discharge than open surgery.[24–27] To examine use in early cancer, two large RCTs were published, KLASS-01[28] and JCOG-0912,[29] confirming the oncologic equivalency of laparoscopic gastrectomy versus open surgery along with the added benefits of a minimally invasive approach. These studies were followed by RCTs for advanced gastric cancer: the CLASS-01,[30] JLSSG0901,[31] KLASS-02,[32] and STOMACH[33] trials. Once again these RCTs revealed technical safety without significant difference in disease-free survival between laparoscopic and open surgery.[30–32] Laparoscopic D2 resection was also confirmed to be equivalent to its counterpart in open surgery.[34] Many studies investigating the benefits of laparoscopic surgery for both early and late cancer have been performed in the East as well as the West, resulting in a wealth of data supporting oncologic equivalency with improved outcomes from MIS including: fewer complications, decreased hospital stay, decreased pain, less blood loss, and faster recovery.[35–49] Patients who had laparoscopic surgery were also significantly more likely to receive adjuvant chemotherapy when indicated.[45]

However, there is a learning curve associated with laparoscopic gastrectomy, with studies determining that 40 to 100 surgeries were needed to achieve decreased operative times.[50–53] Long-term outcomes remained equivalent during this learning stage.[50] After the learning was completed, operative times became comparable to open surgery.[52]

With the advent of robotic surgery, several RCTs investigated outcomes of robotic versus laparoscopic gastric resections. Robotic surgery was found to have fewer postoperative complications, with better LN dissection, faster recovery, and more prompt initiation of adjuvant chemotherapy.[47,54,55] In 2021, a single institution in Korea reviewed its 2000 robotic gastrostomies proving safety and feasibility at a high-volume center with equivalent long- and short-term outcomes.[56] This transition from open to MIS gastrectomy is summarized in **Fig. 1**. Currently, the NCCN guidelines state that laparoscopic or robotic approaches can be considered if the surgeon is experienced in MIS approaches and MIS lymphadenectomy.[9,10] Open surgery is still recommended if the tumor is T4b or there is bulky N2 disease.[9,10]

In regard to reconstruction after gastrectomy, no single method has emerged as superior. Reconstruction after proximal gastrectomy can be achieved with esophagogastrostomy, jejunal interposition, or double-tract reconstruction, a technique that is currently being evaluated in a randomized, prospective trial. Meta-analysis suggests that although esophagogastrostomy carried a higher risk of reflux esophagitis, it had a shorter operating time and hospital stay as well as lower risk of anastomotic stenosis and obstruction when compared with jejunal interposition.[57] Double-tract reconstruction was found to be comparable to esophagogastrostomy with fundoplication in terms of postoperative complications and may help prevent extreme body weight loss.[58] Double-tract reconstruction continues under investigation; however, the KLASS 05 study confirmed the short-term outcomes of laparoscopic proximal gastrectomy with double-tract reconstruction to be comparable to total laparoscopic

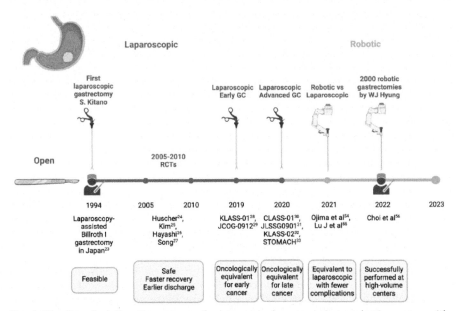

Fig. 1. Timeline depicting the progress from open to laparoscopic to robotic surgery with pertinent studies and conclusions. (Created with BioRender.com.)

gastrectomy.[59] Distal gastrectomy can be reconstructed with Billroth I, Billroth II, or Roux-en-Y. Outcomes from Roux-en-Y and Billroth II are similar, though Billroth II may be associated with a higher incidence of heartburn symptoms.[60] Meta-analysis suggests that complications and overall outcomes are similar between all three methods, though Roux-en-Y carried a lower risk of remnant gastritis.[61] Reconstruction after total gastrectomy can be achieved with Roux-en-Y, jejunal interposition, jejunal pouch, or Billroth II. One study suggested that jejunal pouch may be associated with improved quality of life when compared with Roux-en-Y, though overall both groups had similar outcomes.[62] The optimal method of reconstruction continues to be debated.

Along with the transition to laparoscopic and robotic surgery for gastrectomy, the role of diagnostic laparoscopy (DL) in staging and restaging has been well established. Positive peritoneal cytology was found to be the most predictive preoperative factor of gastric cancer mortality.[63] Therefore, DL allows identification of a population that is at high risk for early recurrence and death. The NCCN guidelines recommend DL for middle- and late-stage disease, and positive cytology as well as gross metastasis should direct care toward initial treatment with systemic therapy.[9,10] After chemotherapy, DL has been shown to be useful in restaging to determine which patients may be considered for subsequent primary tumor resection.[64]

Laparoscopy also has a role in several forms of intraperitoneal chemotherapy, though these remain controversial. Hyperthermic Intraperitoneal Chemotherapy (HIPEC) continues to be under investigation with several RCTs still enrolling.[65] The GASTRIPEC study has been completed and examined therapeutic HIPEC treatment in patients with peritoneal carcinomatosis.[66] They found no difference in overall survival with HIPEC added to treatment compared with cytoreductive surgery and systemic chemotherapy alone; however, progression-free survival and metastasis-free survival were significantly improved by a few months.[66] Pressurized intraperitoneal aerosolized chemotherapy (PIPAC) was initially developed in Germany and uses nebulized chemotherapy injected into the abdomen at high pressure during laparoscopic surgery. No large RCTs have been completed at this time, though PIPAC VEROne is currently recruiting.[67] A systematic literature review suggests a possible survival benefit.[68] Early postoperative intraperitoneal chemotherapy involves installation of chemotherapy via catheters immediately after gastrectomy. Studies have revealed differing results, with a potential for prolonging survival but a higher degree of morbidity.[69,70] A systematic literature review reveals that although limited, the improvement in overall survival for patients with gastric cancers may be statistically significant.[71] Intraperitoneal chemotherapy remains under investigation, and ongoing clinical trials will help to identify its role in gastric cancer treatment.

NEW TECHNIQUES AND TECHNOLOGY

Developments in endoscopic techniques have allowed for safe and effective endoscopic resection of T1a N0 lesions, supported by the NCCN guidelines.[9,10] Endoscopic submucosal dissection compared with surgery was shown to be less expensive with less trauma and faster recovery, but there was no significant difference in overall or disease-specific survival when strict selection criteria were applied.[72,73]

Along with the development of the surgical robot, technology has allowed for near-infrared fluorescence imaging with indocyanine green (ICG) which can be used to improve visualization and identification of LNs. This technique can assist in LN identification and retrieval without adding significant operative time (<10 minutes in one study).[74] The use of this technology has the potential to allow less extensive resections, with more LN retrieval and better staging to guide treatment. It also can play a role in teaching, to help better guide trainees during lymphadenectomy.

GENETICS AND MOLECULAR SUBTYPES

The Cancer Genome Atlas Project proposed 4 molecular subtypes: tumors positive for Epstein–Barr virus, microsatellite unstable tumors (microsatellite instability [MSI]-high), genomically stable tumors, and those with chromosomal instability.[75] This new understanding has led to research investigating subtype-based treatment response and outcome. A secondary analysis of the MAGIC trial revealed that MSI-high patients treated with surgery alone had superior survival compared with patients with microsatellite stable cancers and actually worse survival when treated with chemotherapy.[76] Analysis of the CLASSIC RCT also confirmed that there was no benefit from adjuvant chemotherapy in MSI-high patients over surgery alone.[77] This evidence suggests that patients with MSI-high tumors could go straight to surgery if early or middle stage. As MSI-high cancers respond well to immune checkpoint inhibitors, there are now clinical trials of these agents as preoperative therapy. Preliminary reports indicate high rates of pathologic complete response to immune checkpoint inhibitor therapy.[78] Surgical care will continue to follow scientific discovery as medicine moves toward more molecular and genetic-based treatment models.

Another example of scientific advances determining surgical management is our understanding of the CDH1 gene. Pathogenic mutations in this gene increase the risk of diffuse gastric cancer characterized by SRCs. The current recommendation for patients with pathogenic CDH1 mutations and a family history who are appropriate surgical candidates is total gastrectomy.[79] Minimally invasive approaches are also feasible for prophylactic total gastrectomy.[79]

DISCUSSION

As technological advances have unlocked minimally invasive methods, fundamentals in technique such as negative resection margin and adequate lymphadenectomy continue to apply. MIS approaches have been proven to be oncologically equivalent with improved recovery, and surgery will continue to move toward less invasive techniques for the appropriately selected patient. No one clear method of reconstruction has been deemed superior, and further RCTs are necessary. Endoscopic techniques are now supported for T1a N0 tumor resection. The impact of intraperitoneal chemotherapy is not yet clear and continues to be investigated. ICG imaging of LNs may allow for a more limited LN dissection in the future, though this also requires further study. Given new understanding of genetic drivers and molecular subtypes, surgical management will have to evolve to become a part of personalized and precision cancer care.

SUMMARY

Gastric cancer resection requires a microscopically negative resection margin and D2 lymphadenectomy. Minimally invasive techniques (laparoscopic and robotic) have been proven to be equivalent for oncologic care, yet with faster recovery. Endoscopic resection can be used for T1a N0 tumor resection. Better understanding of hereditary gastric cancer and molecular subtypes has led to specialized recommendations for MSI-high tumors and patients with pathogenic CDH1 mutations. In the future, surgical management will support MIS approaches and personalized cancer care based on subtype.

CLINICS CARE POINTS

- Gastric cancer should be resected with a negative microscopic margin.
- D2 lymph node dissection has been proven superior but should be done by experienced surgeons.
- Minimally invasive techniques have equivalent oncologic outcomes with reduced hospital stay, less pain, less blood loss, faster return to work/life activities, and fewer adhesions.
- Endoscopic resection is supported for T1aN0 cancers that meet appropriate criteria.
- Care is moving toward treatment based on molecular/genetic subtypes, if MSI-high consider taking directly to surgery or enrolling on an immunotherapy trial.
- The current recommended treatment for carriers of pathogenic CDH1 mutations who are appropriate surgical candidates with positive family history is total gastrectomy.

DISCLOSURES

Dr V.E. Strong has recieved speaking honoraria from AstraZeneca.

REFERENCES

1. Bray F, Ferlay J, Soerjomataram I, et al. Global cancer statistics 2018: GLOBO-CAN estimates of incidence and mortality worldwide for 36 cancers in 185 countries. CA A Cancer J Clin 2018;68(6):394–424.
2. Siegel RL, Miller KD, Fuchs HE, et al. Cancer statistics, 2022. CA A Cancer J Clin 2022;72(1):7–33.

3. Anderson WF. Age-Specific Trends in Incidence of Noncardia Gastric Cancer in US Adults. JAMA 2010;303(17):1723.

4. Bickenbach KA, Gonen M, Strong V, et al. Association of Positive Transection Margins with Gastric Cancer Survival and Local Recurrence. Ann Surg Oncol 2013;20(8):2663–8.

5. Kim SH, Karpeh MS, Klimstra DS, et al. Effect of microscopic resection line disease on gastric cancer survival. J Gastrointest Surg 1999;3(1):24–33.

6. Squires MH, Kooby DA, Pawlik TM, et al. Utility of the Proximal Margin Frozen Section for Resection of Gastric Adenocarcinoma: A 7-Institution Study of the US Gastric Cancer Collaborative. Ann Surg Oncol 2014;21(13):4202–10.

7. Spicer J, Benay C, Lee L, et al. Diagnostic Accuracy and Utility of Intraoperative Microscopic Margin Analysis of Gastric and Esophageal Adenocarcinoma. Ann Surg Oncol 2014;21(8):2580–6.

8. McAuliffe JC, Tang LH, Kamrani K, et al. Prevalence of False-Negative Results of Intraoperative Consultation on Surgical Margins During Resection of Gastric and Gastroesophageal Adenocarcinoma. JAMA Surgery 2019;154(2):126.

9. Ajani JA, D'Amico TA, Bentrem DJ, et al. Gastric Cancer, Version 2.2022, NCCN Clinical Practice Guidelines in Oncology. J Natl Compr Cancer Netw 2022;20(2): 167–92.

10. NCCN®. NCCN Guidelines® Gastric Cancer 2. 2023. Available at: https://www. nccn.org/guidelines/guidelines-detail?category=1&id=1434. [Accessed 30 October 2023].

11. Karpeh MS, Leon L, Klimstra D, et al. Lymph node staging in gastric cancer: is location more important than Number? An analysis of 1,038 patients. Ann Surg 2000;232(3):362–71.

12. Woo Y, Goldner B, Ituarte P, et al. Lymphadenectomy with Optimum of 29 Lymph Nodes Retrieved Associated with Improved Survival in Advanced Gastric Cancer: A 25,000-Patient International Database Study. J Am Coll Surg 2017; 224(4):546–55.

13. Japanese Gastric Cancer Treatment Guidelines 2021 (6th edition). Gastric Cancer 2023;26(1):1–25.

14. Cuschieri A, Fayers P, Fielding J, et al. Postoperative morbidity and mortality after D1 and D2 resections for gastric cancer: preliminary results of the MRC randomised controlled surgical trial. The Surgical Cooperative Group. Lancet 1996; 347(9007):995–9.

15. Bonenkamp JJ, Songun I, Hermans J, et al. Randomised comparison of morbidity after D1 and D2 dissection for gastric cancer in 996 Dutch patients. Lancet 1995; 345(8952):745–8.

16. Degiuli M, Reddavid R, Tomatis M, et al. D2 dissection improves disease-specific survival in advanced gastric cancer patients: 15-year follow-up results of the Italian Gastric Cancer Study Group D1 versus D2 randomised controlled trial. Eur J Cancer 2021;150:10–22.

17. Songun I, Putter H, Kranenbarg EM, et al. Surgical treatment of gastric cancer: 15-year follow-up results of the randomised nationwide Dutch D1D2 trial. Lancet Oncol 2010;11(5):439–49.

18. Wu CW, Hsiung CA, Lo SS, et al. Randomized clinical trial of morbidity after D1 and D3 surgery for gastric cancer. Br J Surg 2004;91(3):283–7.

19. Sasako M, Sano T, Yamamoto S, et al. D2 Lymphadenectomy Alone or with Para-aortic Nodal Dissection for Gastric Cancer. N Engl J Med 2008;359(5):453–62.

20. Bencivenga M, Verlato G, Mengardo V, et al. Is There Any Role for Super-Extended Limphadenectomy in Advanced Gastric Cancer? Results of an Observational Study from a Western High Volume Center. J Clin Med 2019;8(11):1799.

21. Gockel I, Pietzka S, Gonner U, et al. Subtotal or total gastrectomy for gastric cancer: impact of the surgical procedure on morbidity and prognosis? analysis of a 10-year experience. Langenbeck's Arch Surg 2005;390(2):148–55.

22. Bozzetti F, Marubini E, Bonfanti G, et al. Total versus subtotal gastrectomy: surgical morbidity and mortality rates in a multicenter Italian randomized trial. The Italian Gastrointestinal Tumor Study Group. Ann Surg 1997;226(5):613–20.

23. Kitano S, Iso Y, Moriyama M, et al. Laparoscopy-assisted Billroth I gastrectomy. Surg Laparosc Endosc 1994;4(2):146–8.

24. Huscher CG, Mingoli A, Sgarzini G, et al. Laparoscopic versus open subtotal gastrectomy for distal gastric cancer: five-year results of a randomized prospective trial. Ann Surg 2005;241(2):232–7.

25. Kim YW, Baik YH, Yun YH, et al. Improved quality of life outcomes after laparoscopy-assisted distal gastrectomy for early gastric cancer: results of a prospective randomized clinical trial. Ann Surg 2008;248(5):721–7.

26. Hayashi H, Ochiai T, Shimada H, et al. Prospective randomized study of open versus laparoscopy-assisted distal gastrectomy with extraperigastric lymph node dissection for early gastric cancer. Surg Endosc 2005;19(9):1172–6.

27. Kim HH, Hyung WJ, Cho GS, et al. Morbidity and mortality of laparoscopic gastrectomy versus open gastrectomy for gastric cancer: an interim report–a phase III multicenter, prospective, randomized Trial (KLASS Trial). Ann Surg 2010; 251(3):417–20.

28. Kim W, Kim HH, Han SU, et al. Decreased Morbidity of Laparoscopic Distal Gastrectomy Compared With Open Distal Gastrectomy for Stage I Gastric Cancer: Short-term Outcomes From a Multicenter Randomized Controlled Trial (KLASS-01). Ann Surg 2016;263(1):28–35.

29. Katai H, Mizusawa J, Katayama H, et al. Survival outcomes after laparoscopy-assisted distal gastrectomy versus open distal gastrectomy with nodal dissection for clinical stage IA or IB gastric cancer (JCOG0912): a multicentre, non-inferiority, phase 3 randomised controlled trial. Lancet Gastroenterol Hepatol 2020;5(2):142–51.

30. Yu J, Huang C, Sun Y, et al. Effect of Laparoscopic vs Open Distal Gastrectomy on 3-Year Disease-Free Survival in Patients With Locally Advanced Gastric Cancer. JAMA 2019;321(20):1983.

31. Inaki N, Etoh T, Ohyama T, et al. A Multi-institutional, Prospective, Phase II Feasibility Study of Laparoscopy-Assisted Distal Gastrectomy with D2 Lymph Node Dissection for Locally Advanced Gastric Cancer (JLSSG0901). World J Surg 2015;39(11):2734–41.

32. Hyung WJ, Yang H-K, Park Y-K, et al. Long-Term Outcomes of Laparoscopic Distal Gastrectomy for Locally Advanced Gastric Cancer: The KLASS-02-RCT Randomized Clinical Trial. J Clin Oncol 2020;38(28):3304–13.

33. Straatman J, Van Der Wielen N, Cuesta MA, et al. Surgical techniques, open versus minimally invasive gastrectomy after chemotherapy (STOMACH trial): study protocol for a randomized controlled trial. Trials 2015;16(1).

34. Shinohara T, Satoh S, Kanaya S, et al. Laparoscopic versus open D2 gastrectomy for advanced gastric cancer: a retrospective cohort study. Surg Endosc 2013; 27(1):286–94.

35. Adachi Y. Laparoscopy-Assisted Billroth I Gastrectomy Compared With Conventional Open Gastrectomy. Arch Surg 2000;135(7):806.

36. Choi SH, Yoon DS, Chi HS, et al. Laparoscopy-assisted radical subtotal gastrectomy for early gastric carcinoma. Yonsei Med J 1996;37(3):174.

37. Tanimura S, Higashino M, Fukunaga Y, et al. Hand-assisted laparoscopic distal gastrectomy with regional lymph node dissection for gastric cancer. Surg Laparosc Endosc Percutaneous Tech 2001;11(3):155–60.

38. Kim H-H, Han S-U, Kim M-C, et al. Effect of Laparoscopic Distal Gastrectomy vs Open Distal Gastrectomy on Long-term Survival Among Patients With Stage I Gastric Cancer. JAMA Oncol 2019;5(4):506.

39. Kitano S, Shiraishi N, Fujii K, et al. A randomized controlled trial comparing open vs laparoscopy-assisted distal gastrectomy for the treatment of early gastric cancer: an interim report. Surgery 2002;131(1 Suppl):S306–11.

40. Lee JH, Han HS, Lee JH. A prospective randomized study comparing open vs laparoscopy-assisted distal gastrectomy in early gastric cancer: early results. Surg Endosc 2005;19(2):168–73.

41. Shimizu S, Uchiyama A, Mizumoto K, et al. Laparoscopically assisted distal gastrectomy for early gastric cancer. Surg Endosc 2000;14(1):27–31.

42. Yano H, Monden T, Kinuta M, et al. The usefulness of laparoscopy-assisted distal gastrectomy in comparison with that of open distal gastrectomy for early gastric cancer. Gastric Cancer 2001;4(2):93–7.

43. Park DJ, Han S-U, Hyung WJ, et al. Long-term outcomes after laparoscopy-assisted gastrectomy for advanced gastric cancer: a large-scale multicenter retrospective study. Surg Endosc 2012;26(6):1548–53.

44. Vinuela EF, Gonen M, Brennan MF, et al. Laparoscopic versus open distal gastrectomy for gastric cancer: a meta-analysis of randomized controlled trials and high-quality nonrandomized studies. Ann Surg 2012;255(3):446–56.

45. Kelly KJ, Selby L, Chou JF, et al. Laparoscopic Versus Open Gastrectomy for Gastric Adenocarcinoma in the West: A Case–Control Study. Ann Surg Oncol 2015;22(11):3590–6.

46. Weber KJ, Reyes CD, Gagner M, et al. Comparison of laparoscopic and open gastrectomy for malignant disease. Surg Endosc 2003;17(6):968–71.

47. Nakauchi M, Vos E, Janjigian YY, et al. Comparison of Long- and Short-term Outcomes in 845 Open and Minimally Invasive Gastrectomies for Gastric Cancer in the United States. Ann Surg Oncol 2021;28(7):3532–44.

48. Varela JE, Hiyashi M, Nguyen T, et al. Comparison of laparoscopic and open gastrectomy for gastric cancer. Am J Surg 2006;192(6):837–42.

49. Van Der Wielen N, Straatman J, Daams F, et al. Open versus minimally invasive total gastrectomy after neoadjuvant chemotherapy: results of a European randomized trial. Gastric Cancer 2021;24(1):258–71.

50. Hu WG, Ma JJ, Zang L, et al. Learning curve and long-term outcomes of laparoscopy-assisted distal gastrectomy for gastric cancer. J Laparoendosc Adv Surg Tech 2014;24(7):487–92.

51. Jung DH, Son S-Y, Park YS, et al. The learning curve associated with laparoscopic total gastrectomy. Gastric Cancer 2016;19(1):264–72.

52. Kunisaki C, Makino H, Yamamoto N, et al. Learning curve for laparoscopy-assisted distal gastrectomy with regional lymph node dissection for early gastric cancer. Surg Laparosc Endosc Percutaneous Tech 2008;18(3):236–41.

53. Zhang X, Tanigawa N. Learning curve of laparoscopic surgery for gastric cancer, a laparoscopic distal gastrectomy-based analysis. Surg Endosc 2009;23(6):1259–64.

54. Ojima T, Nakamura M, Hayata K, et al. Short-term Outcomes of Robotic Gastrectomy vs Laparoscopic Gastrectomy for Patients With Gastric Cancer. JAMA Surgery 2021;156(10):954.

55. Lu J, Zheng CH, Xu BB, et al. Assessment of Robotic Versus Laparoscopic Distal Gastrectomy for Gastric Cancer: A Randomized Controlled Trial. Ann Surg 2021; 273(5):858–67.

56. Choi S, Song JH, Lee S, et al. Trends in clinical outcomes and long-term survival after robotic gastrectomy for gastric cancer: a single high-volume center experience of consecutive 2000 patients. Gastric Cancer 2022;25(1):275–86.

57. Du N, Wu P, Wang P, et al. Reconstruction Methods and Complications of Esophagogastrostomy and Jejunal Interposition in Proximal Gastrectomy for Gastric Cancer: A Meta-Analysis. Gastroenterology Research and Practice 2020; 2020:1–8.

58. Tominaga S, Ojima T, Nakamura M, et al. Esophagogastrostomy With Fundoplication Versus Double-tract Reconstruction After Laparoscopic Proximal Gastrectomy for Gastric Cancer. Surg Laparosc Endosc Percutaneous Tech 2021; 31(5):594–8.

59. Hwang S-H, Park DJ, Kim H-H, et al. Short-Term Outcomes of Laparoscopic Proximal Gastrectomy With Double-Tract Reconstruction Versus Laparoscopic Total Gastrectomy for Upper Early Gastric Cancer: A KLASS 05 Randomized Clinical Trial. Journal of Gastric Cancer 2022;22(2):94.

60. So JB, Rao J, Wong AS, et al. Roux-en-Y or Billroth II Reconstruction After Radical Distal Gastrectomy for Gastric Cancer: A Multicenter Randomized Controlled Trial. Ann Surg 2018;267(2):236–42.

61. Jiang H, Li Y, Wang T. Comparison of Billroth I, Billroth II, and Roux-en-Y reconstructions following distal gastrectomy: A systematic review and network meta-analysis. Cir Esp 2021;99(6):412–20.

62. Chen W, Jiang X, Huang H, et al. Jejunal pouch reconstruction after total gastrectomy is associated with better short-term absorption capacity and quality of life in early-stage gastric cancer patients. BMC Surg 2018;18(1).

63. Bentrem D, Wilton A, Mazumdar M, et al. The Value of Peritoneal Cytology as a Preoperative Predictor in Patients With Gastric Carcinoma Undergoing a Curative Resection. Ann Surg Oncol 2005;12(5):347–53.

64. Cardona K, Zhou Q, Gönen M, et al. Role of Repeat Staging Laparoscopy in Locoregionally Advanced Gastric or Gastroesophageal Cancer after Neoadjuvant Therapy. Ann Surg Oncol 2013;20(2):548–54.

65. Koemans WJ, Van Der Kaaij RT, Boot H, et al. Cytoreductive surgery and hyperthermic intraperitoneal chemotherapy versus palliative systemic chemotherapy in stomach cancer patients with peritoneal dissemination, the study protocol of a multicentre randomised controlled trial (PERISCOPE II). BMC Cancer 2019;19(1).

66. Rau B, Lang H, Königsrainer A, et al. 1376O The effect of hyperthermic intraperitoneal chemotherapy (HIPEC) upon cytoreductive surgery (CRS) in gastric cancer (GC) with synchronous peritoneal metastasis (PM): A randomized multicentre phase III trial (GASTRIPEC-I-trial). Ann Oncol 2021;32:S1040.

67. Casella F, Bencivenga M, Rosati R, et al. Pressurized intraperitoneal aerosol chemotherapy (PIPAC) in multimodal therapy for patients with oligometastatic peritoneal gastric cancer: a randomized multicenter phase III trial PIPAC VER-One. Pleura and Peritoneum 2022;7(3):135–41.

68. Case A, Prosser S, Peters CJ, et al. Pressurised intraperitoneal aerosolised chemotherapy (PIPAC) for gastric cancer with peritoneal metastases: A systematic review by the PIPAC UK collaborative. Crit Rev Oncol Hematol 2022;180:103846.

69. Hultman B, Lind P, Glimelius B, et al. Phase II study of patients with peritoneal carcinomatosis from gastric cancer treated with preoperative systemic chemotherapy followed by peritonectomy and intraperitoneal chemotherapy. Acta Oncologica 2013;52(4):824–30.
70. Kang Y-K, Yook JH, Chang H-M, et al. Enhanced efficacy of postoperative adjuvant chemotherapy in advanced gastric cancer: results from a phase 3 randomized trial (AMC0101). Cancer Chemother Pharmacol 2014;73(1):139–49.
71. Feingold PL, Kwong MLM, Davis JL, et al. Adjuvant intraperitoneal chemotherapy for the treatment of gastric cancer at risk for peritoneal carcinomatosis: A systematic review. J Surg Oncol 2017;115(2):192–201.
72. Liu Q, Ding L, Qiu X, et al. Updated evaluation of endoscopic submucosal dissection versus surgery for early gastric cancer: A systematic review and meta-analysis. Int J Surg 2020;73:28–41.
73. Takizawa K, Ono H, Hasuike N, et al. A nonrandomized, single-arm confirmatory trial of expanded endoscopic submucosal dissection indication for undifferentiated early gastric cancer: Japan Clinical Oncology Group study (JCOG1009/1010). Gastric Cancer 2021;24(2):479–91.
74. Herrera-Almario G, Patane M, Sarkaria I, et al. Initial report of near-infrared fluorescence imaging as an intraoperative adjunct for lymph node harvesting during robot-assisted laparoscopic gastrectomy. J Surg Oncol 2016;113(7):768–70.
75. Cancer Genome Atlas Research N. Comprehensive molecular characterization of gastric adenocarcinoma. Nature 2014;513(7517):202–9.
76. Smyth EC, Wotherspoon A, Peckitt C, et al. Mismatch Repair Deficiency, Microsatellite Instability, and Survival. JAMA Oncol 2017;3(9):1197.
77. Choi YY, Kim H, Shin SJ, et al. Microsatellite Instability and Programmed Cell Death-Ligand 1 Expression in Stage II/III Gastric Cancer: Post Hoc Analysis of the CLASSIC Randomized Controlled study. Ann Surg 2019;270(2):309–16.
78. Andre T, Tougeron D, Piessen G, et al. Neoadjuvant Nivolumab Plus Ipilimumab and Adjuvant Nivolumab in Localized Deficient Mismatch Repair/Microsatellite Instability-High Gastric or Esophagogastric Junction Adenocarcinoma: The GERCOR NEONIPIGA Phase II Study. J Clin Oncol 2023;41(2):255–65.
79. Vos EL, Salo-Mullen EE, Tang LH, et al. Indications for Total Gastrectomy in *CDH1* Mutation Carriers and Outcomes of Risk-Reducing Minimally Invasive and Open Gastrectomies. JAMA Surgery 2020;155(11):1050.

Advances in the Surgical Management of Esophageal Cancer

Smita Sihag, MD, MPH

KEYWORDS

• Esophageal cancer • Esophagectomy • Surgery

KEY POINTS

- In patients at low risk for lymph node involvement, advances in endoscopic therapies have revolutionized the management of early-stage esophageal cancer by offering an organ-sparing approach as an alternative to conventional esophagectomy.
- Adoption of minimally invasive Ivor Lewis esophagectomy (MIE) using laparoscopy and thoracoscopy over the past 10 to 20 years has resulted in significantly lower postoperative morbidity and improved quality of life, along with excellent long-term oncologic outcomes.
- Robotic MIE has improved surgical visualization and has similar outcomes to conventional MIE. Some data suggest that lymphadenectomy may be enhanced with this approach.
- The extent of surgical lymphadenectomy is likely associated with long-term survival, regardless of neoadjuvant therapy, and should be emphasized during esophagectomy.
- Surgical resection in patients with oligometastatic esophageal adenocarcinoma requires further study, but early results indicate a role for this approach in carefully selected patients.

INTRODUCTION

Esophageal cancer is among the top 10 cancers in terms of global incidence and mortality, and less than half of patients present with localized disease.[1] Radical esophagectomy with 2 or 3 field lymphadenectomy remains the mainstay of curative treatment for localized esophageal cancer, often in combination with systemic therapy and/or radiotherapy. Historically, esophageal resection, especially via transthoracic approach, has been associated with high rates of postoperative morbidity and mortality, as well as significant changes in quality of life for patients. This aggressive intervention has been justified, however, by the deadliness of the disease as 5-year survival in patients with localized esophageal cancer remains poor at 30% to 40%.[2] In this article, we describe notable advances in the surgical management of esophageal cancer over the past decade that have led to an improvement in both surgical and oncologic outcomes.

Thoracic Service, Department of Surgery, Memorial Sloan Kettering Cancer Center, 1275 York Avenue, C-881, New York, NY 10065, USA
E-mail address: sihags@mskcc.org

Hematol Oncol Clin N Am 38 (2024) 559–568
https://doi.org/10.1016/j.hoc.2024.03.001
0889-8588/24/© 2024 Elsevier Inc. All rights reserved.

hemonc.theclinics.com

In addition, we discuss new approaches to surgical management currently under investigation that have the potential to offer further benefits to appropriately selected patients. These incremental breakthroughs primarily include advances in endoscopic and minimally invasive techniques, perioperative management protocols, as well as the application of local therapies, including surgery, to oligometastatic disease.

ENDOSCOPIC THERAPIES

Endoscopic techniques have evolved as a critical tool for not only diagnosis and staging, but also the treatment of early esophageal cancers. Advances in endoscopic therapies have revolutionized the management of early-stage esophageal cancer by offering an organ-sparing approach as an alternative to conventional esophagectomy. In patients with esophageal cancer, patient selection for endoscopic therapy is based on the risk of lymph node metastasis, as these procedures do not assess or resect lymph nodes. Factors associated with lymph node metastases include tumor size > 2 cm, high tumor grade or poor differentiation, depth of invasion beyond the mucosa, and the presence of lymphovascular invasion.[3] Patients with none of these factors have a 0% to 5% risk of lymph node metastases and represent ideal candidates for endoscopic treatment based on the most recent NCCN guidelines.[4] Patients with moderate or high risk of occult lymph node involvement are often referred for the consideration of surgical management. In patients with multiple comorbidities and/ or compromised performance status, rendering them high risk for esophagectomy, observation may still be a reasonable strategy. Alternatively, chemoradiotherapy may also be recommended in this patient population if margins are very close or concern for nodal involvement is high, though these approaches require further study to evaluate if survival is enhanced. Overall, the management of these patients may benefit from multidisciplinary discussion in the decision-making.

Endoscopic resection has been described with 2 main approaches: endoscopic mucosal resection (EMR) and endoscopic submucosal dissection (ESD). Both techniques, initially developed in Japan, are designed for the treatment of early-stage esophageal cancers (uT1a or uT1b superficial). The commonly used EMR methods can be grouped into cap-assisted and ligation-assisted categories.[5] A study involving 1000 patients with intramucosal carcinoma who underwent EMR showed that 96% were completely resected, with a 10-year survival rate of 75%. Recurrent or metachronous lesions developed in 15% of patients but the majority (82%) were successfully treated with repeat endoscopic resection.[6]

The ESD technique is designed for the en-bloc resection of larger and deeper superficial lesions of the esophagus. The procedure begins by marking the lesion's parameters with cautery and then creating a submucosal cushion by injecting normal saline. Dissection of the submucosa is then performed after a circumferential incision around the lesion is made, thereby separating it from the muscularis propria. Multiple studies have examined the long-term results of ESD. Rates of curative en-bloc resection for ESD have been reported to be as high as 100% for squamous cell carcinoma, while slightly lower at 95% for adenocarcinoma according to results from a European cohort.[7] Overall, ESD has been associated with higher rates of complete resection irrespective of histology when compared with EMR, as well as lower local recurrence rates.[8] Rates of adverse events appear similar between ESD and EMR in terms of bleeding or stricture formation. However, ESD may be associated with a higher risk of perforation. According to Guidelines from the American Society for Gastrointestinal Endoscopy (ASGE) on ESD for the management of early esophageal cancers, ESD is recommended for patients with early-stage, well-differentiated, nonulcerated cancer greater than 15 to 20 mm, whereas in patients with similar lesions less than 15 to 20 mm, either ESD or EMR is recommended.[9]

MINIMALLY INVASIVE ESOPHAGECTOMY

In the United States, adenocarcinoma is the predominant histology of esophageal cancer, most commonly involving the distal esophagus and gastroesophageal junction.[10] Although tumors in this location can also be resected via a transhiatal or three-hole approach, transthoracic Ivor Lewis esophagectomy is the most frequently recommended operation for this indication. Open Ivor Lewis esophagectomy (ILE) consists of a two-field approach in which the stomach is mobilized and a gastric conduit is created via abdominal laparotomy with the resection of the upper third of the stomach. The patient is then repositioned for right thoracotomy and transthoracic esophageal mobilization with intrathoracic division of the esophagus and anastomosis between the upper thoracic esophagus and the gastric conduit. This approach allows for both thoracic and abdominal lymphadenectomy, as well as the direct visualization of the thoracic periesophageal tissue during dissection.

Outcomes of ILE have traditionally been associated with high rates of postoperative morbidity and mortality, approaching 62% and 4%, respectively.[11] Adoption of minimally invasive Ivor Lewis esophagectomy (MIE) using laparoscopy and thoracoscopy over the past 10 to 20 years, pioneered by Luketich and colleagues, has resulted in significantly lower postoperative morbidity, especially with respect to pulmonary complications, alongside excellent long-term oncologic outcomes.[12–15] Equally importantly, patient-reported outcomes of MIE demonstrate improvements in pain, recovery time, and overall quality of life.[16]

Furthermore, the development of MIE has brought about other important modifications to the way in which esophagectomy is performed. In particular, the routine tubularization of the gastric conduit to a diameter of approximately 4-5 cm and execution of a stapled anastomosis above the level of the azygous vein have potentially led to an improvement in the functional outcomes of patients undergoing esophagectomy in terms of symptoms related to delayed gastric emptying and reflux.[17–19] Consequently, drainage procedures, such as pyloroplasty or pyloromyotomy, which can introduce another point of possible leakage and complication, are now frequently eliminated by many expert esophageal surgeons as they may no longer be necessary and are without proven benefit.[20]

Mckeown or three-hole esophagectomy remains a relevant surgical option for upper and mid-esophageal cancers, long-segment Barrett's disease, and certain benign conditions necessitating near-total esophagectomy. These operations are typically associated with higher rates of anastomotic breakdown and recurrent laryngeal nerve injury as compared with transthoracic approaches. However, minimally invasive Mckeown esophagectomy has reduced the incidence of in-hospital complications in comparison to open Mckeown esophagectomy with a decrease from 63% to 42%, according to a recent NSQIP analysis of 10,000 procedures.[21] As opposed to the Ivor Lewis esophagectomy, this procedure typically begins in the right chest with the complete mobilization of the intrathoracic esophagus, followed by concurrent abdominal and left neck access in the supine position to allow for resection and reconstruction with cervical anastomosis.

ROBOTIC ESOPHAGECTOMY

Robotic-assisted Ivor Lewis esophagectomy (RAMIE) is performed at several centers using the da Vinci XI platform (Intuitive, Atlanta, GA) and is defined as the complete utilization of robotic-assisted laparoscopic and thoracoscopic instrumentation for all aspects of the procedure including the creation of the esophagogastric anastomosis in the chest. Indications for RAMIE are similar to those of Ivor Lewis esophagectomy and can be performed safely following neoadjuvant therapy. Multiple series published over the past decade demonstrate the feasibility, safety, and oncologic efficacy of this technique. Moreover, equivalent outcomes between robotic-assisted and minimally invasive (MIE) esophagectomy have now been demonstrated by high-volume surgeons.[22,23] More recent studies have suggested RAMIE may allow for a more extensive lymph node harvest compared with nonrobotic MIE, and therefore may be associated with oncologic advantages.[24] Robotic Mckeown esophagectomy has also been reviewed in comparison to conventional Mckeown MIE in a meta-analysis that included 8 studies.[25] No differences in anastomotic leak, length of stay, or hospital mortality were identified. In addition to achieving comparable patient outcomes, RAMIE also portends certain benefits to surgeons given the duration and complexity of the operation in terms of better 3-D visualization and ergonomics, which has increased the popularity of the approach over the past 5 to 10 years.

EXTENT OF LYMPHADENECTOMY DURING ESOPHAGECTOMY

The definition and role of radical en bloc esophagectomy, along with the extent of lymphadenectomy, have been topics of debate since the inception of surgery for esophageal cancer. Lymph node dissection of at least 2 fields, including the mediastinal and upper abdominal lymph nodes, however, is justified in all cases of lower esophageal and junctional adenocarcinoma, given the lymph node mapping of these tumors.[26] Several studies have shown that a more extensive lymphadenectomy is associated with superior pathologic staging for prognostic purposes, as the ratio of positive lymph nodes to the total number removed predicts survival in a linear manner.[27–29] Furthermore, higher absolute number of resected lymph nodes leads to better disease-specific survival in patients treated with surgery alone.[30,31] Some controversy has surrounded whether these associations are present for patients treated with neoadjuvant chemoradiotherapy. A retrospective review of the ChemoRadiotherapy for Esophageal cancer followed by Surgery Study (CROSS) trial cohort revealed that, whereas the number of lymph nodes resected was associated with survival in patients treated with surgery alone, it was not associated with survival in patients treated with neoadjuvant chemoradiotherapy.[32] Recent work by our group sought to evaluate this further and determine the extent of lymphadenectomy that optimizes staging and survival in patients with locally advanced EAC treated with neoadjuvant chemoradiotherapy. Using a large retrospective cohort of 778 patients treated at a high-volume cancer center, we found that removing at least 25 lymph nodes was associated with only a 10% risk of missing a positive lymph node, and the optimization of both disease-free and overall survival regardless of treatment response.[33] The greatest survival benefits of a more extensive lymphadenectomy were, in fact, seen in patients with greater downstaging and treatment response. Therefore, our results justify an aggressive approach to lymphadenectomy during esophagectomy and refute the idea that treatment with neoadjuvant chemoradiotherapy precludes the need for more extensive lymph node retrieval. Current NCCN guidelines recommend retrieval of at least 15 lymph nodes during esophagectomy, but acknowledge that patients with greater than 30 lymph nodes removed and examined had the lowest mortality.[4] As discussed above, evolutions in minimally invasive esophageal surgery have enhanced the surgeon's ability to perform a more extensive lymphadenectomy.

ENHANCED RECOVERY AFTER SURGERY PROTOCOLS, PREHABILITATION, AND EARLY NUTRITION

Enhanced recovery after Surgery (ERAS) protocols provide a framework to optimize and standardize perioperative management across several surgical specialties with the goal of improving outcomes. For patients with esophagectomy, ERAS protocols have encompassed a multi-disciplinary approach to reduce physiologic stress and morbidity related to one of the most complex operations performed for the resection of cancer. Evidence-based interventions that are recommended to be incorporated into such protocols are outlined in the ERAS society guidelines, and particularly emphasize the importance of prehabilitation and early nutrition, which are discussed further later in discussion.[34] However, due to limitations in adoption and implementation, as well as heterogeneity between institutional protocols, the critical evaluation of their success has been challenging. Systematic reviews do, however, consistently show a decrease in pulmonary complications and length of hospital stay across studies.[35]

Performance status and frailty are known predictors of surgical outcomes, particularly in elderly patients.[36] Presurgical rehabilitation—or prehabilitation—has emerged as a tool to potentially improve postoperative recovery and outcomes by attempting to optimize preoperative physical and mental functioning in patients with esophagectomy using multimodal regimens of physical, nutritional, and/or psychological interventions. A recent meta-analysis of 1803 patients, 584 from randomized controlled trials and 1219 from observational studies, found that prehabilitation demonstrated reductions in postoperative pneumonia and pulmonary complications in patients from observational studies, but not consistently in randomized studies.[37] However, given the overall low quality of available evidence, further dedicated the prospective evaluation of the efficacy of prehabilitation is warranted to reveal any potential benefits in reducing postoperative morbidity.

Likewise, early implementation of nutritional support protocols may reduce postoperative weight loss and enhance recovery in patients with esophageal cancer that are candidates for esophagectomy. The risk of cancer-associated malnutrition is highest among patients with esophageal cancer and has been repeatedly shown to be an independent risk factor for worse survival in these patients.[38] Such protocols consist of active nutritional counseling starting at diagnosis and over the course of neoadjuvant therapy, as well as the early initiation of feedings via jejunostomy. A retrospective evaluation of 404 patients treated at our center, 217 in the protocol group and 187 in the control group, showed that length of hospital stay, time to oral diet initiation and feeding tube removal, and postoperative weight loss were all significantly reduced in the protocol group.[39]

ESOPHAGECTOMY IN PATIENTS WITH OLIGOMETASTATIC ADENOCARCINOMA

There is emerging evidence that, among carefully selected patients with oligometastatic esophageal or junctional adenocarcinoma, local treatment with esophagectomy and metastasectomy is associated with significantly longer disease-free and overall survival.[40–43] The concept of oligometastasis has been described as an intermediate state of limited metastatic spread that exists before the manifestation of widely metastatic systemic disease.[44] The clinical implication of this idea is that a window of time may exist during which local interventions, such as surgery, may prolong patient survival or even lead to cure in certain carefully selected patients. The diagnosis and establishment of oligometastatic disease in esophagogastric cancer depend heavily on imaging modalities such as positron-emission tomography, which can define the extent of disease with reasonable sensitivity, particularly at the baseline pretreatment timepoint. Staging laparoscopy is an important complement to imaging to assess for peritoneal metastasis that may not be visible on cross-sectional imaging.

In particular, interest in resecting oligometastatic gastric or GEJ cancer has been generated primarily by the German AIO-FLOT3 study.[45] Inclusive of patients with limited metastatic disease, the study demonstrated that selected patients might benefit from surgery, with promising results. In this phase II trial, 252 patients with resectable or metastatic tumors were assigned to 1 of 3 groups: resectable (arm A), limited metastatic (arm B), or extensive metastatic (arm C). Patients in arm A received perioperative FLOT, with surgery after the first 4 cycles of treatment. Patients in arm B received at least 4 cycles of neoadjuvant FLOT and proceeded to surgical resection if restaging showed that the margin-free (R0) resection of the primary tumor and at least a macroscopic complete resection of the metastatic lesions appeared feasible. Patients in arm C were offered FLOT chemotherapy and surgery only if required for palliation. Median OS was 22.9 months (95% CI, 16.5 to upper level not achieved) for arm B, compared with 10.7 months (95% CI, 9.1–12.8) for arm C (HR 0.37; 95% CI, 0.25–0.55; $P < .001$). Median OS was 31.3 months (95% CI, 18.9 to upper level not achieved) for patients who proceeded to surgery, compared with 15.9 months (95% CI, 7.1–22.9) for the other patients. At a minimum, this study demonstrated that patients with limited metastatic disease who undergo surgical resection have longer survival than patients for whom surgery is not an option.

The most important question regarding these findings is: To what extent did surgery contribute to the favorable outcomes of arm B in the AIO-FLOT-3 trial? Because of the lack of randomization, a relevant selection bias may exist. For instance, a difference in preoperative comorbidity was observed between the groups. Patients who underwent surgery had lower rates of comorbidity than patients who did not undergo surgery (50.0% vs 83.3%). The most common reason for patients not to undergo surgery was the investigator's decision that metastatic lesions were unresectable or incurable after neoadjuvant chemotherapy. Conversely, this means that patients who underwent surgery were super-selected. Nevertheless, within these limitations, the considerable survival in the surgical component of arm B remains promising and should be explored further. Of the patients who underwent surgery in arm B (n = 36), 2 (5.6%) underwent transthoracic esophagectomy, 17 (47.2%) underwent transhiatal esophagectomy, 14 (38.9%) underwent gastrectomy, 2 (5.6%) underwent laparotomy without resection, and 1 (2.8%) underwent an unknown type of resection (missing values). Metastasectomy of at least 1 metastatic lesion was performed in 17 of the 36 patients (47.2%) who underwent surgery in arm B. These surgical procedures included D3 lymphadenectomy in 7 patients, peritonectomy in 3, multi-visceral resection in 3, hepatectomy in 3, and adrenalectomy in 1. Among the 18 patients with retroperitoneal lymph node metastases who underwent resection, metastatic lymph node involvement was confirmed in 11 patients, was not assessable in 3 patients who had complete pathologic regression, and could not be confirmed in the other 4 patients. Complete pathologic regression (stage T0) was observed in 6 of the 36 patients (16.7%) in arm B who underwent surgery. Complete regression of resected metastatic lesions, as indicated by fibrotic changes and the absence of malignant cells, was observed in 3 patients (retroperitoneal lymph nodes in 2 patients and liver lesions in 1 patient). Severe postsurgical morbidity (fulfilling the criteria of a serious adverse event) was observed in 3 patients (8.3%) in arm B. There were no in-hospital deaths in arm B.

The favorable results reported in the FLOT3 study have prompted the now ongoing RENAISSANCE FLOT5 study.[46] This is a prospective, multicenter, randomized phase III trial whereby previously untreated patients with limited metastatic disease (retroperitoneal lymph node metastases only or a maximum of one metastatic organ site that is potentially resectable or locally controllable with or without retroperitoneal lymph nodes) receive 4 cycles of FLOT chemotherapy alone or with trastuzumab for patients with HER2-positive disease. Patients without disease progression after 4 cycles are randomized 1:1 to receive additional chemotherapy cycles or surgical resection of the primary tumor and metastatic sites, followed by subsequent chemotherapy. Other studies are concurrently evaluating similar approaches and will likely demonstrate a role for surgery in this setting. The most important challenge is successfully identifying the patients that will benefit from this approach.

CLINICS CARE POINTS

- In patients with superficial esophageal cancers with low risk for lymph node involvement, endoscopic resection with negative margins followed by close surveillance has replaced esophagectomy as the standard of care.
- Minimally invasive esophagectomy is associated with lower morbidity and better quality of life for patients, with equivalent surgical outcomes. This approach should be offered to patients, when feasible, at high-volume centers.
- A greater extent of surgical lymphadenectomy during esophagectomy likely improves long-term survival, regardless of neoadjuvant therapy, and should be emphasized during esophagectomy.
- Local therapy, including surgery, is reasonable to consider in carefully selected patients with oligometastatic esophageal adenocarcinoma.

FUNDING

This research was supported in part by NIH/NCI Cancer Center Support Grant P30 CA008748, which funds institutional core resources.

REFERENCES

1. Sung H, Ferlay J, Siegel RL, et al. Global cancer statistics 2020: GLOBOCAN estimates of incidence and mortality worldwide for 36 cancers in 185 countries. CA Cancer J Clin 2021;71(3):209–49.
2. Esophageal cancer – cancer stat facts, Available at: https://seer.cancer.gov/statfacts/html/esoph.html. Accessed December 27, 2023.
3. Sihag S, De La Torre S, Hsu M, et al. Defining low-risk lesions in early-stage esophageal adenocarcinoma. J Thorac Cardiovasc Surg 2021;162(4):1272–9.
4. Ajani JA, D'Amico TA, Bentrem DJ, et al. Esophageal and esophagogastric junction cancers, version 2.2023, NCCN clinical practice guidelines in oncology. J Natl Compr Cancer Netw 2023;21(4):393–422.
5. Malik S, Sharma G, Sanaka MR, et al. Role of endoscopic therapy in early esophageal cancer. World J Gastroenterol 2018;24(35):3965–73.
6. Pech O, May A, Manner H, et al. Long-term efficacy and safety of endoscopic resection for patients with mucosal adenocarcinoma of the esophagus. Gastroenterology 2014;146(3):652–660 e1.
7. Probst A, Aust D, Markl B, et al. Early esophageal cancer in Europe: endoscopic treatment by endoscopic submucosal dissection. Endoscopy 2015;47(2):113–21.

8. Sun F, Yuan P, Chen T, et al. Efficacy and complication of endoscopic submucosal dissection for superficial esophageal carcinoma: a systematic review and meta-analysis. J Cardiothorac Surg 2014;9:78.

9. Committee Asop, Forbes N, Elhanafi SE, et al, ASGE Standards of Practice Committee Chair. American Society for Gastrointestinal Endoscopy guideline on endoscopic submucosal dissection for the management of early esophageal and gastric cancers: summary and recommendations. Gastrointest Endosc 2023; 98(3):271–84.

10. Patel N, Benipal B. Incidence of esophageal cancer in the United States from 2001-2015: a United States cancer statistics analysis of 50 states. Cureus 2018;10(12):e3709.

11. Sihag S, Kosinski AS, Gaissert HA, et al. Minimally invasive versus open esophagectomy for esophageal cancer: a comparison of early surgical outcomes from the society of thoracic surgeons national database. Ann Thorac Surg 2016; 101(4):1281–8, discussion 8-9.

12. Luketich JD, Pennathur A, Awais O, et al. Outcomes after minimally invasive esophagectomy: review of over 1000 patients. Ann Surg 2012;256(1):95–103.

13. Biere SS, van Berge Henegouwen MI, Maas KW, et al. Minimally invasive versus open oesophagectomy for patients with oesophageal cancer: a multicentre, open-label, randomised controlled trial. Lancet 2012;379(9829):1887–92.

14. Kalff MC, Fransen LFC, de Groot EM, et al, Dutch Upper Gastrointestinal Cancer Audit group. Long-term survival after minimally invasive versus open esophagectomy for esophageal cancer: a nationwide propensity-score matched analysis. Ann Surg 2022;276(6):e749–57.

15. Dyas AR, Stuart CM, Bronsert MR, et al. Minimally invasive surgery is associated with decreased postoperative complications after esophagectomy. J Thorac Cardiovasc Surg 2023;166(1):268–78.

16. Brady JJ, Witek TD, Luketich JD, et al. Patient reported outcomes (PROs) after minimally invasive and open esophagectomy. J Thorac Dis 2020;12(11):6920–4.

17. Zhang J, Wang R, Liu S, et al. Refinement of minimally invasive esophagectomy techniques after 15 years of experience. J Gastrointest Surg 2012;16(9):1768–74.

18. Zhang W, Yu D, Peng J, et al. Gastric-tube versus whole-stomach esophagectomy for esophageal cancer: A systematic review and meta-analysis. PLoS One 2017;12(3):e0173416.

19. Usui H, Fukaya M, Itatsu K, et al. The impact of the location of esophagogastrostomy on acid and duodenogastroesophageal reflux after transthoracic esophagectomy with gastric tube reconstruction and intrathoracic esophagogastrostomy. World J Surg 2018;42(2):599–605.

20. Loo JH, Ng ADR, Chan KS, et al. Outcomes of intraoperative pyloric drainage on delayed gastric emptying following esophagectomy: a systematic review and meta-analysis. J Gastrointest Surg 2023;27(4):823–35.

21. Zheng R, Tham EJH, Rios-Diaz AJ, et al. A 10-year ACS-NSQIP analysis of trends in esophagectomy practices. J Surg Res 2020;256:103–11.

22. Ekeke CN, Kuiper GM, Luketich JD, et al. Comparison of robotic-assisted minimally invasive esophagectomy versus minimally invasive esophagectomy: a propensity-matched study from a single high-volume institution. J Thorac Cardiovasc Surg 2023;166(2):374–382 e1.

23. Zhang Y, Dong D, Cao Y, et al. Robotic versus conventional minimally invasive esophagectomy for esophageal cancer: a meta-analysis. Ann Surg 2023;278(1): 39–50.

24. Tagkalos E, Goense L, Hoppe-Lotichius M, et al. Robot-assisted minimally invasive esophagectomy (RAMIE) compared to conventional minimally invasive esophagectomy (MIE) for esophageal cancer: a propensity-matched analysis. Dis Esophagus 2020;33(4):doz060.

25. Zhou J, Xu J, Chen L, et al. McKeown esophagectomy: robot-assisted versus conventional minimally invasive technique-systematic review and meta-analysis. Dis Esophagus 2022;35(10):doac011.

26. Kurokawa Y, Takeuchi H, Doki Y, et al. Mapping of lymph node metastasis from esophagogastric junction tumors. Ann Surg 2021;274(1):120–7.

27. Lagergren J, Mattsson F, Zylstra J, et al. Extent of lymphadenectomy and prognosis after esophageal cancer surgery. JAMA Surg 2016;151(1):32–9.

28. Sisic L, Blank S, Weichert W, et al. Prognostic impact of lymph node involvement and the extent of lymphadenectomy (LAD) in adenocarcinoma of the esophagogastric junction (AEG). Langenbeck's Arch Surg 2013;398(7):973–81.

29. Ruffato A, Lugaresi M, Mattioli B, et al. Total lymphadenectomy and nodes-based prognostic factors in surgical intervention for esophageal adenocarcinoma. Ann Thorac Surg 2016;101(5):1915–20.

30. Rizk NP, Ishwaran H, Rice TW, et al. Optimum lymphadenectomy for esophageal cancer. Ann Surg 2010;251(1):46–50.

31. Altorki NK, Zhou XK, Stiles B, et al. Total number of resected lymph nodes predicts survival in esophageal cancer. Ann Surg 2008;248(2):221–6.

32. Koen Talsma A, Shapiro J, Looman CW, van Hagen P, Steyerberg EW, van der Gaast A, van Berge Henegouwen MI, Wijnhoven BPL, van Lanschot JJB, CROSS Study Group, Hulshof MCCM, van Laarhoven HWM, Nieuwenhuijzen GAP, Hospers GAP, Bonenkamp JJ, Cuesta MA, Blaisse RJB, Busch ORC, ten Kate FJW, Creemers GJ, Punt CJA, Plukker JTM, Verheul HMW, van Dekken H, van der Sangen MJC, Rozema T, Biermann K, Beukema JC, Piet AHM, van Rij CM, Reinders JG, Tilanus HW. Lymph node retrieval during esophagectomy with and without neoadjuvant chemoradiotherapy: prognostic and therapeutic impact on survival. Ann Surg 2014;260(5):786–92, discussion 92-3.

33. Sihag S, Nobel T, Hsu M, et al. A more extensive lymphadenectomy enhances survival after neoadjuvant chemoradiotherapy in locally advanced esophageal adenocarcinoma. Ann Surg 2022;276(2):312–7.

34. Low DE, Allum W, De Manzoni G, et al. Guidelines for perioperative care in esophagectomy: enhanced recovery after surgery (ERAS((R))) society recommendations. World J Surg 2019;43(2):299–330.

35. Salvans S, Grande L, Dal Cero M, et al. State of the art of enhanced recovery after surgery (ERAS) protocols in esophagogastric cancer surgery: the western experience. Updates Surg 2023;75(2):373–82.

36. Moskovitz AH, Rizk NP, Venkatraman E, et al. Mortality increases for octogenarians undergoing esophagogastrectomy for esophageal cancer. Ann Thorac Surg 2006;82(6):2031–6, discussion 6.

37. An KR, Seijas V, Xu MS, et al. Does prehabilitation before esophagectomy improve postoperative outcomes? A systematic review and meta-analysis. Dis Esophagus 2023;37(3):doad066.

38. Anandavadivelan P, Lagergren P. Cachexia in patients with oesophageal cancer. Nat Rev Clin Oncol 2016;13(3):185–98.

39. Carr RA, Harrington C, Stella C, et al. Early implementation of a perioperative nutrition support pathway for patients undergoing esophagectomy for esophageal cancer. Cancer Med 2022;11(3):592–601.

40. Grimes N, Devlin J, Dunne DF, et al. The role of hepatectomy in the management of metastatic gastric adenocarcinoma: a systematic review. Surg Oncol 2014; 23(4):177–85.
41. Nobel TB, Sihag S, Xing X, et al. Oligometastases after curative esophagectomy are not one size fits all. Ann Thorac Surg 2021;112(6):1775–81.
42. Chiapponi C, Berlth F, Plum PS, et al. Oligometastatic disease in upper gastrointestinal cancer - how to proceed? Visc Med 2017;33(1):31–4.
43. Jung JO, Nienhuser H, Schleussner N, et al. Oligometastatic gastroesophageal adenocarcinoma: molecular pathophysiology and current therapeutic approach. Int J Mol Sci 2020;21(3):951.
44. Reyes DK, Pienta KJ. The biology and treatment of oligometastatic cancer. Oncotarget 2015;6(11):8491–524.
45. Al-Batran SE, Homann N, Pauligk C, et al. Effect of neoadjuvant chemotherapy followed by surgical resection on survival in patients with limited metastatic gastric or gastroesophageal junction cancer: the AIO-FLOT3 trial. JAMA Oncol 2017;3(9):1237–44.
46. Al-Batran SE, Goetze TO, Mueller DW, et al. The RENAISSANCE (AIO-FLOT5) trial: effect of chemotherapy alone vs. chemotherapy followed by surgical resection on survival and quality of life in patients with limited-metastatic adenocarcinoma of the stomach or esophagogastric junction - a phase III trial of the German AIO/CAO-V/CAOGI. BMC Cancer 2017;17(1):893.

Esophagogastric Cancer
The Current Role of Radiation Therapy

Leila T. Tchelebi, MD[a,b,c,*], Karyn A. Goodman, MD[d]

KEYWORDS

- Esophagogastric cancer • Radiation therapy • IMRT • Neoadjuvant

KEY POINTS

- Multimodal therapy, including radiation therapy, is superior to surgery alone for patients with operable esophageal cancer.
- Chemoradiation can be used as definitive therapy in inoperable patients.
- The role of PET-directed treatment, induction chemotherapy, and the ideal radiation dose and treatment technique are under active investigation.

INTRODUCTION

Surgery remains the primary curative therapy for patients with gastroesophageal malignancies; however, the prognosis is poor following surgery alone, with 5 year overall survival (OS) rates of about 30%.[1] As a result, multimodal treatment is warranted for most patients presenting with nonmetastatic disease. While the routine use of radiation therapy in the management of patients with gastric cancer has diminished over the years, it continues to play an important role in the management of patients with cancers of the esophagus and gastroesophageal junction (GEJ).

There are several factors which explain why radiation therapy is of particular benefit for cancers arising from the esophagus. The rich lymphatic supply of the esophagus, coupled with the absence of a serosal layer, permits early microscopic spread of tumor cells beyond the surgical field, and the location of the esophagus within the mediastinum precludes resection with wide surgical margins. Additionally, unlike gastric cancer, esophageal cancer is associated with high rates of local failure of about 20% to 30%, warranting intensified local therapy in its management.[2] Finally,

[a] Northwell, Lake Success, NY, USA; [b] Department of Radiation Medicine, Northern Westchester Hospital, 400 East Main Street, Mount Kisco, NY 10549, USA; [c] Donald and Barbara Zucker School of Medicine at Hofstra/Northwell, Hempstead, NY, USA; [d] Department of Radiation Oncology, Icahn School of Medicine at Mount Sinai, One Gustave L. Levy Place, Box 1128, New York, NY 10029-6574, USA
* Corresponding author. 400 East Main Street, Mount Kisco, NY 10549.
E-mail address: ltchelebi@northwell.edu
Twitter: @LeilaTchelebi (L.T.T.); @KarynAGoodman (K.A.G.)

Hematol Oncol Clin N Am 38 (2024) 569–583
https://doi.org/10.1016/j.hoc.2024.02.001
0889-8588/24/© 2024 Elsevier Inc. All rights reserved.

achieving a pathologic complete response (pCR) to neoadjuvant therapy has been shown to be prognostic for improved local control and OS.[3,4]

Herein, we describe the current role of radiation therapy in the management of patients with esophageal and GEJ cancers. A summary of radiation trials in patients with esophageal cancer is shown in **Table 1**.

DISCUSSION
Operable Patients

Neoadjuvant Chemoradiation versus surgery alone

Long-term results of the landmark Chemoradiotherapy for Oesophageal Cancer Followed by Surgery Study (CROSS) established the superiority of multimodal therapy versus surgery alone for patients with esophageal cancer. In this phase III trial, 368 patients with nonmetastatic T1N1 or T2-3N0-1 squamous cell carcinoma (25%) or adenocarcinoma (75%) of the esophagus or esophagogastric junction were randomized to either upfront surgery or neoadjuvant chemoradiation (41.4 Gy in 23 fractions with concurrent carboplatin–paclitaxel [CP] weekly) followed by surgery.[5] The initial publication reported a significant benefit for the addition of chemoradiation, doubling the median OS from 24.0 months in the surgery group to 49.4 months in the neoadjuvant chemoradiotherapy group ($P = .003$, hazard ratio [HR] 0.657), thus establishing neoadjuvant therapy as standard of care in operable patients.[5] The pCR rates were 23% in patients with adenocarcinoma and 49% in those with squamous cell carcinomas. Ten-year outcomes revealed a persistent OS benefit to neoadjuvant chemoradiation versus surgery alone of 13% (38% vs 25%, $P < .05$). In particular, the 10 year OS was doubled for patients with squamous cell histology (46% vs 23%, $P<.05$).[6] It should be noted that neoadjuvant CRT did not have a negative impact on the postoperative complication rates as compared to patients undergoing surgery alone.[7]

The benefit of neoadjuvant CRT has been confirmed in multiple meta-analyses showing an improvement in OS, locoregional control, and R0 resection rates compared to surgery alone, without a concomitant increase in complication rates.[8,9] In an analysis of patterns of failure among patients treated on the CROSS trial, it was notable that in addition to a significant reduction in locoregional recurrence from 34% to 14%, neoadjuvant chemoradiation also significantly decreased the peritoneal and hematogenous recurrence rates from 14% to 4% and 35% to 29%, respectively. Nonetheless, distant recurrence was still the main cause of cancer mortality.

Neoadjuvant CRT ± induction chemotherapy

Owing to the high rates of distant failure for patients with esophageal cancer of approximately 50%,[10] there have been efforts to intensify neoadjuvant approaches with induction chemotherapy prior to CRT, but results have been mixed. A phase II single-institution study including 126 patients randomized to chemoradiation with or without induction chemotherapy with oxaliplatin/fluorouracil (FU) found no significant difference in median OS to the addition of induction chemotherapy (45.6 vs 43.7 months, $P = .69$).[11] A follow-up study seeking to identity any subsets of patients which might benefit found that the 5 year OS was improved in patients with well or moderately differentiated tumors when induction chemotherapy was added (74% vs 50%, $P =< 0.05$), but there was no benefit in patients with poorly differentiated tumors (31% vs 28%, $P = .04$).[12] Another phase II trial treating 85 patients with esophageal adenocarcinoma to induction chemotherapy (with oxaliplatin/capecitabine) randomized patients to receive subsequent CRT with 1 of 2 regimens (radiation therapy [RT] plus oxaliplatin/capecitabine or RT plus CP) with a primary endpoint of pCR. Only the RT arm including CP passed their predefined pCR criteria for further study.[13]

Table 1
Key trials involving radiation for esophagogastric cancer

Trial	Arms	Primary Outcome(s)	Results
Neoadjuvant CRT versus Surgery Alone			
CROSS	Arm 1: Surgery alone Arm 2: Neoadjuvant CRT (41.4 Gy + carbo/taxol)	mOS	CRT improved mOS: 24 mo vs 49.4 mOS; $P = .003$
Neoadjuvant CRT ± Induction Chemotherapy			
Ajani et al, Phase II	Arm 1: Neoadjuvant CRT (50.4 Gy+5FU/ oxaliplatin) Arm 2: IC (oxaliplatin + FU)→ the same CRT	pCR rate, mOS	No difference in (1) pCR rate: 13% (standard arm) vs 25% (exp arm) ($P = .094$) (2) or mOS 45.62 mo (standard) vs 43.68 mo (exp), $P = .69$)
NEOSCOPE	Arm 1: IC (oxaliplatin/capecitabine) → CRT (45 Gy + carbo/taxol) Arm 2: IC (oxaliplatin/capecitabine) → CRT (45 Gy + oxaliplatin/capecitabine)	Rate of pCR (pCR ≤15% would not warrant further investigation, but pCR ≥35% would)	Only CarPacRT passed the predefined pCR criteria for further investigation.
CALGB 80803	Arm 1: IC (FOLFOX) → CRT (50.4+PET-response directed chemotherapy with FOLFOX for responders or carbo/taxol for nonresponders) Arm 2: IC (carbo/taxol) → CRT (50.4+PET-response directed chemotherapy with carbo/taxol for responders or FOLFOX for non-responders)	pCR rate of PET nonresponders within each induction treatment group	pCR rates for PET nonresponders after induction FOLFOX who crossed over to CP or after induction CP who changed to FOLFOX was 18.0% (95% CI, 7.5–33.5) and 20% (95% CI, 10–33.7), respectively. Median OS: 27.4 mo for PET nonresponders vs 48.8 mo for PET responders ($P = .1$). Median OS not reached for PET responders after induction FOLFOX.
Neoadjuvant Chemotherapy vs Neoadjuvant CRT			
MAGIC	Arm 1: Surgery alone Arm 2: Perioperative ECF (epirubicin/cisplatin/FU)	5 y OS	Perioperative chemotherapy improved 5-y OS (26% vs 23%, $P = .009$)
Burmeister et al, Phase II	Arm 1: Preoperative chemo (cisplatin/FU) Arm 2: Preoperative CRT (35 Gy + cisplatin/FU)	Toxicity, pCR, R0 resection rate	Similar toxicity; improved pCR (31% vs 8%, $P = .01$) rate with CRT); higher rate of R1 resections with chemo vs CRT (11% vs 0%, respectively, $P = .04$)

(continued on next page)

Table 1
(continued)

Trial	Arms	Primary Outcome(s)	Results
POET	Arm 1: Preoperative chemo (cisplatin/FU) Arm 2: Preoperative chemo (cisplatin/FU)→CRT (30 Gy + cisplatin/etoposide)	3 y OS	Nonstatistically significant improvement in 3 y OS with CRT (47.4% for CRT vs 27.7% for chemo alone, $P = .07$)
NeoRes	Arm 1: Preoperative chemo (cisplatin/FU) Arm 2: Preoperative chemo (cisplatin/FU)→CRT (40 Gy + cisplatin/FU)	pCR	Improved pCR rate with CRT (28% vs 9%, $P < .05$)
Neo-AEGIS	Arm 1: Perioperative chemo (MAGIC regimen or FLOT) Arm 2: CRT (41.4 Gy + carbo/taxol)	mOS	No difference between arms (mOS 48 mo chemotherapy arm vs 49.2 mo CRT arm)
Adjuvant RT			
Intergroup-0116	Arm 1: Surgery alone Arm 2: CRT (45 Gy + FU)	mOS	CRT improved mOS (36 mo for CRT vs 27 mo for surgery alone, $P = .005$)
CRITICS	Arm 1: Perioperative chemo (epirubicin/cisplatin or oxaliplatin/capecitabine) Arm 2: Preoperative chemo (as Arm 1) and postop CRT (45 Gy + cisplatin/capecitabine)	mOS	No difference in mOS between arms (43 mo in chemo alone vs 37 mo in CRT arm, $P = .90$)
CALGB 80101	Arm 1: Postoperative FU→CRT (45 Gy + FU)→FU Arm 2: Postoperative ECF (epirubicin/cisplatin/FU)→CRT (45 Gy + FU)→ECF	5 y OS	No difference in 5 y OS between arms (44% in each arm, $P = .69$)
Definitive CRT			
RTOG 85–01	Arm 1: RT alone (50 Gy) Arm 2: CRT (50 Gy + cisplatin/FU)	5 y OS	Improved 5 y OS with CRT vs RT alone (26% vs 0%, respectively, $P < .01$)
Intergroup-0112	Single Arm: FU/cisplatin→CRT (64.8 Gy + FU/cisplatin)	Toxicity	6 deaths occurred, 5 (11%) were treatment related. mOS was only 20 mo.

	Arms	Endpoint	Results
Intergroup-0123	Arm 1: Standard CRT (50.4 Gy + FU/cisplatin) Arm 2: Dose-escalated CRT (64.8 Gy + FU/cisplatin)	2 y OS	No difference in 2 y OS between arms (40% vs 31% for Arm 1 vs Arm 2, respectively, $P > .05$). 11 treatment-related deaths in Arm 2, but 7 occurred before reaching 50.4 Gy
ARTDECO	Arm 1: Standard CRT (50.4 Gy + carbo/taxol) Arm 2: Dose-escalated CRT (61.6 Gy + carbo/taxol)	3 y PFS	No difference in 3 y PFS between arms (52% vs 59% for Arm 1 vs Arm 2, respectively, $P = .08$)
Xu et al	Arm 1: Standard CRT (50.4 Gy + cisplatin/taxol) → cisplatin/ docetaxel Arm 2: Dose-escalated CRT (60 Gy + cisplatin/taxol) → cisplatin/ docetaxel	3 y locoregional PFS	No difference in 3-y locoregional PFS between arms (48.4% vs 57.2% for Arm 1 vs Arm 2, respectively, $P = .98$)
CONCORDE	Arm 1: Standard CRT (50.4 Gy + carbo/taxol) Arm 2: Dose-escalated CRT (59.4 Gy + carbo/taxol)	mOS	No difference in mOS between arms (26 mo vs 28.1 mo for Arm 1 vs Arms 2, respectively, $P = .054$)
SANO	Arm 1: CRT → surgery Arm 2: CRT → active surveillance if cCR	mOS	No difference in mOS between arms (HR = 0.88, 95% upper boundary 1.40, $P = .007$)

Abbreviations: carbo, carboplatin; taxol, paclitaxel; cCR, clinical complete response; CRT, chemoradiation; FOLFOX, folinic acid + fluorouracil + oxaliplatin; FU, fluorouracil; Gy, gray; IC, induction chemotherapy; mOS, median overall survival; OS, overall survival; pCR, pathologic complete response; PFS, progression-free survival.

In addition to eradicating subclinical systemic disease, induction chemotherapy prior to adding radiotherapy allows for assessment of tumor response to chemotherapy, permitting response-adapted treatment. [14]F-fluorodeoxyglucose PET imaging is routinely used in staging esophageal cancer, and utilizing metabolic response to therapy to guide subsequent management has been shown to improve OS in patients.[14] The randomized phase II CALGB 80803 study evaluated whether metabolic response assessment by PET imaging after induction chemotherapy could be used to direct the decision to change chemotherapy during preoperative chemoradiotherapy with the goal of improving pCR and survival outcomes among PET nonresponders.[15] Two-hundred and forty-one patients with esophageal and esophagogastric junction adenocarcinoma were randomly assigned to induction chemotherapy with either FOL-FOX (modified oxaliplatin, leucovorin, and FU), or CP following baseline PET. The change in maximum standardized uptake value (SUV) from baseline after repeat PET following induction chemotherapy was used to guide subsequent management. PET nonresponders (<35% decrease in SUV from baseline) crossed over to the alternative chemotherapy during chemoradiation (50.4 Gy/28 fractions), while PET responders (≥35% decrease in SUV from baseline) continued on the same chemotherapy during chemoradiation. The primary end point was to improve pCR rates in the PET nonresponders to 20%. The pCR rates for PET nonresponders after induction FOLFOX who crossed over to CP ($n = 39$) or after induction CP who changed to FOLFOX ($n = 50$) were 18.0% (95% confidence interval [CI], 7.5–33.5) and 20% (95% CI, 10–33.7), respectively; thus, the efficacy criteria were met for both induction arms. With a median follow-up of 5.2 years, median OS was 48.8 months for PET responders and 27.4 months for nonresponders, which was not statistically significantly different, suggesting that by changing therapy based on PET response, the survival outcomes could also be improved to be closer the survival of the PET responders. For induction FOLFOX patients who were PET responders, median survival was not reached, and 5 year OS was 53%. This study demonstrated that an induction chemotherapy approach using a biomarker such as PET imaging to perform early response assessment allows for tailoring of therapy which improves outcomes in patients who are initially poor responders to induction chemotherapy. In addition, the promising 5 year OS rates suggest that selected patients who are PET responders have improved outcomes with FOLFOX induction followed by chemoradiotherapy using 5 FU and oxaliplatin.

Neoadjuvant chemotherapy versus neoadjuvant CRT

The benefit of neoadjuvant CRT versus neoadjuvant chemotherapy for cancers of the esophagus and GEJ has long been a subject of debate. Prior to the publication of the CROSS trial discussed earlier, the landmark MAGIC trial comparing perioperative chemotherapy (with epirubicin, cisplatin, and FU) with surgery alone showed an OS benefit to perioperative chemotherapy (36% vs 23% at 5 year, $P = .009$).[16] Unlike the CROSS study which included only cancers of the esophagus of GEJ with either squamous cell or adenocarcinoma histology, MAGIC included patients with cancers of the stomach, GEJ, or lower esophagus, thus calling into question the optimal regimen (neoadjuvant CRT vs chemotherapy alone) for patients with lower esophageal and GEJ adenocarcinomas. Subsequently, the landmark FLOT trial compared the perioperative chemotherapy used in MAGIC versus an intensified perioperative chemotherapy regimen (FU, leucovorin, oxaliplatin, docetaxel [FLOT]) in patients with gastric and GEJ adenocarcinoma. The FLOT regimen was associated with an improvement in median OS as compared to the standard arm (50 vs 35 months, respectively, $P = .012$), resulting in FLOT being the preferred perioperative regimen for patients with GEJ adenocarcinoma treated with perioperative chemotherapy alone.

Several randomized trials have questioned the benefit of neoadjuvant CRT versus neoadjuvant chemotherapy alone following the publication of MAGIC and CROSS. None has shown an OS benefit favoring one approach over the other, leaving this question unanswered. Two early randomized trials failed to show an OS benefit to CRT versus neoadjuvant chemotherapy alone, but both were limited by poor accrual.[17,18] While there was no improvement in OS, CRT compared to chemotherapy alone did improve the complete response rate (CRT 31% vs CT 8%, P = .01) and reduced R1 resection rate (CRT 0% vs CT 11%, P = .04).[17] Further, there were fewer locoregional recurrences among patients receiving CRT (18% vs 38%, P = .04) with similar rates of distant metastases (44% vs 29% for CRT vs chemotherapy, respectively, P = .20) and a trend toward improved OS favoring CRT (HR 0.65, 95%, CI, 0.42–1.01, P = .055).[19] The phase II NeoRes study randomized 180 patients with cancer of the esophagus or GEJ to neoadjuvant chemotherapy alone (cisplatin/FU) with or without concurrent radiation (40 Gy/20Fx) followed by surgery. The pCR rate was higher among patients receiving CRT (28% vs 9%), but this did not translate into an improvement in OS (42.2% vs 39.6% at 5 year for patients receiving CRT vs CT alone, respectively, P = .60).[20]

Two additional randomized trials sought to compare the MAGIC regimen to a neoadjuvant CRT approach. TOPGEAR is a phase III trial, which enrolled patients with adenocarcinoma of the stomach or GEJ randomizing them to perioperative chemotherapy alone (with Epirubicin, Cisplatin, 5-Fluorouracil [ECF] or FLOT) or to chemotherapy followed by preoperative CRT (45 Gy + FU).[21] While we await final publication, interim results of the first 120 enrolled patients demonstrated that CRT could be safely delivered preoperatively with an intensified perioperative chemotherapy regimen. Ninety-two percent of patients received their allocated preoperative CRT treatment and similar rates of grade 3 or higher toxicity in each arm (32% for chemotherapy alone vs 30% for CRT).

Neo-AEGIS is the only randomized study directly comparing the CROSS regimen to the MAGIC regimen (use of perioperative FLOT was permitted after publication of FLOT4 study) in patients with adenocarcinoma of the esophagus or GEJ.[22] The trial closed early following a futility analysis. There were no differences in median OS (48.0 months vs 49.2 months for chemotherapy vs CRT, respectively) or disease-free survival (32.4 months vs 24.0 months for chemotherapy vs CRT, respectively), and the patterns of failure were the same between the 2 groups. However, pCR (OR 0.33, 95% CI 0.14–0.81, P = .012) and R0 resection (OR = 0.21, 95% CI 0.08–0.53, P<.05) rates favored trimodality therapy. There were no significant differences among rates of grade 3 or higher toxicity between groups.

While there appears to be equipoise for chemotherapy or chemoradiotherapy as the optimal neoadjuvant treatment approach, the consistent improvement seen in pCR and R0 resection rates, without a concomitant increase in adverse events, highlights the continued role for neoadjuvant CRT in the management of patients with adenocarcinomas of the esophagus or GEJ. Ongoing trials, including TOPGEAR and the German ESOPEC trial (comparing preoperative chemotherapy with FLOT to CROSS chemoradiotherapy), will continue to address this question.

Adjuvant CRT

Adjunctive chemotherapy and radiation therapy in patients undergoing surgery for esophageal cancer should ideally be delivered in the neoadjuvant setting. The potential benefit of neoadjuvant as opposed to adjuvant therapy includes early treatment of micrometastatic disease, optimal selection of patients who would benefit most from surgery given the early development of metastatic disease in some patients, and to allow for nonoperative management in patients with squamous cell cancer achieving a clinical complete response. However, for patients undergoing up front surgery who did not receive chemotherapy and radiation therapy in the neoadjuvant setting, if they were found to have more advanced disease on final pathology as compared to clinical evaluation, there is a role of adjuvant treatment.

Several trials have been conducted to elucidate the optimal adjuvant regimen. The landmark Intergroup-0116 study randomized 559 patients with adenocarcinoma of the stomach or GEJ to surgery alone or postoperative CRT (45 Gy + FU). There was a strong OS benefit to the addition of adjuvant CRT (HR 1.32, 95% CI 1.10–1.60, P = .0046).[23] Overall relapse and local relapse rates were significantly improved with CRT. Given the OS benefit seen with perioperative chemotherapy in the MAGIC trial discussed earlier, the CRITICS study sought to incorporate both treatment strategies (perioperative chemotherapy as in MAGIC with postoperative CRT as in 0116) to determine whether the addition of radiotherapy to postoperative chemotherapy improves survival compared to postoperative chemotherapy alone. The trial randomized 788 patients with adenocarcinoma of the stomach or GEJ all receiving preoperative chemotherapy followed by surgery, to postoperative CRT (45 Gy + capecitabine/cisplatin) or to postoperative chemotherapy (epirubicin/cisplatin/oxaliplatin/capecitabine).[24] Median OS was similar between groups (43 months in the chemotherapy group vs 37 months in the CRT group [HR = 1.01, 95% CI 0.84–1.22, P = .90]). Compliance with the postoperative treatment regimen was poor in both groups (59% in the chemotherapy group and 62% in the CRT group) leading the authors to conclude that future investigations should focus on optimizing preoperative regimens. CALGB 80101 sought to build upon the results of Intergroup-0116 by adding an intensified postoperative adjuvant chemotherapy regimen to CRT. The trial randomized 546 patients with gastric or GEJ adenocarcinoma who had undergone a curative resection to receive either postoperative FU/leuvovorin (LV) before and after CRT (45 Gy/FU) versus ECF before and after CRT.[25] There was no difference in 5 year OS (44% in both arms) or 5 year disease free survival (DFS) (39% in the FU/LV arm vs 37% in the ECF arm, HR = 0.96, 95% CI, 0.77–1.20, P = .94). There were no differences in locoregional recurrences or distant failure between treatment arms.

Inoperable Patients

Definitive CRT

Nonoperative management may be indicated in a number of clinical scenarios. Patients who are not good surgical candidates or who have inoperable disease may be treated with definitive CRT. Further, patients with squamous cell carcinoma achieving a clinical complete response to neoadjuvant therapy may be able to safely forego surgery without compromising survival outcomes. Conducted in the late 1980s, RTOG 85-01 established the superiority of CRT over RT alone for patients with either squamous cell carcinoma (SCC) or adenocarcinoma of the esophagus who do not undergo surgery.[26] Efforts are ongoing to improve upon the results of this trial for patients undergoing definitive CRT without surgery.

Randomized trials have sought to intensify both the RT and the systemic therapy used in the definitive setting. The INT-0122 phase II study sought to increase the RT dose, the chemotherapy dose, the number of chemotherapy cycles, and added induction chemotherapy to the regimen used on RTOG 85-01.[27] Treatment-related mortality was high (9%) and thought to be due to the intensified chemotherapy regimen used. The follow-up study, INT-0123, intensified only the RT. The trial enrolled 236 patients with either SCC or adenocarcinoma of the esophagus and randomized them to either standard-dose RT (50.4 Gy) or high-dose RT (64.8 Gy) with concurrent FU/cisplatin.[28]

There was no benefit in 2 year OS for dose-escalated RT (31% vs 40% for standard-dose vs high-dose RT, respectively) or locoregional failure (56% vs 52% for standard-dose vs high-dose RT, respectively, $P = .71$). There were 11 deaths in the dose-escalated arm; however, 7 of these occurred in patients who received 50.4 Gy or less, leaving the benefit of dose escalation unanswered. Moreover, the radiotherapy techniques used in this study were not as conformal as more modern treatments using intensity-modulated radiotherapy (IMRT). Thus, a criticism of this study was that the radiation therapy was potentially associated with more toxicity, especially when delivering higher doses.

There have been further attempts at dose escalation, all of which have similarly failed to show a benefit to higher doses of radiation in the definitive setting for this disease. ARTDECO randomized patients with inoperable esophageal cancer to standard (50.4 Gy) or dose-escalated (61.6 Gy) RT, using IMRT planning, with concurrent CP. The primary end point of 3 year local progression- free survival (PFS) was not improved with dose escalation (52% and 59% for the standard- vs high-dose arms, respectively, $P = .08$).[29] There was no benefit to dose escalation in either histologic subgroup (SCC or adenocarcinoma). A Chinese phase III randomized study comparing standard (50 Gy) to dose-escalated (60 Gy) radiation, with concurrent cisplatin/docetaxel, for SCC patients also failed to find a benefit to dose escalation and found higher rates of pneumonitis in the dose-escalated arm.[30] Similarly, the CONCORDE trial comparing standard- (50.4 Gy) to high-dose (59.4 Gy) RT using only an IMRT approach with concurrent CP failed to show a benefit to dose escalation in inoperable SCC of the esophagus.[31]

Despite the failure of dose escalation in patients with SCC of the esophagus, there appears to be a role for definitive CRT in the management of these patients with standard-dose RT. In the aforementioned CROSS trial, 49% of patients with SCC achieved a pCR to neoadjuvant CRT, at a dose of 41.4 Gy with concurrent carboplatin/paclitaxel.[5] Two randomized studies comparing neoadjuvant CRT followed by surgery to CRT alone found no OS benefit to surgery in patients with esophageal SCC.[32,33] The recent SANO trial, only available in abstract form, was a noninferiority trial randomizing patients with esophageal cancer (either histology) to active surveillance versus surgery if a complete clinical response to neoadjuvant CRT was achieved. At a median follow-up of 34 months, there was no difference in OS between groups (HR = 0.88, 95% upper boundary 1.40, $P = .007$), but short-term quality of life was significantly improved in the active surveillance arm.[34] The final article and long-term results of this trial will clarify the role of surgery in patients achieving a complete response to neoadjuvant CRT, in particular for patients with SCC histology.

Role of Immunotherapy

Despite the curative intent of neoadjuvant CRT followed by surgery for esophageal cancer, the rates of recurrence, particularly among patients who do not achieve a complete pathologic response, remain high. Studies have thus sought to intensify therapy with the addition of immunotherapy either prior to or following resection, with promising results.

In the neoadjuvant setting, PERFECT was a single-arm phase II feasibility study assessing the feasibility and efficacy of delivering neoadjuvant CRT (per the CROSS regimen) with concurrent atezolizumab, a programmed-death ligand-1 (PD-L1) inhibitor.[35] The pCR rate was 25%. There was no statistically significant difference in survival between the PERFECT cohort and a propensity score-matched neoadjuvant CRT cohort (29.7 vs 34.3 months, respectively, $P = .43$). On exploratory biomarker analysis, there was higher baseline expression of interferon gamma (IFNγ) among responders to neoadjuvant CRT-atezolizumab, leading the authors to conclude that further study into an IFNγ signature and PD-L1 expression as potential biomarkers for prediction of response to neoadjuvant PD-L1 therapy is warranted. The initial safety run-in report of EA2174, a phase II/III study of perioperative nivolumab (given with neoadjuvant CRT), found that there was no increased toxicity from the addition of nivolumab to neoadjuvant CRT.[36]

Immunotherapy has also been studied in the adjuvant setting. Checkmate 577 was a phase III trial which enrolled 1085 patients with esophageal or GEJ cancer who had residual pathologic disease following neoadjuvant CRT and randomized them to receive adjuvant nivolumab versus placebo.[37] After a median follow-up of 24.4 months, the median DFS was significantly higher among patients receiving adjuvant nivolumab (22.4 vs 11.0 months, P<.001). Adverse events that were treatment-related were more common with nivolumab than with placebo, including grade 3 or 4 events (in 13% vs 6%, respectively).

Radiation Therapy Technique

Efforts are ongoing to optimize the radiation dose and delivery technique in patients with esophageal cancer. Patients should be simulated supine, with arms raised, on a custom immobilization device. They should be nil per os for 3 hours prior to simulation and treatment. Provided there are no contrast allergies, intravenous and oral contrast should be administered and diagnostic imaging, such as PET/CT, should be fused with the simulation CT to assist with target volume delineation. It is recommended that a motion management technique, such as 4D CT, is utilized to account for organ motion. The clinical target volume should include both gross disease and at-risk nodal volumes, which depend on the primary tumor location as per the expert consensus contouring guidelines for IMRT in esophageal cancer.[38] In addition, a generous superior and inferior anatomic margin around the esophagus is recommended due to the rich lymphatic system and absent serosal layer which allows for early subclinical tumor spread along the length of the esophagus. An analysis of the patterns of failure for patients in the CROSS trial with respect to radiation target volumes found that only 5% of locoregional recurrences occurred within the target volumes, 2% were at the border of the treatment volume, and 6% were out-of-field.[39] Of note, neoadjuvant CRT also reduced the rate of peritoneal carcinomatosis (14% with CRT vs 4% in surgery alone arm, P<.001) which the authors postulate was due to a reduction in microscopic residual disease following surgery in patients treated with neoadjuvant CRT.

The recommended radiation dose depends on the clinical scenario. Currently, doses in the range of 41.4 Gy (as per CROSS) to 50.4 Gy (as per CALGB 80803) are utilized in the neoadjuvant setting. For definitive treatment, 50.4 Gy is recommended given the failure of dose escalation to show an improvement in patient outcomes, as described earlier, even when utilizing highly conformal IMRT planning. For patients with cancer of the cervical esophagus, however, who are anatomically unable to undergo surgery, doses in the range of 60 to 66 Gy are considered, but this dose escalation remains a subject of active debate.[40,41]

The potential benefit of proton therapy versus photon therapy has been studied in an effort to reduce side effects from treatment. A phase IIB trial of photons using IMRT versus proton therapy in patients receiving neoadjuvant CRT to 50.4 Gy found that the total toxicity burden was significantly reduced with proton therapy (2.3 times higher with photons vs protons) with no difference in 3 year OS (44.5% in both arms).[42] A meta-analysis of 45 studies (31 of which were dosimetric comparisons) comparing proton to photon therapy found that treatment with protons resulted in reduced rates of grade 2 or higher radiation pneumonitis and pericardial effusion and grade 4 or higher lymphocytopenia. The authors also found an improvement in OS with protons (HR, 1.31; 95% CI, 1.07 to 1.61; I^2 = 11%), but given the heterogeneity of studied included in this meta-analysis, these findings must be interpreted with caution. The ongoing phase III randomized controlled trial, NRG-GI006, is seeking to definitively answer the question of whether there is a benefit to protons therapy over IMRT in patients with esophageal cancer.

FUTURE DIRECTIONS

Trials are ongoing to determine the optimal treatment approach in patients with esophageal and GEJ cancer and to improve upon the results described heretofore. We await final survival results from TOPGEAR, discussed earlier (NCT01924819). ESOPEC is a prospective randomized phase III trial comparing perioperative chemotherapy using the FLOT regimen (FU/LV/oxaliplatin/docetaxel) to neoadjuvant CRT per CROSS in patients with adenocarcinoma of the esophagus (NCT02509286) with a primary end point of OS.[43] RACE is a randomized phase III trial investigating the role of induction chemotherapy with FLOT followed by CRT versus preoperative FLOT alone in patients with potentially resectable GEJ adenocarcinoma with the primary end point of PFS (NCT04375605).[44] POWERRANGER is a randomized phase III trial comparing neoadjuvant chemotherapy (using FLOT) versus neoadjuvant CRT with a primary outcome measure of compliance and pathologic response rates (NCT01404156). SCOPE-2 is seeking to determine whether dose escalation to 60 Gy improves survival compared to standard doses of RT and whether PET-response directed therapy with switching the chemotherapy backbone in nonresponders (similar to CALGB 80803) improves outcomes in patients with esophageal cancer (either histology).[45]

SUMMARY

Radiation therapy is an effective treatment modality in the management of patients with esophageal cancer regardless of tumor location (proximal, middle, or distal esophagus) or histology (squamous cell vs adenocarcinoma). The addition of neoadjuvant CRT to surgery in patients who are surgical candidates has consistently shown a benefit in terms of locoregional recurrence, pathologic downstaging, and OS. For patients who are not surgical candidates, CRT has a role as definitive treatment. Studies are ongoing to assess the role of PET-directed treatment, the potential benefit of proton therapy, the role of induction chemotherapy, the earlier incorporation of immunotherapy, and the ideal radiation therapy dose, as well as the role of active surveillance among patients achieving a complete clinical response to neoadjuvant therapy.

CLINICS CARE POINTS

- Neoadjuvant chemoradiation improves survival compared to surgery alone for patients with operable esophageal cancer.

- The role of induction chemotherapy remains to be elucidated but available data show promising outcomes for patients receiving induction chemotherapy followed by PET-directed CRT.

- While there remains equipoise as to the optimal neoadjuvant regimen, neoadjuvant CRT has consistently shown a benefit in pathologic downstaging of patients as compared to other neoadjuvant approaches.

- Adjuvant immunotherapy after preoperative chemoradiation and surgery has been shown to improve disease-free survival in patients who did not achieve a pathologic completer response.
- Patients with esophageal cancer who do not receive neoadjuvant therapy benefit from adjuvant treatment but the optimal regimen remains under investigation.
- Definitive CRT is a standard option for patients with esophageal cancer who are medically inoperable or have unresectable disease, and dose escalation beyond 5040 cGy has not been shown to add any benefit.
- The role of immunotherapy in the neoadjuvant setting for patients with localized esophagogastric cancer is being studied.

REFERENCES

1. Njei B, McCarty TR, Birk JW. Trends in esophageal cancer survival in United States adults from 1973 to 2009: A SEER database analysis. J Gastroenterol Hepatol 2016;31(6):1141–6.
2. Pape M, Vissers PAJ, Beerepoot L, et al. Treatment patterns and overall survival for recurrent esophageal or gastroesophageal junctional cancer: A nationwide European population-based study. J Clin Oncol 2021;39(3_suppl):186.
3. Urba SG, Orringer MB, Turrisi A, et al. Randomized trial of preoperative chemoradiation versus surgery alone in patients with locoregional esophageal carcinoma. J Clin Oncol 2001;19(2):305–13.
4. Shapiro J, van Lanschot JJB, Hulshof MCCM, et al. Neoadjuvant chemoradiotherapy plus surgery versus surgery alone for oesophageal or junctional cancer (CROSS): long-term results of a randomised controlled trial. Lancet Oncol 2015;16(9):1090–8.
5. van Hagen P, Hulshof MC, van Lanschot JJ, et al. Preoperative chemoradiotherapy for esophageal or junctional cancer. N Engl J Med 2012;366(22):2074–84.
6. Eyck BM, JJBv Lanschot, Hulshof MCCM, et al. Ten-Year Outcome of Neoadjuvant Chemoradiotherapy Plus Surgery for Esophageal Cancer: The Randomized Controlled CROSS Trial. J Clin Oncol 2021;39(18):1995–2004.
7. Nederlof N, Slaman AE, van Hagen P, et al. Using the Comprehensive Complication Index to Assess the Impact of Neoadjuvant Chemoradiotherapy on Complication Severity After Esophagectomy for Cancer. Ann Surg Oncol 2016;23(12):3964–71.
8. Feng H, Zhao Y, Jing T, et al. Traditional and cumulative meta-analysis: Chemoradiotherapy followed by surgery versus surgery alone for resectable esophageal carcinoma. Mol Clin Oncol 2018;8(2):342–51.
9. Liu B, Bo Y, Wang K, et al. Concurrent neoadjuvant chemoradiotherapy could improve survival outcomes for patients with esophageal cancer: a meta-analysis based on random clinical trials. Oncotarget 2017;8(12):20410–7.
10. Kavanagh B, Anscher M, Leopold K, et al. Patterns of failure following combined modality therapy for esophageal cancer, 1984–1990. Int J Radiat Oncol Biol Phys 1992;24(4):633–42.
11. Ajani JA, Xiao L, Roth JA, et al. A phase II randomized trial of induction chemotherapy versus no induction chemotherapy followed by preoperative chemoradiation in patients with esophageal cancer. Ann Oncol 2013;24(11):2844–9.
12. Shimodaira Y, Slack RS, Harada K, et al. Influence of induction chemotherapy in trimodality therapy-eligible oesophageal cancer patients: secondary analysis of a randomised trial. Br J Cancer 2018;118(3):331–7.

13. Mukherjee S, Hurt CN, Gwynne S, et al. NEOSCOPE: A randomised phase II study of induction chemotherapy followed by oxaliplatin/capecitabine or carboplatin/paclitaxel based pre-operative chemoradiation for resectable oesophageal adenocarcinoma. Article. European Journal of Cancer 2017;74:38–46.
14. Lordick F, Ott K, Krause B-J, et al. PET to assess early metabolic response and to guide treatment of adenocarcinoma of the oesophagogastric junction: the MUNICON phase II trial. Lancet Oncol 2007;8(9):797–805.
15. Goodman KA, Ou F-S, Hall NC, et al. Randomized Phase II Study of PET Response–Adapted Combined Modality Therapy for Esophageal Cancer: Mature Results of the CALGB 80803 (Alliance) Trial. J Clin Oncol 2021;39(25):2803–15.
16. Cunningham D, Allum WH, Stenning SP, et al. Perioperative chemotherapy versus surgery alone for resectable gastroesophageal cancer. N Engl J Med 2006; 355(1):11–20.
17. Burmeister BH, Thomas JM, Burmeister EA, et al. Is concurrent radiation therapy required in patients receiving preoperative chemotherapy for adenocarcinoma of the oesophagus? A randomised phase II trial. European Journal of Cancer 2011; 47(3):354–60.
18. Stahl M, Walz MK, Stuschke M, et al. Phase III Comparison of Preoperative Chemotherapy Compared With Chemoradiotherapy in Patients With Locally Advanced Adenocarcinoma of the Esophagogastric Junction. J Clin Oncol 2009;27(6):851–6.
19. Stahl M, Walz MK, Riera-Knorrenschild J, et al. Preoperative chemotherapy versus chemoradiotherapy in locally advanced adenocarcinomas of the oesophagogastric junction (POET): Long-term results of a controlled randomised trial. European journal of cancer (Oxford, England : 1990) 2017;81:183–90.
20. von Dobeln GA, Klevebro F, Jacobsen AB, et al. Neoadjuvant chemotherapy versus neoadjuvant chemoradiotherapy for cancer of the esophagus or gastroesophageal junction: long-term results of a randomized clinical trial. Dis Esophagus 2019;32(2). https://doi.org/10.1093/dote/doy078.
21. Leong T, Smithers BM, Haustermans K, et al. TOPGEAR: A Randomized, Phase III Trial of Perioperative ECF Chemotherapy with or Without Preoperative Chemoradiation for Resectable Gastric Cancer: Interim Results from an International, Intergroup Trial of the AGITG, TROG, EORTC and CCTG. Ann Surg Oncol 2017;24(8):2252–8.
22. Reynolds JV, Preston SR, O'Neill B, et al. Trimodality therapy versus perioperative chemotherapy in the management of locally advanced adenocarcinoma of the oesophagus and oesophagogastric junction (Neo-AEGIS): an open-label, randomised, phase 3 trial. The Lancet Gastroenterology & Hepatology 2023;8(11): 1015–27.
23. Smalley SR, Benedetti JK, Haller DG, et al. Updated analysis of SWOG-directed intergroup study 0116: a phase III trial of adjuvant radiochemotherapy versus observation after curative gastric cancer resection. J Clin Oncol 2012;30(19): 2327–33.
24. Cats A, Jansen EPM, van Grieken NCT, et al. Chemotherapy versus chemoradiotherapy after surgery and preoperative chemotherapy for resectable gastric cancer (CRITICS): an international, open-label, randomised phase 3 trial. Lancet Oncol 2018;19(5):616–28.
25. Fuchs CS, Enzinger PC, Meyerhardt J, et al. Adjuvant chemoradiotlherapy with epirubicin, cisplatin, and fluorouracil compared with adjuvant chemoradiotherapy with fluorouracil and leucovorin after curative resection of gastric cancer: Results from CALGB 80101 (Alliance). Article. J Clin Oncol 2017;35(32):3671–7.

26. Cooper JS, Guo MD, Herskovic A, et al. Chemoradiotherapy of locally advanced esophageal cancer: Long-term follow-up of a prospective randomized trial (RTOG 85-01). Article. JAMA 1999;281(17):1623–7.

27. Minsky BD, Neuberg D, Kelsen DP, et al. Neoadjuvant chemotherapy plus concurrent chemotherapy and high-dose radiation for squamous cell carcinoma of the esophagus: a preliminary analysis of the phase II intergroup trial 0122. J Clin Oncol 1996;14(1):149–55.

28. Minsky BD, Pajak TF, Ginsberg RJ, et al. INT 0123 (Radiation Therapy Oncology Group 94-05) phase III trial of combined-modality therapy for esophageal cancer: high-dose versus standard-dose radiation therapy. J Clin Oncol 2002;20(5): 1167–74.

29. Hulshof M, Geijsen ED, Rozema T, et al. Randomized Study on Dose Escalation in Definitive Chemoradiation for Patients With Locally Advanced Esophageal Cancer (ARTDECO Study). J Clin Oncol 2021;39(25):2816–24.

30. Xu Y, Dong B, Zhu W, et al. A Phase III Multicenter Randomized Clinical Trial of 60 Gy versus 50 Gy Radiation Dose in Concurrent Chemoradiotherapy for Inoperable Esophageal Squamous Cell Carcinoma. Clin Cancer Res 2022;28(9): 1792–9.

31. You J, Zhu S, Li J, et al. High-Dose Versus Standard-Dose Intensity-Modulated Radiotherapy With Concurrent Paclitaxel Plus Carboplatin for Patients With Thoracic Esophageal Squamous Cell Carcinoma: A Randomized, Multicenter, Open-Label, Phase 3 Superiority Trial. Int J Radiat Oncol Biol Phys 2023; 115(5):1129–37.

32. Stahl M, Stuschke M, Lehmann N, et al. Chemoradiation with and without surgery in patients with locally advanced squamous cell carcinoma of the esophagus. J Clin Oncol 2005;23(10):2310–7.

33. Bedenne L, Michel P, Bouche O, et al. Chemoradiation followed by surgery compared with chemoradiation alone in squamous cancer of the esophagus: FFCD 9102. J Clin Oncol 2007;25(10):1160–8.

34. Eyck BM, van der Wilk BJ, Noordman BJ, et al. Updated protocol of the SANO trial: a stepped-wedge cluster randomised trial comparing surgery with active surveillance after neoadjuvant chemoradiotherapy for oesophageal cancer. Trials 2021;22(1):345.

35. van den Ende T, de Clercq NC, van Berge Henegouwen MI, et al. Neoadjuvant Chemoradiotherapy Combined with Atezolizumab for Resectable Esophageal Adenocarcinoma: A Single-arm Phase II Feasibility Trial (PERFECT). Clin Cancer Res 2021;27(12):3351–9.

36. Eads JR, Weitz M, Catalano PJ, et al. A phase II/III study of perioperative nivolumab and ipilimumab in patients (pts) with locoregional esophageal (E) and gastroesophageal junction (GEJ) adenocarcinoma: Results of a safety run-in— A trial of the ECOG-ACRIN Cancer Research Group (EA2174). J Clin Oncol 2021;39(15_suppl):4064.

37. Kelly RJ, Ajani JA, Kuzdzal J, et al. Adjuvant Nivolumab in Resected Esophageal or Gastroesophageal Junction Cancer. N Engl J Med 2021;384(13):1191–203.

38. Wu AJ, Bosch WR, Chang DT, et al. Expert Consensus Contouring Guidelines for Intensity Modulated Radiation Therapy in Esophageal and Gastroesophageal Junction Cancer. Int J Radiat Oncol Biol Phys 2015;92(4):911–20.

39. Oppedijk V, Avd Gaast, JJBv Lanschot, et al. Patterns of Recurrence After Surgery Alone Versus Preoperative Chemoradiotherapy and Surgery in the CROSS Trials. J Clin Oncol 2014;32(5):385–91.

40. Burmeister BH, Dickie G, Smithers BM, et al. Thirty-four Patients With Carcinoma of the Cervical Esophagus Treated With Chemoradiation Therapy. Arch Otolaryngol Head Neck Surg 2000;126(2):205–8.

41. Hoeben A, Polak J, Van De Voorde L, et al. Cervical esophageal cancer: a gap in cancer knowledge. Ann Oncol 2016;27(9):1664–74.

42. Lin SH, Hobbs BP, Verma V, et al. Randomized Phase IIB Trial of Proton Beam Therapy Versus Intensity-Modulated Radiation Therapy for Locally Advanced Esophageal Cancer. J Clin Oncol 2020;38(14):1569–79.

43. Hoeppner J, Lordick F, Brunner T, et al. ESOPEC: prospective randomized controlled multicenter phase III trial comparing perioperative chemotherapy (FLOT protocol) to neoadjuvant chemoradiation (CROSS protocol) in patients with adenocarcinoma of the esophagus (NCT02509286). BMC Cancer 2016; 16:503.

44. Lorenzen S, Biederstädt A, Ronellenfitsch U, et al. RACE-trial: neoadjuvant radiochemotherapy versus chemotherapy for patients with locally advanced, potentially resectable adenocarcinoma of the gastroesophageal junction - a randomized phase III joint study of the AIO, ARO and DGAV. BMC Cancer 2020;20(1):886.

45. Bridges S, Thomas B, Radhakrishna G, et al. SCOPE 2 – Still Answering the Unanswered Questions in Oesophageal Radiotherapy? SCOPE 2: a Randomised Phase II/III Trial to Study Radiotherapy Dose Escalation in Patients with Oesophageal Cancer Treated with Definitive Chemoradiation with an Embedded Phase II Trial for Patients with a Poor Early Response using Positron Emission Tomography/Computed Tomography. Clin Oncol 2022;34(7):e269–80.

Advances in Human Epidermal Growth Factor Receptor 2-Targeted Therapy in Upper Gastrointestinal Cancers

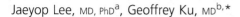

Jaeyop Lee, MD, PhD[a], Geoffrey Ku, MD[b],*

KEYWORDS

- HER2 • Esophagogastric cancer • Trastuzumab • Antibody drug conjugate
- Immune modulation • Immunotherapy • Targeted therapy

KEY POINTS

- Trastuzumab for Gastric Cancer (ToGA) Trial Significance: The ToGA trial established trastuzumab as the first human epidermal growth factor receptor 2 (HER2)-targeted therapy for advanced HER2-positive esophagogastric (EG) cancer.
- Decade-Long Interval: Many subsequent HER2-targeted approaches failed despite the ToGA trial's success. This highlights the complexity and challenges in advancing treatment strategies for HER2-positive EG cancer.
- KEYNOTE-811 Trial Breakthrough: The KEYNOTE-811 trial showcased the benefits of combining immune checkpoint blockade with HER2-targeting, opening new avenues for enhancing treatment efficacy in HER2-positive cases.
- Impact of T-DXd: The introduction of trastuzumab deruxtecan (T-DXd) demonstrated the potential of innovative drug technologies to improve treatment outcomes in patients who progressed after first-line HER2-targeted therapy.
- Review's Focus on Progress and Challenges: This review will focus on trials currently underway investigating promising and novel HER2-targeted therapeutic strategies, including first-in-class and first-in-human agents.

INTRODUCTION

By now, the human epidermal growth factor receptor 2 (HER2) is a well-known and well-validated biomarker and target in a growing list of solid tumors, which notably include gastroesophageal junction (GEJ) and gastric adenocarcinoma.

In 2010, the pivotal Trastuzumab for Gastric Cancer (ToGA) study established a clear role for the addition of trastuzumab, the prototypical anti-HER2 antibody, to

[a] Department of Medicine, Memorial Sloan Kettering Cancer Center, New York, NY, USA;
[b] Gastrointestinal Oncology Service, Department of Medicine, Memorial Sloan Kettering Cancer Center, New York, NY, USA
* Corresponding author.
E-mail address: kug@mskcc.org

Hematol Oncol Clin N Am 38 (2024) 585–598
https://doi.org/10.1016/j.hoc.2024.02.005
0889-8588/24/© 2024 Elsevier Inc. All rights reserved.

chemotherapy in the first-line treatment of advanced GEJ/gastric cancer[1] After a frustrating span of nearly a decade where subsequent phase III studies failed to establish benefit for any other anti-HER2 strategies, the last several years have seen the results of several positive phase II/III studies, which have significantly moved the field forward.

In this review article, we will focus on the principles of HER2 assessment, phase III evaluations in the last decade, and ongoing and promising studies of novel therapies.

Human Epidermal Growth Factor Receptor 2

HER2 is encoded by the *ERBB2* gene, which is a critical member of the epidermal growth factor receptor (EGFR) family that also includes EGFR (*ERBB1*), HER3 (*ERBB3*), and HER4 (*ERBB4*).[2] This family plays a fundamental role in various cellular functions, including growth, differentiation, and survival. HER2 is unique among these receptors due to its ability to remain in an active conformation without the need for ligand binding, thus functioning as an "orphan receptor."

The HER receptors typically form homodimers or heterodimers upon activation, which leads to the autophosphorylation of specific tyrosine residues in the cytoplasmic domain and downstream signaling cascade activation. For HER2, the dimerization, either as homodimers or more commonly as heterodimers with other HER family members, is a pivotal step in the activation of downstream RAS/mitogen activated protein kinase (MAPK)[3] and PI3K/Akt/mTOR pathways.[4] HER2/HER2 or HER2/EGFR dimerization leads to the initiation of the former pathway, while HER2/HER3 dimerization is one of the most potent drivers of the latter, a key player in cell survival and anti-apoptotic mechanisms.

In esophagogastric (EG) cancers, the amplification of the *ERBB2* gene and the resultant overexpression of the HER2 protein are associated with aggressive tumor behavior[5] and poor prognosis.[6] The heterodimerization of HER2 with other EGFR family members in these cancers suggests a complex network of signaling that drives tumorigenesis and progression.[7] Understanding the nuances of these interactions and the resultant signaling pathways is crucial for the development of targeted therapies and improving patient outcomes in HER2+ EG cancers.

Navigating Through Human Epidermal Growth Factor Receptor 2 Screening and Diagnostic Challenges

HER2 expression, a vital parameter in delineating therapeutic pathways, is often assessed through immunohistochemistry (IHC) and/or in situ hybridization (ISH) methodologies. According to the American Society of Clinical Oncology/College of American Pathologists (ASCO/CAP) guidelines, a sequential testing approach is recommended for HER2 testing. The guidelines suggest first performing IHC testing, followed by ISH if the IHC results show a score of 2+ (equivocal), as previously established by Rüschoff/Hoffmann.[8,9] For tumors with an IHC score of 0 or 1+ (negative), or 3+ (positive), additional ISH testing is generally not needed as these scores are considered conclusive for the absence or presence of HER2 overexpression, respectively. For IHC 2+, ISH positivity is determined by an ERBB2:CEP17 ratio of ≥ 2 or an average ERBB2 copy number ≥ 6 signals per cell. Conversely, HER2 is deemed negative for IHC 2+ with negative ISH findings.

This sequential testing strategy helps in accurately determining HER2 status, which is crucial for guiding appropriate treatment. This evaluation should be conducted at the initial diagnosis of EG adenocarcinoma with clinical or radiographic indications of advanced or progressive disease. This classification has been established after seeing patients with HER2 IHC 3+ or HER2 2+ plus ISH positivity experienced the most benefit from HER2-directed therapy in the ToGA trial, which will be discussed later.

The prevalence of HER2+ disease in EG cancers approximates 20%,[10–13] with the ToGA trial indicating a higher rate of HER2+ tumors originating at the GEJ or gastric cardia (approximately 30%) compared to distal gastric sites (approximately 15%).[1] A HER2+ status is also more commonly observed in intestinal subtypes (30%), Barrett-related dysplasia (24%), cases with chromosomal instability,[14] and low tumor mutational burden.[15] In the authors' anecdotal experience, HER2 positivity and mismatch repair protein (MMR) deficiency (dMMR)/microsatellite instability (MSI) are almost always mutually exclusive, that is, virtually no HER2-positive tumors are dMMR/MSI.

Determining HER2 positivity in EG cancers presents unique challenges due to the heterogeneous nature of HER2 expression across tissue samples.[8,16] This heterogeneity is more pronounced in gastric cancers compared to breast or colorectal cancers, with variations not only in intensity but also in the distribution of HER2 along different cellular axes, from the apical to the basolateral and from the cytosol to the membrane. Additionally, there can be discordance between immunohistochemistry (IHC) and *in situ* hybridization (ISH) results in these cancers.[16,17] This complexity in HER2 staining patterns makes it imperative that HER2 IHC be reviewed by an experienced pathologist to ensure accurate interpretation.

The evaluation of small tissue samples for HER2 testing in EG cancers is particularly challenging. To obtain a reliable analysis, it is recommended to use primary tumor specimens or multiple biopsies from either primary or metastatic lesions, rather than relying solely on fine needle aspiration samples.[18] This approach is critical because of the spatial heterogeneity of HER2 expression in these tumors.[19] Furthermore, for cases where traditional tissue sampling is not feasible, alternative methods for HER2 detection including cell-free DNA (cfDNA) are being actively explored to offer more options for accurate diagnosis.

First-line therapy for advanced human epidermal growth factor receptor 2+ esophagogastric cancer

Pioneering advances: the Trastuzumab for Gastric Cancer trial. The landmark ToGA trial, conducted by Bang and colleagues,[1] established the clinical utility of HER2-directed therapy as a first-line intervention for unresectable, locally advanced, recurrent, or metastatic gastric/GEJ cancers. This phase III study randomized 584 patients, whose tumors were defined as being HER2 positive based on criteria of HER2 IHC 3+ or fluorescence in situ hybridization (FISH) positive, to receive standard chemotherapy (fluorouracil or capecitabine plus cisplatin) with or without trastuzumab, the antibody against HER2. The intent-to-treat analysis revealed a statistically significant improvement in median overall survival (OS) in the investigational arm (13.8 vs 11.1 months, hazard ratio [HR] 0.74, $P = 0046$). Subsequent exploratory analyses, employing the Hoffman and colleagues criteria for HER2+ cases (IHC 3+ or IHC 2+/FISH positive), revealed an improvement in median overall survival (OS) to 16 months in the trastuzumab arm versus 11.8 months in the chemotherapy-only arm (HR 0.65; 95% CI 0.51–0.83). Notably, this therapeutic advantage was observed irrespective of geographic origin (European, 23.6%; Asian, 23.9%) and HER2 heterogeneity, as evidenced by the fact that 50.3% of tumor samples had less than 30% stained cells.[20] Similarly, tumors characterized by an IHC score of 0 or 1+—despite FISH positivity—failed to exhibit a substantial therapeutic advantage upon the incorporation of trastuzumab, with an OS of 10 months compared to 8.7 months in the control group (HR = 1.07). These results underscore the rationale for the contemporary definition of HER2 positivity. Nevertheless, it is worth noting that in the rare situation of an IHC 3+ tumor without ERBB2 gene amplification, patients experience a short progression-free survival (PFS) on first-line trastuzumab/chemotherapy.[21]

The decade-long gap after Trastuzumab for Gastric Cancer. Although the ToGA trial established HER2 as a validated biomarker in EG cancer, raising hopes for the study of other novel HER2-targeted treatments that were already established in HER2-positive breast cancer, it would be another decade before the next regimen would be approved for this subgroup.

The LOGiC trial,[22] a phase III study published in 2015, sought to augment the effects of chemotherapy by adding lapatinib, a small molecule tyrosine kinase inhibitor (TKI) of EGFR and HER2, in patients with *HER2*-amplified disease. Lapatinib had been approved for HER2+ breast cancer[23] and with significant preclinical data showing preclinical efficacy in upper gastrointestinal (GI) cancers.[24] However, the trial failed to demonstrate a statistically significant improvement in OS for the investigational arm (12.2 vs 10.5 months, HR 0.91, $P = .3492$) regardless of IHC scores. Although not powered for subgroup analysis, it was noted that Asian patients younger than 60 years of age, who predominantly had gastric cancer, may have benefited more than the Western patients. Similarly, the HELOISE trial,[25] a phase IIIb study, which aimed to enhance the cytotoxic effects of trastuzumab by administering higher doses, was negative for the higher dose trastuzumab experimental arm (median OS 10.6 vs 12.5 months, HR, 1.24; $P = .2401$).

In 2018, the phase III JACOB trial[26] evaluated pertuzumab in combination with trastuzumab/chemotherapy. Pertuzumab is an inhibitory antibody that acts by binding the dimerization-domain of HER2, while trastuzumab is a direct inhibitor by binding the sub-domain IV of HER2. While this combination is part of the gold-standard in the management of HER2+ breast cancer,[27] there was no significant difference in OS observed between the pertuzumab-treated or control groups (17.5 vs 14.2 months, HR 0.84,$P = .057$), despite a numerical improvement in overall response rate (ORR) (56.7% vs 48.3%, $P = .026$) and PFS (8.5 vs 7.0 months, HR 0.73, $P = .0001$); because of the hierarchical testing procedure in this study, statistical significance for PFS and ORR could not be formally assessed. It remains plausible that this was a "near-miss" and that a slightly larger study may have been better powered to detect a statistically significant difference in OS. Nevertheless, further evaluation of pertuzumab in gastric cancer ceased.

In the second-line and later, there were also several negative trials. The phase III TyTAN[28] trial in 2014 aimed to evaluate the efficacy of lapatinib combined with paclitaxel compared to paclitaxel alone in advanced gastric cancers in Asian patients with HER2- amplified disease (regardless of IHC status). Despite failing to show a significant overall benefit compared to paclitaxel alone, a hypothesis-generating observation was the significant OS benefit in the subgroup of patients with IHC 3+ disease (14.0 vs 7.6 months; HR 0.59, $P = 0176$). This result suggested that HER2 inhibition is most effective in patients with high target expression. The majority of patients in the study (57%) had a non-intestinal subtype, commonly associated with lower HER2 IHC scores, which may have blunted the drug's response.

Trastuzumab emtansine (T-DM1), an antibody-drug conjugate (ADC) or trastuzumab plus a microtubule inhibitor known for its success in breast cancer,[29] was evaluated in HER2-positive EG cancers in the GATSBY trial.[30] This phase II/III study compared T-DM1 to docetaxel or paclitaxel in previously treated patients with advanced HER2-positive EG cancer. Unfortunately, T-DM1 failed to show significant benefit in OS or PFS. Potential reasons for its lack of efficacy include poor drug internalization and release, suboptimal activity in gastric cancers, increased emtansine efflux, or resistance leading to downregulation of HER2 surface protein.[21,31]

A complementary strategy of continuing trastuzumab beyond progression was evaluated in the randomized phase II T-ACT trial,[31] which randomized 91 patients to paclitaxel with or without trastuzumab. There was no improvement in the primary endpoint of PFS or secondary endpoints of ORR and OS. However, it provided key insights into resistance mechanisms. Approximately 69% of 16 patients who had tissue available for testing exhibited downregulation or loss of HER2 protein expression post-first-line treatment, suggesting downregulation of HER2 expression as an adaptive resistance mechanism. Circulating HER2 DNA amplification was detected in only 60% of assayed patients. Patients exhibiting IHC 0 also had an associated negative cfDNA and ISH status, pointing to a genomic-level loss of HER2 amplification consistent with prior findings.[32,33]

Recent developments: immune checkpoint inhibitors and KEYNOTE-811. The advent of immune checkpoint inhibitors (ICIs) has reinvigorated the therapeutic landscape. Two single-center phase II trials added pembrolizumab to trastuzumab/chemotherapy with promising efficacy and safety. These findings paved the way for the KEYNOTE-811 trial,[34] a randomized, double-blind, placebo-controlled phase III study. An interim analysis revealed a statistically and clinically significant improvement in the ORR to 74.4% in the pembrolizumab arm compared to 51.9% in the placebo arm, which led to its FDA approval in May 2021 for all patients irrespective of programmed death-ligand 1 (PD-L1) status. Notably, this was the first FDA approval in oncology for a combination based on an improvement in ORR alone.

Very recently, updated results from the third interim analysis from March 2023 were published.[35] This analysis confirmed an improvement in the co-primary endpoint of median PFS (10.0 vs 8.1 months, HR 0.72, $P = 0.0002$). The other co-primary endpoint, OS, is numerically improved (20.0 vs 16.8 months, HR 0.83) but was not statistically significant. At this time, patients will continue to be followed for this outcome. This updated analysis also revealed that benefit was restricted only to tumors with PD-L1 combined positive score (CPS) ≥ 1 (85% of the patient population). In fact, in patients whose tumor PD-L1 CPS was <1, the HR for PFS was 1.03 (95% CI 0.65–1.64), while the HR for OS was 1.41 (95% CI 0.90–2.20). The point estimate for the HR for OS suggesting harm from the addition of pembrolizumab to standard therapy is concerning. But this could be related to undetermined imbalance in the small number of patients with PD-L1 CPS <1 tumors. Additional follow-up and further biomarker evaluation of this subgroup will be important to try to understand this initial observation.

Human epidermal growth factor receptor 2-targeted therapies as second-line treatment or later
The impact of trastuzumab deruxtecan in human epidermal growth factor receptor 2+ esophagogastric cancers. Trastuzumab deruxtecan (T-DXd)[36] is a groundbreaking treatment for HER2-positive breast cancer as a second-line therapy.[37,38] T-DXd is an antibody-drug conjugate (ADC) that combines trastuzumab and deruxtecan with a cleavable peptide linker. Its multifaceted mechanism includes HER2 receptor dimerization blocking, antibody-dependent cell cytotoxicity activation, payload release in lysosomes, and targeted chemotherapy delivery with a bystander effect.[39,40] Notably, T-DXd remains effective in patients with prior HER2-targeted therapies and works across varying HER2 expression levels in EG cancers.

The DESTINY-Gastric01 trial, a critical Phase II study led by Shitara and colleagues,[41] assessed T-DXd's efficacy and safety in Japanese and South Korean patients with advanced HER2-positive gastric/GEJ cancer. This trial achieved its primary endpoint, demonstrating a remarkable increase in ORR with 51% of the patients responding to T-DXd compared to only 14% who received the physician's choice of treatment. Furthermore, significant improvements were seen in OS, a secondary endpoint, with the T-DXd group showing OS of 12.5 months versus 8.4 months (HR 0.59, P = .01). PFS was numerically improved in the T-DXd group (5.6 months vs 3.5 months, HR 0.47) but the study was not designed to formally evaluate this outcome. In a subset analysis, greater efficacy was seen in patients with HER2 IHC 3+ compared to those with HER2 IHC 2+/ISH+, an observation that warrants close attention in ongoing studies. A subsequent exploratory analysis by Shitara and colleagues[42] further highlighted that patients who had received ICIs prior to the trial benefitted more in terms of ORR (65.9% vs 42.7%) and OS (16.6 vs 10.3 months), underlining the potential synergistic effect of combining ICIs with HER2 targeting.

Building on these findings, the single-arm DESTINY-Gastric02 trial[43] was conducted with patients from the United States and Europe. Patients received T-DXd as second-line therapy and, notably, had to have pre-treatment biopsies following progression on first-line trastuzumab-based therapy confirming retention of HER2 positivity. This study mirrored the positive results of DESTINY-Gastric01, with a 42% response rate to T-DXd, an OS of 12.1 months, and PFS of 5.6 months. Notably, a higher ORR was also observed in HER2 IHC 3+ versus IHC 2+/ISH + cancers (47.1% vs 10.0%).

These studies have successfully established T-DXd as a valuable addition to the HER2-targeted treatment arsenal, leading to its approval by the FDA in the U.S., by the European Medicines Agency and in Japan. Possible explanations include that T-DXd retains killing activity in lower IHC score lesions,[37] potentially due to its cleavable linker, more potent cytotoxic payload, and higher payload ratio (3.8 in T-DM1 vs 8 in T-DXd).[44,45]

Novel anti-human epidermal growth factor receptor 2 therapies

Tucatinib is an HER2-selective tyrosine kinase inhibitor and has shown significant efficacy in treating patients with HER2+ metastatic breast cancer,[46] particularly those who have previously undergone HER2-directed therapies. The drug is also able to cross the blood-brain barrier and has shown activity in breast cancer patients with central nervous system metastases. In GI cancers, its effectiveness was further established in the MOUNTAINEER trial,[47] where tucatinib combined with trastuzumab became the first approved anti-HER2 regimen for HER2+ RAS wild-type metastatic colorectal cancer. Building on this success, the phase II/III MOUNTAINEER-02 trial (NCT04499924) was launched to evaluate the combination of ramucirumab/paclitaxel with or without tucatinib in the second-line treatment of HER2-positive gastric cancer. However, as of August 2023, enrollment has stopped.

Disitamab vedotin (RC-48) is a novel humanized anti-HER2 immunoglobulin (Ig) G1 antibody (ie, hertuzumab) conjugated to a microtubule inhibitor, monomethyl auristatin E (MMAE) through a cleavable linker.[48] Its mechanism of action is by inhibiting the HER2 signaling pathway, inducing cytotoxicity through its payload both on target and to bystander cells. Recent findings from a phase II trial showed its effectiveness as ≥third-line treatment in Chinese patients with advanced HER2+ gastric/GEJ cancers, achieving an ORR of 24.8%, median PFS of 4.1 months, and median OS of 7.9 months.[49,50] This trial was notable for including patients with HER2 IHC scores 2 and 3 irrespective of their ISH status. Patients with IHC 2+ and negative ISH had an ORR of 16.7%, slightly lower than the conventional HER2+ group (26.3%). The most common treatment-related adverse events (TRAEs) included grade leukopenia (52%), anemia (49.6%), increased aspartate aminotransferase (AST) (43.2%), and alopecia (53.6%). The ongoing phase III trial RC48-007 (NCT04714190) aims to further establish its efficacy as a third-line treatment against standard care in HER2+ gastric/ GEJ cancer patients. The study seeks to enroll 351 patients and is estimated to complete accrual at the end of December 2023.

Margetuximab, a new monoclonal antibody targeting HER2, features an optimized Fc region enhancing its binding to CD16 A on natural killer (NK) cells and increasing antibody-dependent cellular cytotoxicity (ADCC)-mediated cell death. It proved safe and tolerable as a single agent in various advanced cancers, mainly causing grade 1 to 2 constitutional symptoms as TRAEs.[51]

The CP-MGAH22 to 05 phase Ib/II trial assessed margetuximab combined with pembrolizumab in advanced HER2+ EG cancer patients previously treated with trastuzumab and chemotherapy.[52] The trial included HER2 amplification and PD-L1 combined positive score (CPS) analysis. This combination achieved an 18% ORR overall with subgroup analyses showing that those with HER2 IHC 3+ or PD-L1 CPS $\geq$1 trended toward greater benefit compared to HER2 IHC 2+ (ORR 24% vs 0%) or PD-L1 CPS <1 (33% vs 7%). The highest response (60% ORR) was seen in HER2 amplied, HER2 IHC 3+ and PD-L1 CPS $\geq$1 group.

Building on these findings, the MAHOGANY trial[53] (NCT04082364) explored margetuximab plus chemotherapy with retifanlimab (MG012, a novel anti-PD-1 humanized monoclonal antibody) or tebotelimab (MGD013, a novel bispecific antibody targeting PD-1 and LAG3) in HER2+ advanced gastric/GEJ cancer, focusing on first-line treatments. However, the study was closed in February 2022 after enrolling 82 patients.

Zanidatamab (ZW25) is a humanized, IgG isotype-like, bispecific monoclonal antibody directed against the juxtamembrane domain (ECD4) and the dimerization domain (ECD2) of HER2. This unique biparatopic binding mechanism results in several therapeutic actions[54–56]: it causes HER2-receptor clustering, internalization, and downregulation, effectively inhibiting both growth factor-dependent and growth factor-independent tumor cell proliferation. Additionally, zanidatamab activates ADCC, along with complement-dependent cytotoxicity, attacking the cancer cells through multiple pathways.

A first-in-human phase I dose-escalation demonstrated its safety and tolerability in patients with either HER2-expressing or HER2-amplified advanced solid tumors of any kind, with common treatment-related adverse events (TRAEs) being diarrhea (52%) and infusion reactions (34%), both grade 1 or 2.[56] A subsequent phase II trial evaluating its efficacy when combined with chemotherapy in first-line treatment for advanced HER2+ EG cancers demonstrated a remarkable antitumor effect with a 75% confirmed ORR (cORR) and 89% disease control rate (DCR).[57] The proposed phase III regimen of zanidatamab with CAPOX or 5FU/cisplatin had a 94% cORR and a 100% DCR from a cohort of 16 patients. Median overall PFS across all treatment groups was 12.0 months.[58] Most common TRAEs (grade 1 to 3) were diarrhea, which was manageable with loperamide in an outpatient setting. No grade $\geq$3 adverse infusion reactions or cardiac events were noted.

These outcomes prompted the HERIZON-GEA-01 trial[59] (NCT05152147), which is a phase III study comparing trastuzumab and chemotherapy to zanidatamab in combination with chemotherapy with or without tislelizumab, a humanized IgG4 anti-PD1 monoclonal antibody designed to minimize binding to FcgR on macrophages, as first-line treatment in patients with advanced HER2+ EG cancers. Primary endpoints are PFS and OS, results of which may place zanidatamab not only as a new first-line treatment option but also as a new HER2-targeted treatment modality.

Evorpacept (ALX148) is a high-affinity antibody that binds to the "do-not-eat-me" surface protein CD47, which is expressed on many cell types and signals macrophages not to phagocytose them. Binding of evorpacept on CD47+ cancer cells inhibits such signal and promotes their elimination by phagocytosis through a concerted activity of a concurrent targeted drug such as trastuzumab.[60]

ASPEN-01 was a dose-escalation with dose-expansion phase I trial to determine the safety and tolerability of evorpacept. In the dose-expansion cohort of 19 patients with previously treated HER2+ gastric/GEJ cancers, including those that have progressed on trastuzumab, the evorpacept with trastuzumab doublet showed an 21.1% ORR with 8.7 months duration of response (DOR), and 8.1 months median OS.[61] Following this, the safety and activity of evorpacept in combination with trastuzumab, ramucirumab plus paclitaxel was evaluated. There were no dose-limiting toxicities and the maximum tolerated dose was not reached. ORR in this group was 73.3% and a median DOR that was not reached at 7.7 months median follow-up. Median PFS was 9.8 months, median OS was not reached, and the estimated OS at 1 year was 70%.[62]

Subsequently, the ASPEN-06 trial was launched, which is a randomized phase II/III trial evaluating evorpacept in combination with trastuzumab/ramucirumab/paclitaxel as second-line or later-line treatment for patients with advanced HER2+ gastric/GEJ cancers. Interim analysis showed a 52% cORR in patients receiving evorpacept, many of whom had previously progressed on T-DXd and checkpoint inhibitors. This was significantly higher than the 22% in the control arm. The median DOR was not reached in the investigational arm, while the control group's was 7.4 months.[63] Final results of the randomized phase II portion of the study—whose primary endpoint is ORR—are anticipated in the second quarter of 2024. Notably, this was the first randomized trial in HER2+ EG cancer where prior treatment with ICI and T-DXd was permitted as well as the first study to highlight a positive result for any CD47 blocker, and consequently establishing it as a potential first-in-class immunotherapy modality. For now, the phase III portion of the study, where the primary endpoint is OS, is anticipated to begin accrual in late 2024.

Trastuzumab deruxtecan is further being explored in 2 ongoing trials: DESTINY-Gastric03 (NCT04379596) and DESTINY-Gastric04 (NCT04704934). DESTINY-Gastric03, a phase I/IIb multicenter trial, is evaluating T-DXd combined with fluoropyrimidine-based regimens with or without an ICI as a first-line and second-line treatment. Early results, as reported by Janjigian and colleagues,[64] show significant responses in 5 out of 7 heavily pretreated, trastuzumab-refractory, and fluoropyrimidine-refractory HER2+ patients. Meanwhile, DESTINY-Gastric04, a phase III trial, is conducting a head-to-head comparison of T-DXd with ramucirumab/paclitaxel as second-line therapy, aiming to definitively establish T-DXd's role as a second-line HER2-directed treatment.

Human epidermal growth factor receptor 2-targeted therapies in the adjuvant and neoadjuvant setting

For localized, operable esophageal gastric cancer (EGC), the prevailing treatment approach, irrespective of HER2 presence, is typically either preoperative chemoradiotherapy or perioperative chemotherapy followed by surgery, as guided by the findings of the CROSS[65] and FLOT4[66] studies. Attempts to enhance these treatment frameworks by incorporating anti-HER2 therapies have been made. While initial phase II trials appeared promising, no phase III randomized trials have yet shown a definitive advantage.

The exploration of trastuzumab in adjuvant and neoadjuvant settings for EG cancer has been a focal point in recent clinical trials. The Radiation Therapy Oncology Group (RTOG) 1010 trial,[67] a phase III study, investigated the addition of trastuzumab to the

CROSS regimen (carboplatin/paclitaxel with concurrent radiation) in a neoadjuvant context. However, this trial did not demonstrate significant improvements in pathologic complete responses (pCRs), disease-free survival or OS. Similarly, the PET-RARCA trial,[68] a phase II/III study, compared the FLOT regimen with and without trastuzumab and pertuzumab. The phase II results indicated a significant increase in pCR rates and lymph node negativity with the addition of trastuzumab and pertuzumab (35% vs 12%). Despite these encouraging findings, the trial did not progress to phase III, influenced partly by the negative outcomes of the JACOB trial. The European Organization for Research and Treatment of Cancer (EORTC) 1203 INNOVATION trial,[69] which also terminated early due to slow accrual, examined the combination of trastuzumab and pertuzumab with chemotherapy, but it did not show a significant difference in major pathologic response. The final report and OS results are awaited to potentially identify patient subgroups that could benefit from this combination therapy.

These trials highlight the complexity of optimizing treatment strategies for HER2+ EG cancers and emphasize the need to refine patient selection and biomarkers, a better understanding of tumor heterogeneity, and investigate new treatment avenues as well as mechanisms of HER2 treatment resistance.

SUMMARY

The research landscape for HER2-positive EG cancer has significantly advanced in the last 5 years, with notable progress in HER2-targeted therapies. These treatments, effective even after initial progression on trastuzumab, underscore the importance of the HER2 pathway in disease management and progression. Their favorable safety profiles, characterized by tolerability and manageable side effects, highlight their potential for ongoing research.

Variations in outcomes with different treatments, such as trastuzumab and T-DXd, emphasize the need for optimized drug delivery, particularly in antibody-drug conjugates (ADCs), which is an active area of ongoing trials.

The emergence of ICIs has revolutionized the approach to HER2-positive EG cancers, highlighting the significant role of the immune system. This has spurred new strategies to enhance the antitumor effects of immune cells, leading to innovative immunotherapy approaches that modify both myeloid and lymphoid cell functions. Analyzing biopsies and non-invasive samples before and after treatment will be crucial for understanding the interaction between the immune system and HER2+ EG cancer.

Concurrently, efforts are being made to improve the detection of HER2 amplification and protein overexpression over time, along with tracking other relevant biomarkers. This is the key in understanding the biology and evolution of the disease, predicting treatment response, and elucidating mechanisms of resistance to HER2-targeted therapies.

Overall, the ongoing and dedicated research in this field reflects the scientific community's commitment to combat HER2+ EG cancers. This dedication is leading to better treatment options and a deeper understanding of the disease.

CLINICS CARE POINTS

- Verification of HER2 Status: The verification of HER2 expression or amplification in metastatic EG adenocarcinomas is critical. Given the histological heterogeneity, accurate determination of HER2 status via IHC and/or FISH by an experienced pathologist is essential.

- Caution with Novel Diagnostic Technologies: The utilization of novel methodologies, such as cfDNA for HER2 status assessment, should be approached with caution, as these techniques lack validation in the clinical practice context.

- Combination Therapy with Immune Checkpoint Inhibitors: The integration of immune checkpoint inhibitors with HER2-targeted therapies necessitates judicious patient selection, particularly based on PD-L1 status, to optimize therapeutic outcomes while mitigating risks. Exclusion of immune checkpoint blockade is advised for PD-L1 CPS <1 in metastatic EG adenocarcinomas as first-line therapy, in light of recent insights from the KEYNOTE-811 trial.

- Continuation of HER2-Directed Therapy Post-Progression: For patients who progress following first-line trastuzumab, continuation with second-line trastuzumab-deruxtecan (T-DXd) where approved, or enrollment in clinical trials including T-DXd, is recommended.

- Clinical Trial Participation: Clinicians are urged to advocate for eligible patient participation in clinical trials exploring innovative HER2-targeted therapies and combinations, thereby fostering the evolution of treatment paradigms for HER2-positive EG cancers.

REFERENCES

1. Bang Y-J, Van Cutsem E, Feyereislova A, et al. Trastuzumab in combination with chemotherapy versus chemotherapy alone for treatment of HER2-positive advanced gastric or gastro-oesophageal junction cancer (ToGA): a phase 3, open-label, randomised controlled trial. Lancet 2010;376:687–97.
2. Rubin I, Yarden Y. The basic biology of HER2. Ann Oncol 2001;12:S3–8.
3. Yarden Y, Pines G. The ERBB network: at last, cancer therapy meets systems biology. Nat Rev Cancer 2012;12:553–63.
4. Faber AC, Li D, Song Y, et al. Differential induction of apoptosis in HER2 and EGFR addicted cancers following PI3K inhibition. Proc Natl Acad Sci USA 2009;106:19503–8.
5. Shiraishi N, Sato K, Yasuda K, et al. Multivariate prognostic study on large gastric cancer. J Surg Oncol 2007;96:14–8.
6. Kato S, Okamura R, Baumgartner JM, et al. Analysis of Circulating Tumor DNA and Clinical Correlates in Patients with Esophageal, Gastroesophageal Junction, and Gastric Adenocarcinoma. Clin Cancer Res 2018;24:6248–56.
7. Jørgensen JT, Hersom M. HER2 as a Prognostic Marker in Gastric Cancer - A Systematic Analysis of Data from the Literature. J Cancer 2012;3:137–44.
8. Hofmann M, Stoss O, Shi D, et al. Assessment of a HER2 scoring system for gastric cancer: results from a validation study. Histopathology 2008;52:797–805.
9. Rüschoff J, Hanna W, Bilous M, et al. HER2 testing in gastric cancer: a practical approach. Mod Pathol 2012;25:637–50.
10. Janjigian YY, Werner D, Pauligk C, et al. Prognosis of metastatic gastric and gastroesophageal junction cancer by HER2 status: a European and USA International collaborative analysis. Ann Oncol 2012;23:2656–62.
11. Moelans CB, van Diest PJ, Milne ANA, et al. Her-2/neu testing and therapy in gastroesophageal adenocarcinoma. Pathol Res Int 2010;2011:674182.
12. Chua TC, Merrett ND. Clinicopathologic factors associated with HER2-positive gastric cancer and its impact on survival outcomes—A systematic review. Int J Cancer 2012;130:2845–56.
13. Gómez-Martin C, Garralda E, Echarri MJ, et al. HER2/neu testing for anti-HER2-based therapies in patients with unresectable and/or metastatic gastric cancer. J Clin Pathol 2012;65:751–7.

14. Hisamatsu Y, Oki E, Otsu H, et al. Effect of EGFR and p-AKT Overexpression on Chromosomal Instability in Gastric Cancer. Ann Surg Oncol 2016;23:1986–92.
15. Kim HR, Ahn S, Jo H, et al. The Impact of Tumor Mutation Burden on the Effect of Frontline Trastuzumab Plus Chemotherapy in Human Epidermal Growth Factor Receptor 2-Positive Advanced Gastric Cancers. Front Oncol 2021;11:792340.
16. Haffner I, Schierle K, Raimúndez E, et al. HER2 Expression, Test Deviations, and Their Impact on Survival in Metastatic Gastric Cancer: Results From the Prospective Multicenter VARIANZ Study. J Clin Oncol 2021;39:1468–78.
17. Huemer F, Weiss L, Regitnig P, et al. Local and Central Evaluation of HER2 Positivity and Clinical Outcome in Advanced Gastric and Gastroesophageal Cancer—Results from the AGMT GASTRIC-5 Registry. J Clin Med 2020;9:935.
18. Bartley AN, Washington MK, Colasacco C, et al. HER2 Testing and Clinical Decision Making in Gastroesophageal Adenocarcinoma: Guideline From the College of American Pathologists, American Society for Clinical Pathology, and the American Society of Clinical Oncology. J Clin Oncol 2017;35:446–64.
19. Fusco N, Rocco EG, Del Conte C, et al. HER2 in gastric cancer: a digital image analysis in pre-neoplastic, primary and metastatic lesions. Mod Pathol 2013;26: 816–24.
20. Van Cutsem E, Nordlinger B, Adam R, et al. Towards a pan-European consensus on the treatment of patients with colorectal liver metastases. Eur J Cancer 2006; 42:2212–21.
21. Janjigian YY, Sanchez-Vega F, Jonsson P, et al. Genetic Predictors of Response to Systemic Therapy in Esophagogastric Cancer. Cancer Discov 2018;8:49–58.
22. Hecht JR, Bang YJ, Qin SK, et al. Lapatinib in Combination With Capecitabine Plus Oxaliplatin in Human Epidermal Growth Factor Receptor 2–Positive Advanced or Metastatic Gastric, Esophageal, or Gastroesophageal Adenocarcinoma: TRIO-013/LOGiC—A Randomized Phase III Trial. J Clin Oncol 2016;34: 443–51.
23. Blackwell KL, Burstein HJ, Storniolo AM, et al. Overall Survival Benefit With Lapatinib in Combination With Trastuzumab for Patients With Human Epidermal Growth Factor Receptor 2–Positive Metastatic Breast Cancer: Final Results From the EGF104900 Study. J Clin Oncol 2012;30:2585–92.
24. Wainberg ZA, Anghel A, Desai AJ, et al. Lapatinib, a dual EGFR and HER2 kinase inhibitor, selectively inhibits HER2-amplified human gastric cancer cells and is synergistic with trastuzumab in vitro and in vivo. Clin Cancer Res 2010;16: 1509–19.
25. Shah MA, Xu RH, Bang YJ, et al. HELOISE: Phase IIIb Randomized Multicenter Study Comparing Standard-of-Care and Higher-Dose Trastuzumab Regimens Combined With Chemotherapy as First-Line Therapy in Patients With Human Epidermal Growth Factor Receptor 2–Positive Metastatic Gastric or Gastroesophageal Junction Adenocarcinoma. J Clin Oncol 2017. https://doi.org/10.1200/JCO. 2016.71.6852.
26. Tabernero J, Hoff PM, Shen L, et al. Pertuzumab plus trastuzumab and chemotherapy for HER2-positive metastatic gastric or gastro-oesophageal junction cancer (JACOB): final analysis of a double-blind, randomised, placebo-controlled phase 3 study. Lancet Oncol 2018;19:1372–84.
27. Swain SM, Miles D, Kim SB, et al. Pertuzumab, trastuzumab, and docetaxel for HER2-positive metastatic breast cancer (CLEOPATRA): end-of-study results from a double-blind, randomised, placebo-controlled, phase 3 study. Lancet Oncol 2020;21:519–30.

28. Satoh T, Xu RH, Chung HC, et al. Lapatinib Plus Paclitaxel Versus Paclitaxel Alone in the Second-Line Treatment of HER2-Amplified Advanced Gastric Cancer in Asian Populations: TyTAN—A Randomized, Phase III Study. J Clin Oncol 2014; 32:2039–49.

29. Diéras V, Miles D, Verma S, et al. Trastuzumab emtansine versus capecitabine plus lapatinib in patients with previously treated HER2-positive advanced breast cancer (EMILIA): a descriptive analysis of final overall survival results from a randomised, open-label, phase 3 trial. Lancet Oncol 2017;18:732–42.

30. Thuss-Patience PC, Shah MA, Ohtsu A, et al. Trastuzumab emtansine versus taxane use for previously treated HER2-positive locally advanced or metastatic gastric or gastro-oesophageal junction adenocarcinoma (GATSBY): an international randomised, open-label, adaptive, phase 2/3 study. Lancet Oncol 2017; 18:640–53.

31. Makiyama A, Sukawa Y, Kashiwada T, et al. Randomized, Phase II Study of Trastuzumab Beyond Progression in Patients With HER2-Positive Advanced Gastric or Gastroesophageal Junction Cancer: WJOG7112G (T-ACT Study). J Clin Oncol 2020;38:1919–27.

32. Saeki H, Oki E, Kashiwada T, et al. Re-evaluation of HER2 status in patients with HER2-positive advanced or recurrent gastric cancer refractory to trastuzumab (KSCC1604). Eur J Cancer 2018;105:41–9.

33. Seo S, Ryu MH, Park YS, et al. Loss of HER2 positivity after anti-HER2 chemotherapy in HER2-positive gastric cancer patients: results of the GASTric cancer HER2 reassessment study 3 (GASTHER3). Gastric Cancer 2019;22:527–35.

34. Janjigian YY, Kawazoe A, Yañez P, et al. The KEYNOTE-811 trial of dual PD-1 and HER2 blockade in HER2-positive gastric cancer. Nature 2021;600:727–30.

35. Janjigian YY, Kawazoe A, Bai Y, et al. Pembrolizumab plus trastuzumab and chemotherapy for HER2-positive gastric or gastro-oesophageal junction adenocarcinoma: interim analyses from the phase 3 KEYNOTE-811 randomised placebo-controlled trial. Lancet 2023;0.

36. Ogitani Y, Aida T, Hagihara K, et al. DS-8201a, A Novel HER2-Targeting ADC with a Novel DNA Topoisomerase I Inhibitor, Demonstrates a Promising Antitumor Efficacy with Differentiation from T-DM1. Clin Cancer Res 2016;22:5097–108.

37. Modi S, Jacot W, Yamashita T, et al. Trastuzumab Deruxtecan in Previously Treated HER2-Low Advanced Breast Cancer. N Engl J Med 2022;387:9–20.

38. André F, Hee Park Y, Kim SB, et al. Trastuzumab deruxtecan versus treatment of physician's choice in patients with HER2-positive metastatic breast cancer (DESTINY-Breast02): a randomised, open-label, multicentre, phase 3 trial. Lancet 2023;401:1773–85.

39. Doi T, Shitara K, Naito Y, et al. Safety, pharmacokinetics, and antitumour activity of trastuzumab deruxtecan (DS-8201), a HER2-targeting antibody–drug conjugate, in patients with advanced breast and gastric or gastro-oesophageal tumours: a phase 1 dose-escalation study. Lancet Oncol 2017;18:1512–22.

40. Ogitani Y, Hagihara K, Oitate M, et al. Bystander killing effect of DS-8201a, a novel anti-human epidermal growth factor receptor 2 antibody-drug conjugate, in tumors with human epidermal growth factor receptor 2 heterogeneity. Cancer Sci 2016;107:1039–46.

41. Shitara K, Bang YJ, Iwasa S, et al. Trastuzumab Deruxtecan in Previously Treated HER2-Positive Gastric Cancer. N Engl J Med 2020;382:2419–30.

42. Shitara K, Bang YJ, Iwasa S, et al. Exploratory analysis of the impact of prior immune checkpoint inhibitor (ICI) on trastuzumab deruxtecan (T-DXd; DS-8201) clinical outcomes and biomarkers (BM) in DESTINY-Gastric01 (DG-01), a

randomized, phase 2, multicenter, open-label study in patients (pts) with HER2+ advanced gastric or gastroesophageal junction adenocarcinoma. J Clin Oncol 2022;40:322.

43. Van Cutsem E, di Bartolomeo M, Smyth E, et al. Trastuzumab deruxtecan in patients in the USA and Europe with HER2-positive advanced gastric or gastroesophageal junction cancer with disease progression on or after a trastuzumab-containing regimen (DESTINY-Gastric02): primary and updated analyses from a single-arm, phase 2 study. Lancet Oncol 2023;24:744–56.

44. Nakada T, Sugihara K, Jikoh T, et al. The Latest Research and Development into the Antibody-Drug Conjugate, [fam-] Trastuzumab Deruxtecan (DS-8201a), for HER2 Cancer Therapy. Chem Pharm Bull (Tokyo) 2019;67:173–85.

45. Marcoux J, Champion T, Colas O, et al. Native mass spectrometry and ion mobility characterization of trastuzumab emtansine, a lysine-linked antibody drug conjugate. Protein Sci Publ Protein Soc 2015;24:1210–23.

46. Murthy RK, Loi S, Okines A, et al. Tucatinib, Trastuzumab, and Capecitabine for HER2-Positive Metastatic Breast Cancer. N Engl J Med 2020;382:597–609.

47. Strickler JH, Nakamura Y, Yoshino T, et al. MOUNTAINEER-02: Phase II/III study of tucatinib, trastuzumab, ramucirumab, and paclitaxel in previously treated HER2+ gastric or gastroesophageal junction adenocarcinoma—Trial in Progress. J Clin Oncol 2021;39:TPS252.

48. Jiang J, Li S, Shan X, et al. Preclinical safety profile of disitamab vedotin : a novel anti-HER2 antibody conjugated with MMAE. Toxicol Lett 2020;324:30–7.

49. Peng Z, Liu T, Wei J, et al. Efficacy and safety of a novel anti-HER2 therapeutic antibody RC48 in patients with HER2-overexpressing, locally advanced or metastatic gastric or gastroesophageal junction cancer: a single-arm phase II study. Cancer Commun Lond Engl 2021;41:1173–82.

50. Xu Y, Wang Y, Gong J, et al. Phase I study of the recombinant humanized anti-HER2 monoclonal antibody–MMAE conjugate RC48-ADC in patients with HER2-positive advanced solid tumors. Gastric Cancer 2021;24:913–25.

51. Bang YJ, Giaccone G, Im SA, et al. First-in-human phase 1 study of margetuximab (MGAH22), an Fc-modified chimeric monoclonal antibody, in patients with HER2-positive advanced solid tumors. Ann Oncol 2017;28:855–61.

52. Catenacci DVT, Kang YK, Park H, et al. Margetuximab plus pembrolizumab in patients with previously treated, HER2-positive gastro-oesophageal adenocarcinoma (CP-MGAH22–05): a single-arm, phase 1b–2 trial. Lancet Oncol 2020;21: 1066–76.

53. Catenacci DV, Rosales M, Chung HC, et al. MAHOGANY: margetuximab combination in HER2+ unresectable/metastatic gastric/gastroesophageal junction adenocarcinoma. Future Oncol Lond Engl 2021;17:1155–64.

54. Weisser NE, Sanches M, Escobar-Cabrera E, et al. An anti-HER2 biparatopic antibody that induces unique HER2 clustering and complement-dependent cytotoxicity. Nat Commun 2023;14:1394.

55. Proctor JR, Gartner EM, Gray TE, et al. Population pharmacokinetics of zanidatamab, an anti-HER2 biparatopic antibody, in patients with advanced or metastatic cancer. Cancer Chemother Pharmacol 2022;90:399–408.

56. Meric-Bernstam F, Beeram M, Hamilton E, et al. Zanidatamab, a novel bispecific antibody, for the treatment of locally advanced or metastatic HER2-expressing or HER2-amplified cancers: a phase 1, dose-escalation and expansion study. Lancet Oncol 2022;23:1558–70.

57. Ku G, Elimova E, Denlinger C, et al. 1380P Phase (Ph) II study of zanidatamab + chemotherapy (chemo) in first-line (1L) HER2 expressing gastroesophageal adenocarcinoma (GEA). Ann Oncol 2021;32:S1044–5.

58. Elimova E, Ajani JA, Burris III HA, et al. Zanidatamab + chemotherapy as first-line treatment for HER2-expressing metastatic gastroesophageal adenocarcinoma (mGEA). J Clin Oncol 2023;41:347.

59. Tabernero J, Shen L, Elimova E, et al. HERIZON-GEA-01: Zanidatamab + chemo ± tislelizumab for 1L treatment of HER2-positive gastroesophageal adenocarcinoma. Future Oncol 2022;18:3255–66.

60. Lakhani NJ, Chow LQM, Gainor JF, et al. Evorpacept alone and in combination with pembrolizumab or trastuzumab in patients with advanced solid tumours (ASPEN-01): a first-in-human, open-label, multicentre, phase 1 dose-escalation and dose-expansion study. Lancet Oncol 2021;22:1740–51.

61. Lee K-W, Chung H, Kim TM, et al. 498 Evorpacept (ALX148), a CD47 myeloid checkpoint inhibitor, in patients with head and neck squamous cell carcinoma (HNSCC) and with gastric/gastroesophageal cancer (GC); ASPEN-01. J. Immunother. Cancer 2021;9.

62. Chung H, Lee K, Kim W, et al. SO-31 ASPEN-01: A phase 1 study of ALX148, a CD47 blocker, in combination with trastuzumab, ramucirumab and paclitaxel in patients with second-line HER2-positive advanced gastric or gastroesophageal junction cancer. Ann Oncol 2021;32:S215–6.

63. ALX Oncology Reports Positive Interim Phase 2 ASPEN-06 Clinical Trial Results of Evorpacept for the Treatment of Advanced HER2-Positive Gastric Cancer – ALX Oncology. https://ir.alxoncology.com/news-releases/news-release-details/alx-oncology-reports-positive-interim-phase-2-aspen-06-clinical/.

64. Janjigian YY, Oh DY, Rha SY, et al. Dose-escalation and dose-expansion study of trastuzumab deruxtecan (T-DXd) monotherapy and combinations in patients (pts) with advanced/metastatic HER2+ gastric cancer (GC)/gastroesophageal junction adenocarcinoma (GEJA): DESTINY-Gastric03. J Clin Oncol 2022;40:295.

65. van Hagen P, Hulshof MCCM, van Lanschot JJB, et al. Preoperative Chemoradiotherapy for Esophageal or Junctional Cancer. N Engl J Med 2012;366:2074–84.

66. Al-Batran S-E, Homann N, Pauligk C, et al. Perioperative chemotherapy with fluorouracil plus leucovorin, oxaliplatin, and docetaxel versus fluorouracil or capecitabine plus cisplatin and epirubicin for locally advanced, resectable gastric or gastro-oesophageal junction adenocarcinoma (FLOT4): a randomised, phase 2/3 trial. Lancet 2019;393:1948–57.

67. Safran HP, Winter K, Ilson DH, et al. Trastuzumab with trimodality treatment for oesophageal adenocarcinoma with HER2 overexpression (NRG Oncology/RTOG 1010): a multicentre, randomised, phase 3 trial. Lancet Oncol 2022;23:259–69.

68. Hofheinz R-D, Merx K, Haag GM, et al. FLOT Versus FLOT/Trastuzumab/Pertuzumab Perioperative Therapy of Human Epidermal Growth Factor Receptor 2–Positive Resectable Esophagogastric Adenocarcinoma: A Randomized Phase II Trial of the AIO EGA Study Group. J Clin Oncol 2022;40:3750–61.

69. Wagner AD, Grabsch HI, Mauer M, et al. Integration of trastuzumab (T), with or without pertuzumab (P), into perioperative chemotherapy (CT) of HER-2 positive gastric (GC) and esophagogastric junction cancer (EGJC): First results of the EORTC 1203 INNOVATION study, in collaboration with the Korean Cancer Study Group, and the Dutch Upper GI Cancer group. J Clin Oncol 2023;41:4057.

Advances in Immunotherapy in Esophagogastric Cancer

Khalid Jazieh, MBBS*, Harry Yoon, MD, Mojun Zhu, MD

KEYWORDS

- Immunotherapy • Immune checkpoint inhibitor • PD-1 • PD-L1 • Esophageal
- Gastroesophageal • Cancer • Malignancy

KEY POINTS

- The role of anti-PD-1 therapy in treating advanced esophagogastric cancers has evolved from being used in cases refractory to multiple lines of therapy to being an effective first-line management, typically in combination with chemotherapy or anti-CTLA-4 therapy.
- Adding anti-PD-1 therapy in combination with chemotherapy or chemoradiotherapy demonstrated promising results in some patients with localized esophagogastric cancer.
- Immune-checkpoint inhibitor-based therapy appears to be particularly effective in esophagogastric adenocarcinoma with high levels of microsatellite instability.

BACKGROUND

Immune checkpoint inhibitors (ICIs) targeting the PD-1/PD-L1 axis are rapidly transforming the treatment of esophagogastric cancer comprising esophageal squamous cell carcinoma (ESCC), esophageal adenocarcinoma (EA), and gastric and gastroesophageal junction adenocarcinoma (GEA). Since pembrolizumab, an anti-PD-1 therapy, received its first approval from the US Food and Drug Administration (FDA) specifically for esophagogastric cancer in 2017[1,2], anti-PD-1 therapy has swiftly made its way from the palliative to curative-intent setting. This progress has improved clinical outcomes of many patients, but it is not without controversies. In November 2023, the FDA amended its 2021 approval of pembrolizumab for HER2-positive GEA to restrict its use to PD-L1-expressing tumors only,[3] underscoring the importance of biomarker-driven analysis that help better define patients who can benefit from ICI. To date, PD-L1 expression, tumor histology, and microsatellite instability (MSI) appear to be the most important factors that select patients who meaningfully benefit from anti-PD-1/-L1 therapy in esophagogastric cancer.[4]

PD-L1 protein expression has been established as a predictive biomarker for anti-PD-1/-L1 therapy across multiple, although not all, tumor types.[5] It is expressed on

Division of Medical Oncology, Mayo Clinic, 200 First Street Southwest, Rochester, MN 55905, USA
* Corresponding author. 200 First Street Southwest, Rochester, MN 55905, USA
E-mail address: jazieh.khalid@mayo.edu
Twitter: @kjazieh (K.J.)

Hematol Oncol Clin N Am 38 (2024) 599–616
https://doi.org/10.1016/j.hoc.2024.02.002
0889-8588/24/© 2024 Elsevier Inc. All rights reserved.

the surface of tumor and immune cells[5] and is detected in approximately 40% of esophagogastric cancers.[6] It binds to PD-1, which are surface receptors expressed by many lymphocytes particularly T cells, to predominantly suppress immune response,[7–9] underlying the mechanism of action of anti-PD-1/-L1 therapy. In clinical trials, PD-L1 expression is assessed by immunohistochemistry (IHC) studies and quantified using the tumor proportion score (TPS) or the combined positive score (CPS). In contrast to TPS, CPS accounts for PD-L1 expression on immune cells in addition to tumor cells.

ICI response also appears to differ according to tumor histology demonstrating a larger magnitude of survival benefit in ESCC than EA/GEA.[4] In line with this, the prevalence of high PD-L1 expression (eg, TPS $\geq$ 1% or CPS $\geq$ 10) in phase 3 study populations has generally been higher in ESCC than EA/GEA.[4] Additionally, ESCC and EA/GEA have distinct genetic signatures.[10,11]

Unsurprisingly, MSI is the strongest predictor for ICI response in EA/GEA.[4] About 4% to 25% and less than 4% of EA/GEA and ESCC have high levels of MSI (MSI-H), respectively.[12] These tumors possess deficient DNA mismatch repair mechanisms (MMRs) and can be identified by MSI polymerase chain reaction or MMR IHC testing, which were shown to be highly concordant.[13] MSI-H tumors tend to be characterized by increased neoantigen load and enriched immune cell infiltration and can display dramatic response to ICI across tumor types.[14] Additionally, high tumor mutational burden, which correlates strongly with MSI-H in GEA, has been reported to predict favorable response to anti-PD-1.[15–17]

CURRENT EVIDENCE
Management of Advanced Esophageal Adenocarcinoma/Gastroesophageal Junction Adenocarcinoma

The first FDA approval of ICI in esophagogastric cancer was based on the phase 2, single-arm KEYNOTE-059 trial, which evaluated pembrolizumab in patients with metastatic GEA that had progressed on $\geq$2 lines of therapy (**Table 1**).[1] Patients with PD-L1 positive tumors (CPS $\geq$1 vs < 1) had a higher objective response rate (ORR). However, a planned voluntary withdrawal of this indication was announced in 2021 because it did not meet its postmarketing requirement of demonstrating an overall survival (OS) benefit in a phase 3 study.[18]

Three phase 3 studies further evaluated anti-PD-1/-L1 in previously treated GEA. In the third-line setting, the Asia-based, ATTRACTION-2 trial has been the only comparison, to date, of immunotherapy in GEA with placebo alone; this trial reported improved OS with nivolumab versus placebo regardless of PD-L1 expression.[19] The JAVELIN Gastric 300 trial that evaluated avelumab versus physician's choice of chemotherapy did not meet its primary endpoint of OS, and subgroup analysis did not find tumor cell PD-L1 expression favoring either treatment arm.[20] Of note, in both trials, the percentage of patients with tumors evaluable for PD-L1 expression was modest and CPS was not assessed. In the second-line setting, the KEYNOTE-061 trial that evaluated pembrolizumab versus paclitaxel did not demonstrate improved OS or progression-free survival (PFS) in GEA with CPS $\geq$1.[21] However, post hoc analysis demonstrated numerically improved OS with pembrolizumab in patients with CPS $\geq$10 or MSI-H.

These promising data accelerated clinical trials to investigate first-line therapy with ICI. The KEYNOTE-062 trial was the first fully published phase 3 study that evaluated first-line use of anti-PD-1. It randomized HER2-negative GEA patients with CPS $\geq$1 to receive pembrolizumab monotherapy, pembrolizumab plus chemotherapy, or placebo plus chemotherapy. It showed that pembrolizumab was statistically noninferior

Table 1
Clinical trials of immunotherapy in advanced esophagogastric adenocarcinoma

Trial Name	Phase	Eligibility	Intervention	Control	Primary Endpoint	PFS	OS
First line							
KEYNOTE-062 (Shitara et al,[22] 2020)	3	GEA with CPS ≥1	Pembrolizumab	Placebo + chemotherapy	OS and PFS in CPS ≥1 or ≥10	CPS ≥1: HR 1.66, 95% CI 1.37–2.01, P not available; CPS ≥10: HR 1.10, 95% CI 0.79–1.51, P not available	CPS ≥1: HR 0.91, 99.2% CI 0.69–1.18, noninferiority margin 1.2; CPS ≥10: HR 0.69, 95% CI 0.49–0.97, P not available
			Pembrolizumab + chemotherapy	Placebo + chemotherapy	OS and PFS in CPS ≥1 or ≥10	CPS ≥1: HR 0.84, 95% CI 0.70–1.02, P = .04; CPS ≥10: HR 0.73, 95% CI 0.53–1.00, P not available	CPS ≥1: HR 0.85, 95% CI 0.7–1.03, P = .05; CPS ≥10: HR 0.85, 95% CI 0.62–1.17, P = .16
CHECKMATE-649 (Janjigian et al,[24] 2021)	3	EA/GEA regardless of PD-L1	Nivolumab + chemotherapy	Chemotherapy alone	OS and PFS in CPS ≥5	HR 0.68, 98% CI 0.56–0.81, P < .0001	HR 0.71, 98.4% CI 0.59–0.86, P < .0001
ATTRACTION-4 (Kang et al,[29] 2022)	3	GEA regardless of PD-L1	Nivolumab + chemotherapy	Placebo + chemotherapy	OS and PFS	HR 0.68, 98.51% CI 0.51–0.90, P = .0007	HR 0.90, 95% CI 0.75–1.08, P = .26
KEYNOTE-859 (Rha et al,[23] 2023)	3	GEA regardless of PD-L1	Pembrolizumab + chemotherapy	Placebo + chemotherapy	OS in ITT, CPS ≥1, or CPS ≥10	ITT: HR 0.76, 95% CI 0.67–0.85, P < .0001; CPS ≥1: HR 0.72, 95% CI 0.63–0.82, P < .0001); CPS ≥10: HR 0.62, 95% CI 0.51–0.76, P < .0001	ITT: HR 0.78, 95% CI 0.70–0.87, P < .0001; CPS ≥1: HR 0.74, 95% CI 0.65–0.84, P < .0001; CPS ≥10: HR 0.65, 95% CI 0.53–0.79, P < .0001

(continued on next page)

Table 1
(continued)

Trial Name	Phase	Eligibility	Intervention	Control	Primary Endpoint	PFS	OS
ORIENT-16 (Xu et al,[33] 2023)	3	GEA regardless of PD-L1	Sintilimab + chemotherapy	Placebo + chemotherapy	OS in ITT or CPS ≥5	ITT: HR 0.64, 95% CI 0.52–0.77, P<.001; CPS ≥5: HR 0.63, 95% CI 0.49–0.81, P <.001	ITT: HR 0.77, 95% CI 0.63–0.94, P = .009; CPS ≥5: HR 0.66, 95% CI 0.63–0.94, P = .009
RATIONALE-305 (Moehler et al,[34] 2023, abstract only)	3	GEA regardless of PD-L1	Tislelizumab + chemotherapy	Placebo + chemotherapy	OS in ITT or TAP ≥5%	ITT: HR 0.78, 95% CI 0.67–0.90, P not available; Not available	ITT: HR 0.80, 95% CI 0.70–0.92, P = .0011; TAP ≥5%: HR 0.71, 95% CI 0.58–0.86, P not available
JAVELIN Gastric 100 (Moehler et al,[36] 2020)	3	GEA regardless of PD-L1	Maintenance avelumab after chemotherapy	Continued chemotherapy	OS after induction chemotherapy in ITT TPS ≥1%	ITT: HR 1.04, 95% CI 0.85–1.28, P not available; TPS ≥1%: HR 1.04, 95% CI, 0.53–2.02, P not available	ITT: HR 0.91, 95% CI 0.74–1.11, P = .1779; TPS ≥1%: HR 1.13, 0.57–2.23, P = .6352
Second line							
KEYNOTE-061 (Shitara et al,[21] 2018)	3	GEA with CPS ≥1	Pembrolizumab	Paclitaxel	OS and PFS	HR 1.27, 95% CI 1.03–1.57, P not available	HR 0.82, 95% CI 0.66–1.03, P = .0421
Third line							
ATTRACTION-2 (Kang et al,[19] 2017)	3	GEA regardless of PD-L1 (≥2 prior lines of therapy)	Nivolumab	Placebo	OS	HR 0.60, 95% CI 0.49–0.75, P <.0001	HR 0.63, 95% CI 0.51–0.78, P <.0001

					ORR and safety	Median PFS	Median OS
KEYNOTE-059 (Fuchs et al,[1] 2018)	2	GEA regardless of PD-L1 (≥2 prior lines of therapy)	Pembrolizumab	N/A		Median PFS 2.0 mo (95% CI 2.0–2.1)	Median OS 5.6 mo (95% CI 4.3–6.9)
JAVELIN Gastric 300 (Bang et al,[20] 2018)	3	GEA regardless of PD-L1 (2 prior lines of therapy)	Avelumab	Chemotherapy	OS	HR 1.73, 95% CI 1.4–2.2, $P > .99$	HR 1.1, 95% CI 0.9–1.4, $P = .81$

Abbreviations: CI, confidence interval; CPS, combined positive score; EA, esophageal adenocarcinoma; GEA, gastric and gastroesophageal junction adenocarcinoma; HR, hazard ratio; ITT, intention-to-treat; ORR, objective response rate; OS, overall survival; PFS, progression-free survival; TAP, tumor area positivity; TPS, tumor proportion score.

to chemotherapy for OS, but the survival curves crossed with early death and disease progression noted in some patients who received pembrolizumab monotherapy.[22] The trial also failed to show superiority of pembrolizumab plus chemotherapy to chemotherapy for OS in patients with CPS ≥1 or ≥10, although a numerical improvement in OS was observed. The subsequent phase 3, KEYNOTE-859 trial, which had twice the sample size, recently reported significantly improved OS with the addition of pembrolizumab (vs placebo) to chemotherapy in the intention-to-treat (ITT) population, CPS of ≥1 population, and CPS of ≥10 population with greater survival benefit noted in patients with higher CPS.[23] The proportion of patients with CPS ≥10 (~35%) and patients who received subsequent therapy (~50%) was similar in KEYNOTE-062 and KEYNOTE-859, respectively, but KEYNOTE-859 accrued more patients who were treated in Asia, had gastric adenocarcinoma, or received oxaliplatin-containing chemotherapy (KEYNOTE-062 allowed cisplatin-containing chemotherapy only).

The addition of nivolumab to oxaliplatin-containing chemotherapy (vs chemotherapy alone) improved outcomes in patients with HER2-negative GEA and EA based on the open-label, CHECKMATE-649 trial, which enrolled globally and indiscriminately of CPS.[24] The primary endpoints of this study were OS and PFS, each in patients with CPS ≥5 with planned, subsequent hierarchical OS analysis in the CPS ≥1 population and all only if superiority of OS was demonstrated in the CPS ≥5 population. It was designed for final PFS and interim OS analyses to be assessed after a minimum 12 month follow-up and final OS analysis after a minimum 24 month follow-up. The first results showed significantly improved PFS and OS in the CPS ≥5 population (hazard ratio [HR] 0.71), and significantly improved OS in CPS ≥1 (HR 0.77) and all randomized patients (HR 0.80) after 13.1 months of median follow-up for OS in the nivolumab plus chemotherapy arm.[24] This led to FDA approval of first-line use of this combination regardless of PD-L1 expression.[25] About 60% and 80% of all randomized patients had CPS ≥5 and ≥ 1, respectively. Further analysis demonstrated improved OS in CPS ≥ 10, ≥5, and ≥1 with HR of 0.66, 0.69, and 0.74, respectively. In CPS < 10, <5, and <1, the OS HRs were 0.91, 0.94, and 0.95, respectively.[26] A study that attempted to reconstruct unreported Kaplan–Meier plots of the CPS subgroups did not find significant improved PFS or OS in CPS 1 to 4 (OS, HR 0.950; 95% confidence interval [CI] 0.747 to 1.209; P = .678; PFS, HR 0.958; 95% CI 0.743 to 1.236; P = .743).[27] The National Comprehensive Cancer Network granted Category 1 and Category 2B recommendation to first-line nivolumab plus chemotherapy in patients with CPS ≥5 and CPS less than 5, respectively.[28] Importantly, CHECKMATE-649 further showed that nivolumab plus ipilimumab, an ICI targeting CTLA-4, did not improve OS in CPS ≥5 compared with chemotherapy.[26] In fact, early death and disease progression was noted in patients who received ICI alone, consistent with the trend previously observed in KEYNOTE-062.

In the placebo-controlled, Asia-based ATTRACTION-4 trial, the combination of nivolumab and chemotherapy did not significantly improve OS in the ITT population regardless of PD-L1 expression (CPS not assessed).[29] Although the proportion of patients with TPS ≥1% was similar (~16%) in both ATTRACTION-4 and CHECKMATE-649, more patients in ATTRACTION-4 received subsequent therapy (72% vs 39%) that may at least partly explain the favorable OS in both treatment arms reported in this study.

The KEYNOTE-811 trial evaluated pembrolizumab versus placebo plus trastuzumab and chemotherapy in HER2-positive GEA. In an early interim analysis that included a subset of patients, a 22% difference in response rates was observed between arms, which led the FDA and guidelines committees to approve pembrolizumab in this indication regardless of PD-L1 expression status.[30] A survival analysis was recently reported.[31] The response rates in the full population showed a difference of 12.8% between arms. Pembrolizumab significantly improved PFS in the ITT and CPS ≥ 1 population, and OS only in the CPS ≥ 1 population in the prespecified third interim analysis, leading to FDA amendment restricting its use to patients with HER2-positive, CPS ≥ 1 GEA (initial approval indiscriminate of CPS).[31,32]

In addition, 2 other placebo-controlled phase 3 clinical trials that investigated anti-PD-1 plus chemotherapy as a first-line therapy for HER2-negative GEA were recently reported. ORIENT-16, a China-based trial, demonstrated that the addition of sintilimab to chemotherapy improved OS in all randomized patients (stratified HR 0.77) and the CPS ≥ 5 population (HR 0.66).[33] It met these 2 dual primary endpoints. Of note, the primary endpoint of the PD-L1-positive population was amended from CPS ≥ 10 to ≥ 5 after enrollment completion based on the results of CHECKMATE-649. About 61% and 44% of all randomized patients had CPS ≥ 5 and ≥ 10, respectively. RATIONALE-305, a global study with 75% of its patients treated in Asia, also met its dual primary endpoints: the addition of tislelizumab to chemotherapy improved OS in the ITT population (HR 0.80) and the PD-L1 positive cohort (HR 0.71).[34] This study assessed PD-L1 expression using tumor area positivity (TAP) that accounts for both tumor and immune cell expression of PD-L1.[35] The cutoff for positive PD-L1 expression was TAP $\geq 5\%$ and about 55% of all randomized patients met these criteria. The final analysis of RATIONALE-305 is yet to be reported in a full study.

The role of ICI maintenance was examined in the JAVELIN Gastric 100 phase 3, global trial.[36] It randomized patients with HER2-negative GEA without progressive disease after 12 weeks of first-line chemotherapy to receive avelumab versus the same chemotherapy. Neither OS nor PFS was significantly improved with avelumab in the entire population studied or in TPS $\geq 1\%$. Interestingly, early death was again noted with avelumab monotherapy.

Management of Advanced Esophageal Squamous Cell Carcinoma

Multiple anti-PD-1 agents have demonstrated efficacy in advanced ESCC (**Table 2**). Anti-PD-1 appears to be more efficacious than chemotherapy in patients with previously treated ESCC that is ICI-naïve based on 2 phase 3 trials. KEYNOTE-181 showed that second-line pembrolizumab (vs investigator's choice of chemotherapy) improved OS in the CPS ≥ 10 population: patients with ESCC or treated in Asia benefitted the most.[37] Accordingly, pembrolizumab is approved as a second-line therapy for advanced ESCC with CPS ≥ 10 by the FDA.[38] ATTRACTION-3 enrolled only patients with advanced ESCC who had received one line of therapy with a primary endpoint of OS in the ITT population regardless of PD-L1 expression.[39] Nivolumab (vs investigator's choice of chemotherapy) improved OS in the ITT population leading to its FDA approval in ESCC irrespective of PD-L1 expression,[40] although OS benefit appeared to be enriched in the TPS $\geq 1\%$ (vs TPS $<1\%$) subgroup. In ATTRACTION-3, approximately 96% of patients were Asian, ~48% had TPS $\geq 1\%$, and ~56% received subsequent therapy. Interestingly, the nivolumab arm had numerically shorter median PFS but significantly longer median OS than the control, with early death noted in some patients, suggesting that the beneficial impact of ICI may be complex and not limited to the short term.[41]

First-line anti-PD-1 in combination with chemotherapy is effective in ESCC evidenced by multiple phase 3 studies.[42–45] The placebo-controlled, phase 3 KEYNOTE-590 was the first global trial to report significantly improved OS and PFS with the addition of pembrolizumab to chemotherapy in advanced esophageal cancer.[42] Patients with CPS ≥ 10 (51%, vs CPS <10) and ESCC (73%, vs EA) appeared to benefit the most

Table 2
Clinical trials of immunotherapy in advanced esophageal squamous cell carcinoma

Trial Name	Phase	Eligibility	Intervention	Control	Primary Endpoint	PFS	OS
First line							
KEYNOTE-590 (Sun et al,[42] 2021)	3	ESCC and GEA regardless of PD-L1	Pembrolizumab + chemotherapy	Placebo + chemotherapy	OS in CPS ≥10 ESCC; OS and PFS in ESCC, CPS ≥10, or ITT	CPS ≥10 ESCC: HR 0.53, 95% CI 0.40–0.69, P not available ESCC: HR 0.65, 95% CI 0.54–0.78, P <.0001 CPS ≥10: HT 0.51, 95% CI 0.41–0.65, P <.0001 ITT: HR 0.65, 95% CI 0.55–0.76, P <.0001	CPS ≥10 ESCC: HR 0.57, 95% CI 0.43–0.75, P <.0001 ESCC: HR 0.72, 95% CI 0.60–0.88, P = .0006 CPS ≥10: HR 0.62, 95% CI 0.49–0.78, P <.0001 ITT: HR 0.73, 95% CI 0.62–0.86, P <.0001
CHECKMATE-648 (Doki et al,[43] 2022)	3	ESCC regardless of PD-L1	Nivolumab + chemotherapy	Chemotherapy alone	OS and PFS in TPS ≥1% or ITT	TPS ≥1%: HR 0.65, 98.5% CI 0.46–0.92, P = .002 ITT: HR 0.81, 95% CI 0.54–1.04, P = .04	TPS ≥1%: HR 0.54, 99.5% CI 0.37–0.80, P < .001 ITT: HR 0.74, 99.1% CI 0.58–0.96, P = .002
			Nivolumab + ipilimumab	Chemotherapy alone	OS and PFS in TPS ≥1% or ITT	TPS ≥1%: HR 1.02, 95% CI 0.73–1.43, P = .90 ITT: HR 1.26, 95% CI 1.04–1.52, P not tested	TPS ≥1%: HR 0.64, 98.6% CI 0.46–0.90, P = .001 ITT: HR 0.78, 98.2% CI 0.62–0.98, P = .01
ORIENT-15 (Lu et al,[45] 2022)	3	ESCC regardless of PD-L1	Sintilimab + chemotherapy	Placebo + chemotherapy	OS in CPS ≥10 or ITT	CPS ≥10: HR 0.58, 95% CI 0.45–0.75, P <.001 ITT: HR 0.56, 95% CI 0.46–0.68, P <.001	CPS ≥10: HR 0.64, 95% CI 0.48–0.85, P = .002 ITT: HR 0.63, 95% CI 0.51–0.78, P <.001

Study	Phase	Population	Treatment	Control	Endpoint		
RATIONALE-306 (Xu et al,[44] 2023)	3	ESCC regardless of PD-L1	Tislelizumab + chemotherapy	Placebo + chemotherapy	OS	HR 0.62, 95% CI 0.52–0.75, P <.0001	HR 0.66, 95% CI 0.54–0.80, P < .0001
Second line							
ATTRACTION-3 (Kato et al,[39] 2019)	3	ESCC regardless of PD-L1	Nivolumab	Chemotherapy	OS	HR 1.08, 95% CI 0.87–1.34, P not available	HR 0.77, 95% CI 0.62–0.96, P =.019
KEYNOTE-181 (Kojima et al,[37] 2020)	3	EA and ESCC regardless of PD-L1	Pembrolizumab	Chemotherapy	OS in CPS ≥10, ESCC, or ITT	CPS ≥10: HR 0.73, 95% CI 0.54–0.97, P not available; ESCC: HR 0.92, 95% CI 0.75–1.13, P not available; ITT: HR 1.11, 95% CI 0.94–1.31, P not available	CPS ≥10: HR 0.69, 95% CI 0.52–0.93, P = .0074; ESCC: HR 0.78, 95% CI 0.63–0.96, P = .0095; ITT: HR 0.89, 95% CI 0.75–1.05, P = .0560
ORIENT-2 (Xu et al,[85] 2022)	2	ESCC regardless of PD-L1	Sintilimab	Chemotherapy	OS	HR 1.00, 95% CI 0.72–1.39, P = .979	HR 0.70, 95% CI 0.50–0.97, P = .032
RATIONALE-302 (Shen et al,[86] 2022)	3	ESCC regardless of PD-L1	Tislelizumab	Chemotherapy	OS	HR 0.83, 95% CI 0.67–1.01, P not available	HR 0.70, 95% CI 0.57–0.85, P = .0001

Abbreviations: CI, confidence interval; CPS, combined positive score; EA, esophageal adenocarcinoma; ESCC, esophageal squamous cell cancer; GEA, gastric and gastroesophageal junction adenocarcinoma; HR, hazard ratio; ITT, intention-to-treat; OS, overall survival; PFS, progression-free survival; TPS, tumor proportion score.

with early diverging OS curves based on prespecified subgroup analysis. The proportion of patients who received treatment in Asia (53%) or subsequent therapy (46%) was similar in both arms. This led to FDA approval of pembrolizumab plus chemotherapy as a first-line therapy in advanced esophagogastric cancer regardless of PD-L1 expression.[46]

The open-label, global CHECKMATE-648 trial randomized patients with ESCC regardless of PD-L1 expression to receive nivolumab plus chemotherapy, nivolumab plus ipilimumab, or chemotherapy alone.[43] Similarly distributed in all 3 treatment arms, approximately 71% of patients were Asian and 49% had TPS ≥1%. Compared with chemotherapy alone, nivolumab-containing regimens improved OS with greater benefits seen in TPS ≥1% tumors, leading to FDA approval of nivolumab plus chemotherapy or ipilimumab as first-line therapies for advanced ESCC irrespective of PD-L1 expression.[47] The best median OS and response rates were observed in the nivolumab plus chemotherapy arm. Early death was noted in some patients who received nivolumab plus ipilimumab compared with chemotherapy alone, but this trend was not seen with nivolumab plus chemotherapy.

The placebo-controlled RATIONALE-306 trial, which is the third global trial to address this question, was the first to substantially allow for investigator-choice chemotherapy and thus provided insights on whether the cooperativity of anti-PD-1 therapy might differ according to chemotherapy backbone. The trial showed that first-line anti-PD-1 tislelizumab plus platinum-based chemotherapy (vs chemotherapy) significantly improved OS in the whole population. Similar efficacy was observed regardless of chemotherapy backbone (platinum plus fluoropyrimidine vs platinum plus paclitaxel).[44] Similar to RATIONALE-305, this study assessed PD-L1 expression using TAP.[35] Post hoc analysis demonstrated numerically improved efficacy in subgroups with TAP ≥10% (vs 10%), CPS ≥10 (vs <10), and PD-L1-expressing tumor cell ≥1% (vs <1%), respectively, and did not find significant interaction between treatment and PD-L1 expression.

Management of Localized Esophagogastric Cancer

Incorporating ICI to multimodality therapy for localized esophagogastric cancer is currently being investigated, with positive findings in the post-trimodality setting. The CHECKMATE-577 trial that enrolled both ESCC (29%) and GEA (71%) is the first phase 3 study to report improved disease-free survival with nivolumab maintenance versus placebo in patients with residual disease following trimodality therapy consisting of chemoradiotherapy and surgery.[48] The phase 3, Asia-based ATTRACTION-5 trial that enrolled GEA exclusively regardless of PD-L1 expression, however, did not meet its primary endpoint of improved relapse-free survival (RFS) by adding nivolumab (vs placebo) to adjuvant chemotherapy following at least gastrectomy with D2 lymphadenectomy. Of note, subgroup analysis suggested that patients with TPS ≥1% (vs <1%) had improved RFS from this approach (HR 0.33; 95% CI 0.14–0.75).[49]

In resectable GEA, the phase 2/3 DANTE trial showed that the addition of perioperative anti-PD-L1 atezolizumab to chemotherapy followed by atezolizumab maintenance led to a higher pathologic complete response (pCR) rate in patients who were treated in the phase 2 portion of the study.[50] The phase 3 MATTERHORN trial with a similar design that evaluated the addition of anti-PD-1 durvalumab to chemotherapy also announced improved pCR rates (19% vs 7%; OR 3.08; $P < .00001$), a secondary endpoint of the study.[51] It remains to be determined whether improved pCR rates will translate to long-term survival benefits in these trials. In the same space, the phase 3, KEYNOTE-585 trial evaluated perioperative pembrolizumab versus placebo plus chemotherapy. At a prespecified interim analysis, it failed to meet its primary endpoint of event-free survival (EFS) despite meeting the other primary endpoint of pCR rate.[52] The last primary endpoint, OS, was not tested as EFS superiority was not reached.

The feasibility and safety of adding anti-PD-1/-L1 to chemotherapy or chemoradiotherapy in resectable GEA has been established.[53–57] A positive signal of combining ICI with chemoradiotherapy[58] has been reported in at least some patients and supports further investigation of this approach, which will be evaluated by the EA2174 trial.[59]

Management of High Levels of Microsatellite Instability Esophagogastric Cancer

Anti-PD-1 plus anti-CTLA-4 showed great antitumor activity in resectable MSI-H GEA in 2 single-arm phase 2 studies. The GERCOR NEONIPIGA trial demonstrated a pCR of 59% (17/29) in patients who underwent surgery with neoadjuvant nivolumab plus ipilimumab followed by adjuvant nivolumab.[60] Pathologic tumor regression was seen in patients with CPS 0 to 5. Interestingly, 3 patients did not undergo surgery because they were considered to have complete clinical response. The INFINITY trial evaluated a similar ICI combination, durvalumab plus tremelimumab, followed by either surgery or active surveillance. In 15 patients who underwent surgery, a pCR rate of 60% was reported and preoperative circulating tumor DNA was undetectable in those with pCR.[61] In advanced MSI-H GEA, ICI also appears effective in both first-line and refractory setting based on subgroup analysis of several clinical trials with reported ORR ranging 45.8% to 70%.[15,26,62] Within the small MSI-H subgroups in KEYNOTE-062 and CHECKMATE-649, first-line ICI-containing regimens appeared more effective than chemotherapy alone.[22,26]

Immune Checkpoint Inhibitor Under Investigation

ICI targeting other inhibitory checkpoints such as CTLA-4, lymphocyte activation gene 3 (LAG-3), T cell immunoglobulin and mucin domain-containing protein 3 (TIM-3), and T cell immunoreceptor with Ig and ITIM domains (TIGIT) are currently under investigation. CTLA-4 is thought to regulate immune response predominantly in lymph nodes and functions differently from PD-1.[63,64] Yet, the combination of anti-CTLA-4 and anti-PD-1 demonstrated limited efficacy in metastatic, non-MSI-H GEA in both first-line and refractory settings.[26,65] LAG-3 that is expressed by 25% to 88% of gastric cancers[66,67] may be associated with prognosis and response to anti-PD-1 therapy in this disease.[68,69] The efficacy of anti-LAG-3 plus anti-PD-1 appears limited based on currently available data.[70–72] TIM-3 can curtail T-cell cytotoxicity through trogocytosis[73] and appears upregulated in tumors after progression on anti-PD-1.[74] In an upcoming clinical trial, anti-TIM-3 will be investigated in combination with anti-PD-1 in the presence and absence of irinotecan in ESCC (NCT04641871). Anti-TIGIT therapy, which appears to synergize with anti-PD-1/-L1 therapy,[75] has demonstrated encouraging antitumor activity in combination with anti-PD-1 and chemotherapy.[76] The phase 3 STAR-221 trial will evaluate whether anti-TIGIT further improves on the combination of anti-PD-1 and oxaliplatin-containing chemotherapy in metastatic GEA (NCT05568095).

DISCUSSION

Anti-PD-1 therapy in combination with fluoropyrimidine- and platinum-containing chemotherapy in the first-line setting in metastatic ESCC and EA/GEA, as well as adjuvant anti-PD-1 therapy after trimodality therapy in localized EA/GEA, has been approved by regulatory agencies in many parts of the world. Although these approvals vary with respect to PD-L1 expression and specific anti-PD-1 therapy, a few important trends are emerging. First, patients with ESCC appear to benefit more from anti-PD-1 therapy compared to patients with EA/GEA.[4] Second, in patients with EA/GEA, the magnitude of clinical benefit with the addition of anti-PD-1 to chemotherapy appears to increase with higher PD-L1 expression[23,24] Third, tumors which generate potent neo-antigens such as MSI-H GEA have emerged as a distinct subset which are exquisitely sensitive to anti-PD-1/-L1 and other ICI. For these patients, further transformative treatment approaches can be considered such as organ preservation in patients with localized disease and curative-intent therapy in those with distant metastases. To elucidate molecular mechanisms underlying these observations, we must support translational research that dissects the tumor immune microenvironment to better understand its composition and dynamics. For instance, data suggest that anti-PD-1 therapy may promote tumor progression by potentiating immunosuppressive regulatory T cells,[77–79] which is one potential explanation for the early progression observed in some patients who were treated with ICI alone. Thus, delineating the precise target and action of anti-PD-1 and other ICI is key to advance patient care and therapeutic development.

Further development of immunotherapy in esophagogastric cancer is ongoing. Novel immunotherapy such as bispecific antibodies (BsAb), cellular therapy, and oncolytic virotherapy are currently under investigation. BsAb engages dual targets simultaneously, which can be 2 molecules on a cell membrane (eg, PD-1 and TIGIT on a T cell) or 2 different types of cells.[80] In EA/GEA, clinical trials with BsAb-targeting CD3 plus HER2 and CD3 plus claudin 18.2, respectively, are underway (NCT03448042, NCT06005493). Cellular therapy such as chimeric antigen receptor T-cell therapy targeting claudin 18.2 has demonstrated promising activity in GEA,[81,82] while oncolytic virotherapy has shown interesting signals in ESCC.[83,84]

SUMMARY

Immunotherapy in esophagogastric cancer is an evolving field. ICI-containing regimens have become a cornerstone in management of advanced esophagogastric cancer and may have a role in the treatment of localized disease.

CLINICS CARE POINTS

- Anti-PD-1 therapy in combination with chemotherapy is an effective first-line therapy in advanced, PD-L1-expressing esophagogastric adenocarcinoma.
- Anti-PD-1 therapy in combination with chemotherapy or anti-CTLA-4 therapy is effective first-line therapies in advanced esophageal squamous cell carcinoma.
- Anti-PD-1 therapy in combination with chemotherapy or chemoradiotherapy may be a promising approach in some patients with localized esophagogastric cancer.
- Anti-PD-1 therapy alone or in combination with chemotherapy or anti-CTLA-4 therapy appears to be effective in esophagogastric adenocarcinoma with high levels of microsatellite instability.

DISCLOSURE

H. Yoon: Consulting or Advisory Role or Research: Merck (to Institution), Beigene (to Institution), BMS (to Institution), Elevation Oncol, Astellas, AstraZeneca (to Institution), LSK BioPharma (to Institution), ALX Oncol, OncXerna, Novartis (to Institution); Amgen (to Institution); Roche/Genentech (to Institution), Lilly/ImClone (to Institution), and CARsgen (to Institution).

REFERENCES

1. Fuchs CS, Doi T, Jang RW, et al. Safety and Efficacy of Pembrolizumab Monotherapy in Patients With Previously Treated Advanced Gastric and Gastroesophageal Junction Cancer: Phase 2 Clinical KEYNOTE-059 Trial. JAMA Oncol 2018;4(5): e180013.

2. FDA grants accelerated approval to pembrolizumab for advanced gastric cancer | FDA. Available at: https://www.fda.gov/drugs/resources-information-approved-drugs/fda-grants-accelerated-approval-pembrolizumab-advanced-gastric-cancer. [Accessed 26 November 2023].

3. FDA amends pembrolizumab's gastric cancer indication | FDA. Available at: https://www.fda.gov/drugs/resources-information-approved-drugs/fda-amends-pembrolizumabs-gastric-cancer-indication. [Accessed 26 November 2023].

4. Yoon HH, Jin Z, Kour O, et al. Association of PD-L1 Expression and Other Variables With Benefit From Immune Checkpoint Inhibition in Advanced Gastroesophageal Cancer: Systematic Review and Meta-analysis of 17 Phase 3 Randomized Clinical Trials. JAMA Oncol 2022;8(10):1456–65.

5. Herbst RS, Soria JC, Kowanetz M, et al. Predictive correlates of response to the anti-PD-L1 antibody MPDL3280A in cancer patients. Nature 2014;515(7528): 563–7.

6. Zhou KI, Peterson B, Serritella A, et al. Spatial and temporal heterogeneity of pd-l1 expression and tumor mutational burden in gastroesophageal adenocarcinoma at baseline diagnosis and after chemotherapy. Clin Cancer Res 2020; 26(24):6453–63.

7. Patsoukis N, Wang Q, Strauss L, et al. Revisiting the PD-1 pathway. Sci Adv 2020; 6(38):eabd2712.

8. Dong H, Zhu G, Tamada K, et al. B7-H1, a third member of the B7 family, co-stimulates T-cell proliferation and interleukin-10 secretion. Nat Med 1999;5(12): 1365–9.

9. Ishida Y, Agata Y, Shibahara K, et al. Induced expression of PD-1, a novel member of the immunoglobulin gene superfamily, upon programmed cell death. EMBO J 1992;11(11):3887–95.

10. Kim J, Bowlby R, Mungall AJ, et al. Integrated genomic characterization of oesophageal carcinoma. Nature 2017;541(7636):169–75.

11. Bass AJ, Thorsson V, Shmulevich I, et al. Comprehensive molecular characterization of gastric adenocarcinoma. Nature 2014;513(7517):202–9.

12. Zhu M, Jin Z, Hubbard JM. Management of Non-Colorectal Digestive Cancers with Microsatellite Instability. Cancers 2021;13(4):651.

13. Ye M, Ru G, Yuan H, et al. Concordance between microsatellite instability and mismatch repair protein expression in colorectal cancer and their clinicopathological characteristics: a retrospective analysis of 502 cases. Front Oncol 2023; 13:1178772.

14. Le DT, Uram JN, Wang H, et al. PD-1 Blockade in Tumors with Mismatch-Repair Deficiency. N Engl J Med 2015;372(26):2509–20.

15. Marabelle A, Le DT, Ascierto PA, et al. Efficacy of Pembrolizumab in Patients With Noncolorectal High Microsatellite Instability/Mismatch Repair-Deficient Cancer: Results From the Phase II KEYNOTE-158 Study. J Clin Oncol 2020;38(1):1–10.

16. Janjigian YY, Sanchez-Vega F, Jonsson P, et al. Genetic predictors of response to systemic therapy in esophagogastric cancer. Cancer Discov 2018;8(1):49–58.

17. Salem ME, Puccini A, Grothey A, et al. Landscape of tumor mutation load, mismatch repair deficiency, and PD-L1 expression in a large patient cohort of gastrointestinal cancers. Mol Cancer Res 2018;16(5):805–12.

18. Merck Provides Update on KEYTRUDA® (pembrolizumab) Indication in Third-Line Gastric Cancer in the US - Merck.com. Available at: https://www.merck.com/news/merck-provides-update-on-keytruda-pembrolizumab-indication-in-third-line-gastric-cancer-in-the-us/. [Accessed 26 November 2023].

19. Kang YK, Boku N, Satoh T, et al. Nivolumab in patients with advanced gastric or gastro-oesophageal junction cancer refractory to, or intolerant of, at least two previous chemotherapy regimens (ONO-4538-12, ATTRACTION-2): a randomised, double-blind, placebo-controlled, phase 3 trial. Lancet 2017; 390(10111):2461–71.

20. Bang YJ, Yañez Ruiz E, Van Cutsem E, et al. Phase III, randomised trial of avelumab versus physician's choice of chemotherapy as third-line treatment of patients with advanced gastric or gastro-oesophageal junction cancer: Primary analysis of JAVELIN Gastric 300. Ann Oncol 2018;29(10):2052–60.

21. Shitara K, Özgüroğlu M, Bang YJ, et al. Pembrolizumab versus paclitaxel for previously treated, advanced gastric or gastro-oesophageal junction cancer (KEYNOTE-061): a randomised, open-label, controlled, phase 3 trial. Lancet 2018; 392(10142):123–33.

22. Shitara K, Van Cutsem E, Bang YJ, et al. Efficacy and Safety of Pembrolizumab or Pembrolizumab Plus Chemotherapy vs Chemotherapy Alone for Patients With First-line, Advanced Gastric Cancer: The KEYNOTE-062 Phase 3 Randomized Clinical Trial. JAMA Oncol 2020;6(10):1571–80.

23. Rha SY, Oh DY, Yañez P, et al. Pembrolizumab plus chemotherapy versus placebo plus chemotherapy for HER2-negative advanced gastric cancer (KEYNOTE-859): a multicentre, randomised, double-blind, phase 3 trial. Lancet Oncol 2023;24(11):1181–95.

24. Janjigian YY, Shitara K, Moehler M, et al. First-line nivolumab plus chemotherapy versus chemotherapy alone for advanced gastric, gastro-oesophageal junction, and oesophageal adenocarcinoma (CheckMate 649): a randomised, open-label, phase 3 trial. Lancet 2021;398(10294):27–40.

25. FDA approves nivolumab in combination with chemotherapy for metastatic gastric cancer and esophageal adenocarcinoma | FDA. Available at: https://www.fda.gov/drugs/resources-information-approved-drugs/fda-approves-nivolumab-combination-chemotherapy-metastatic-gastric-cancer-and-esophageal. [Accessed 29 November 2023].

26. Shitara K, Ajani JA, Moehler M, et al. Nivolumab plus chemotherapy or ipilimumab in gastro-oesophageal cancer. Nature 2022;603(7903):942–8.

27. Zhao JJ, Yap DWT, Chan YH, et al. Low Programmed Death-Ligand 1–Expressing Subgroup Outcomes of First-Line Immune Checkpoint Inhibitors in Gastric or Esophageal Adenocarcinoma. J Clin Oncol 2022;40(4):392–402.

28. Aggarwal S, Hang L, McMillian N, et al. NCCN Guidelines Version 3.2023 Esophageal and Esophagogastric Junction Cancers. 2023. Available at: https://www.nccn.org/home/. [Accessed 29 November 2023].

29. Kang YK, Chen LT, Ryu MH, et al. Nivolumab plus chemotherapy versus placebo plus chemotherapy in patients with HER2-negative, untreated, unresectable advanced or recurrent gastric or gastro-oesophageal junction cancer (ATTRACTION-4): a randomised, multicentre, double-blind, placebo-controlled, phase 3 trial. Lancet Oncol 2022;23(2):234–47.

30. Janjigian YY, Kawazoe A, Yañez P, et al. The KEYNOTE-811 trial of dual PD-1 and HER2 blockade in HER2-positive gastric cancer. Nature 2021;600(7890):727–30.

31. Janjigian YY, Kawazoe A, Bai Y, et al. Pembrolizumab plus trastuzumab and chemotherapy for HER2-positive gastric or gastro-oesophageal junction adenocarcinoma: interim analyses from the phase 3 KEYNOTE-811 randomised placebo-controlled trial. Lancet 2023;0(0). https://doi.org/10.1016/S0140-6736(23)02033-0.

32. FDA amends pembrolizumab's gastric cancer indication | FDA. Available at: https://www.fda.gov/drugs/resources-information-approved-drugs/fda-amends-pembrolizumabs-gastric-cancer-indication. [Accessed 28 November 2023].

33. Xu J, Jiang H, Pan Y, et al. Sintilimab Plus Chemotherapy for Unresectable Gastric or Gastroesophageal Junction Cancer: The ORIENT-16 Randomized Clinical Trial. JAMA 2023;330(21):2064–74.

34. Xu RH, Oh DY, Kato K, et al. Tislelizumab plus chemotherapy versus placebo plus chemotherapy as first-line treatment of advanced gastric or gastroesophageal junction adenocarcinoma: final analysis results of the RATIONALE-305 study. Milan, Spain: ESMO Congress; 2023.

35. Chao Y, Yang S, Zhang Y, et al. 154P Investigation of PD-L1 expression and tislelizumab efficacy in gastroesophageal adenocarcinoma using a novel tumor and immune cell score with VENTANA PD-L1 (SP263) assay and Combined Positive Score (CPS). Ann Oncol 2020;31:S300.

36. Moehler M, Dvorkin M, Boku N, et al. Phase III Trial of Avelumab Maintenance after First-Line Induction Chemotherapy Versus Continuation of Chemotherapy in Patients with Gastric Cancers: Results from JAVELIN Gastric 100. J Clin Oncol 2021;39(9):966–77.

37. Kojima T, Shah MA, Muro K, et al. Randomized phase III KEYNOTE-181 study of pembrolizumab versus chemotherapy in advanced esophageal cancer. J Clin Oncol 2020;38(35):4138–48.

38. FDA approves pembrolizumab for advanced esophageal squamous cell cancer | FDA. Available at: https://www.fda.gov/drugs/resources-information-approved-drugs/fda-approves-pembrolizumab-advanced-esophageal-squamous-cell-cancer. [Accessed 26 November 2023].

39. Kato K, Cho BC, Takahashi M, et al. Nivolumab versus chemotherapy in patients with advanced oesophageal squamous cell carcinoma refractory or intolerant to previous chemotherapy (ATTRACTION-3): a multicentre, randomised, open-label, phase 3 trial. Lancet Oncol 2019;20(11):1506–17.

40. FDA approves nivolumab for esophageal squamous cell carcinoma | FDA. Available at: https://www.fda.gov/drugs/drug-approvals-and-databases/fda-approves-nivolumab-esophageal-squamous-cell-carcinoma. [Accessed 26 November 2023].

41. Yoon HH, Dong H, Shi Q. Impact of PD-1 Blockade in Nonresponders: Pitfalls and Promise. Clin Cancer Res 2022;28(15):3173–5.

42. Sun JM, Shen L, Shah MA, et al. Pembrolizumab plus chemotherapy versus chemotherapy alone for first-line treatment of advanced oesophageal cancer (KEYNOTE-590): a randomised, placebo-controlled, phase 3 study. Lancet 2021;398(10302):759–71.

43. Doki Y, Ajani JA, Kato K, et al. Nivolumab Combination Therapy in Advanced Esophageal Squamous-Cell Carcinoma. N Engl J Med 2022;386(5):449–62.

44. Xu J, Kato K, Raymond E, et al. Tislelizumab plus chemotherapy versus placebo plus chemotherapy as first-line treatment for advanced or metastatic oesophageal squamous cell carcinoma (RATIONALE-306): a global, randomised, placebo-controlled, phase 3 study. Lancet Oncol 2023;24(5):483–95.

45. Lu Z, Wang J, Shu Y, et al. Sintilimab versus placebo in combination with chemotherapy as first line treatment for locally advanced or metastatic oesophageal squamous cell carcinoma (ORIENT-15): multicentre, randomised, double blind, phase 3 trial. BMJ 2022;377. https://doi.org/10.1136/BMJ-2021-068714.

46. FDA approves pembrolizumab for esophageal or GEJ carcinoma | FDA. Available at: https://www.fda.gov/drugs/resources-information-approved-drugs/fda-approves-pembrolizumab-esophageal-or-gej-carcinoma. [Accessed 28 November 2023].

47. FDA approves Opdivo in combination with chemotherapy and Opdivo in combination with Yervoy for first-line esophageal squamous cell carcinoma indications | FDA. Available at: https://www.fda.gov/drugs/resources-information-approved-drugs/fda-approves-opdivo-combination-chemotherapy-and-opdivo-combination-yervoy-first-line-esophageal. [Accessed 26 November 2023].

48. Kelly RJ, Ajani JA, Kuzdzal J, et al. Adjuvant Nivolumab in Resected Esophageal or Gastroesophageal Junction Cancer. N Engl J Med 2021;384(13):1191–203.

49. Terashima M, Kang YK, Kim YW, et al. ATTRACTION-5: A phase 3 study of nivolumab plus chemotherapy as postoperative adjuvant treatment for pathological stage III (pStage III) gastric or gastroesophageal junction (G/GEJ) cancer. J Clin Oncol 2023;41(16_suppl):4000.

50. Lorenzen S, Götze TO, Thuss-Patience P, et al. Perioperative Atezolizumab Plus Fluorouracil, Leucovorin, Oxaliplatin, and Docetaxel for Resectable Esophagogastric Cancer: Interim Results From the Randomized, Multicenter, Phase II/III DANTE/IKF-s633 Trial. J Clin Oncol 2023;14. https://doi.org/10.1200/JCO.23.00975. JCO2300975.

51. Janjigian YY, Al-Batran S, Wainberg Z, et al. LBA73 - Pathological complete response (pCR) to durvalumab plus 5-fluorouracil, leucovorin, oxaliplatin and docetaxel (FLOT) in resectable gastric and gastroesophageal junction cancer (GC/GEJC): Interim results of the global, phase III MATTERHORN study. ESMO Congress 2023.

52. Merck Provides Update on Phase 3 KEYNOTE-585 Trial in Locally Advanced Resectable Gastric and Gastroesophageal Junction (GEJ) Adenocarcinoma - Merck.com. Available at: https://www.merck.com/news/merck-provides-update-on-phase-3-keynote-585-trial-in-locally-advanced-resectable-gastric-and-gastroesophageal-junction-gej-adenocarcinoma/. [Accessed 26 November 2023].

53. Li H, Deng J, Ge S, et al. Phase II study of perioperative toripalimab in combination with FLOT in patients with locally advanced resectable gastric/gastroesophageal junction (GEJ) adenocarcinoma. J Clin Oncol 2021;39(15_suppl):4050.

54. Van Den Ende T, De Clercq NC, Van Berge Henegouwen MI, et al. Neoadjuvant Chemoradiotherapy Combined with Atezolizumab for Resectable Esophageal Adenocarcinoma: A Single-arm Phase II Feasibility Trial (PERFECT). Clin Cancer Res 2021;27(12):3351–9.

55. Zhu M, Chen C, Foster NR, et al. Pembrolizumab in Combination with Neoadjuvant Chemoradiotherapy for Patients with Resectable Adenocarcinoma of the Gastroesophageal Junction. Clin Cancer Res 2022;28(14):3021–31. COMBINATION-WITH-NEOADJUVANT.

56. Li N, Li Z, Fu Q, et al. Phase II study of sintilimab combined with FLOT regimen for neoadjuvant treatment of gastric or gastroesophageal junction (GEJ) adenocarcinoma. J Clin Oncol 2021;39(3_suppl):216.

57. Tang Z, Wang Y, Liu D, et al. The Neo-PLANET phase II trial of neoadjuvant camrelizumab plus concurrent chemoradiotherapy in locally advanced adenocarcinoma of stomach or gastroesophageal junction. Nat Commun 2022;13(1):1–11.

58. Rodriguez-Ruiz ME, Rodriguez I, Garasa S, et al. Abscopal effects of radiotherapy are enhanced by combined immunostimulatory mAbs and are dependent on CD8 T cells and crosspriming. Cancer Res 2016;76(20):5994–6005.

59. Eads JR, Weitz M, Gibson MK, et al. A phase II/III study of perioperative nivolumab and ipilimumab in patients (pts) with locoregional esophageal (E) and gastroesophageal junction (GEJ) adenocarcinoma: A trial of the ECOG-ACRIN Cancer Research Group (EA2174). J Clin Oncol 2020;38(15_suppl):TPS4651.

60. André T, Tougeron D, Piessen G, et al. Neoadjuvant Nivolumab Plus Ipilimumab and Adjuvant Nivolumab in Localized Deficient Mismatch Repair/Microsatellite Instability-High Gastric or Esophagogastric Junction Adenocarcinoma: The GERCOR NEONIPIGA Phase II Study. J Clin Oncol 2023;41(2):255–65.

61. Pietrantonio F, Raimondi A, Lonardi S, et al. INFINITY: A multicentre, single-arm, multi-cohort, phase II trial of tremelimumab and durvalumab as neoadjuvant treatment of patients with microsatellite instability-high (MSI) resectable gastric or gastroesophageal junction adenocarcinoma (GAC/GEJAC). J Clin Oncol 2023;41(4_suppl):358.

62. Chao J, Fuchs CS, Shitara K, et al. Assessment of Pembrolizumab Therapy for the Treatment of Microsatellite Instability–High Gastric or Gastroesophageal Junction Cancer Among Patients in the KEYNOTE-059, KEYNOTE-061, and KEYNOTE-062 Clinical Trials. JAMA Oncol 2021;7(6):895–902.

63. Krummel MF, Allison JP. CD28 and CTLA-4 have opposing effects on the response of T cells to stimulation. J Exp Med 1995;182(2):459–65.

64. Buchbinder EI, Desai A. CTLA-4 and PD-1 Pathways: Similarities, Differences, and Implications of Their Inhibition. Am J Clin Oncol 2016;39(1):98–106.

65. Kelly RJ, Lee J, Bang YJ, et al. Safety and efficacy of durvalumab and tremelimumab alone or in combination in patients with advanced gastric and gastroesophageal junction adenocarcinoma. Clin Cancer Res 2020;26(4):846–54.

66. Lee SJ, Byeon SJ, Lee J, et al. LAG3 in Solid Tumors as a Potential Novel Immunotherapy Target. J Immunother 2019;42(8):279–83.

67. Chen F, Sherwood T, Costa A De, et al. Immunohistochemistry analyses of LAG-3 expression across different tumor types and co-expression with PD-1. J Clin Oncol 2020;38(15_suppl):e15086.

68. Tsugaru K, Boku N, Kudo-Saito C, et al. LAG3-related factors to predict response to nivolumab monotherapy in advanced gastric cancer (WJOG10417GTR study). J Clin Oncol 2023;41(4_suppl):425.

69. Ulase D, Behrens HM, Krüger S, et al. LAG3 in gastric cancer: it's complicated. J Cancer Res Clin Oncol 2023;149(12):10797.

70. Yamaguchi K, Kang YK, Oh DY, et al. Phase I study of BI 754091 plus BI 754111 in Asian patients with gastric/gastroesophageal junction or esophageal cancer. J Clin Oncol 2021;39(3_suppl):212.

71. Feeney K, Kelly R, Lipton LR, et al. CA224-060: A randomized, open label, phase II trial of relatlimab (anti-LAG-3) and nivolumab with chemotherapy versus nivolumab with chemotherapy as first-line treatment in patients with gastric or gastroesophageal junction adenocarcinoma. J Clin Oncol 2019;37(15_suppl):TPS4143.

72. Rha SY, Miller WH, de Miguel MJ, et al. Phase 1 trial of the anti-LAG3 antibody favezelimab plus pembrolizumab in advanced gastric cancer. J Clin Oncol 2023;41(4_suppl):394.

73. Pagliano O, Morrison RM, Chauvin JM, et al. Tim-3 mediates T cell trogocytosis to limit antitumor immunity. J Clin Invest 2022;132(9). https://doi.org/10.1172/JCI152864.

74. Koyama S, Akbay EA, Li YY, et al. Adaptive resistance to therapeutic PD-1 blockade is associated with upregulation of alternative immune checkpoints. Nat Commun 2016;7(1):1–9.

75. Banta KL, Xu X, Chitre AS, et al. Mechanistic convergence of the TIGIT and PD-1 inhibitory pathways necessitates co-blockade to optimize anti-tumor CD8+ T cell responses. Immunity 2022;55(3):512–26.e9.

76. Janjigian YY, Oh DY, Pelster M, et al. EDGE-Gastric Arm A1: Phase 2 study of domvanalimab, zimberelimab, and FOLFOX in first-line (1L) advanced gastro-esophageal cancer. J Clin Oncol 2023;41(36_suppl):433248.

77. Kamada T, Togashi Y, Tay C, et al. PD-1+ regulatory T cells amplified by PD-1 blockade promote hyperprogression of cancer. Proc Natl Acad Sci U S A 2019;116(20):9999–10008.

78. Kumagai S, Togashi Y, Kamada T, et al. The PD-1 expression balance between effector and regulatory T cells predicts the clinical efficacy of PD-1 blockade therapies. Nat Immunol 2020;21(11):1346–58.

79. Eschweiler S, Clarke J, Ramírez-Suástegui C, et al. Intratumoral follicular regulatory T cells curtail anti-PD-1 treatment efficacy. Nat Immunol 2021;22(8):1052–63.

80. Blanco B, Domínguez-Alonso C, Alvarez-Vallina L. Bispecific Immunomodulatory Antibodies for Cancer Immunotherapy. Clin Cancer Res 2021;27(20):5457–64.

81. Zhan X, Wang B, Li Z, et al. Phase I trial of Claudin 18.2-specific chimeric antigen receptor T cells for advanced gastric and pancreatic adenocarcinoma. J Clin Oncol 2019;37(15_suppl):2509.

82. Botta GP, Becerra CR, Jin Z, et al. Multicenter phase Ib trial in the U.S. of salvage CT041 CLDN18.2-specific chimeric antigen receptor T-cell therapy for patients with advanced gastric and pancreatic adenocarcinoma. J Clin Oncol 2022; 40(16_suppl):2538.

83. Xia ZJ, Chang JH, Zhang L, et al. [Phase III randomized clinical trial of intratumoral injection of E1B gene-deleted adenovirus (H101) combined with cisplatin-based chemotherapy in treating squamous cell cancer of head and neck or esophagus]. Ai zheng = Chinese J cancer 2004;23(12):1666–70.

84. Shirakawa Y, Tazawa H, Tanabe S, et al. Phase I dose-escalation study of endoscopic intratumoral injection of OBP-301 (Telomelysin) with radiotherapy in oesophageal cancer patients unfit for standard treatments. Eur J Cancer 2021;153:98–108.

85. Xu J, Li Y, Fan Q, et al. Clinical and biomarker analyses of sintilimab versus chemotherapy as second-line therapy for advanced or metastatic esophageal squamous cell carcinoma: a randomized, open-label phase 2 study (ORIENT-2). Nat Commun 2022;13(1):1–12.

86. Shen L, Kato K, Kim SB, et al. Tislelizumab versus chemotherapy as second-line treatment for advanced or metastatic esophageal squamous cell carcinoma (RATIONALE-302): a randomized phase III study. J Clin Oncol 2022;71. https://doi.org/10.1200/JCO.21.01926.

Advances in Systemic Therapy in Pancreatic Cancer

Kenneth H. Yu, MD, MSc

KEYWORDS

- Pancreatic adenocarcinoma • DNA damage repair • Mismatch repair
- Kirsten rat sarcoma viral oncogene homolog (*KRAS*) • Immunotherapy
- poly(adenosine diphosphate-ribose) polymerase (PARP)

KEY POINTS

- New cytotoxic chemotherapy regimens have changed the landscape for the treatment of pancreatic adenocarcinoma (PDAC).
- Next-generation sequencing identifies patients responsive to targeted and immune-based therapies.
- Experimental targeted and immune-based approaches may impact treatment paradigms in the future.

INTRODUCTION

Pancreatic ductal adenocarcinoma (PDAC) is the 3rd leading cause of cancer mortality in the US, with an estimated 60,050 new cases diagnosed and 50,550 deaths in 2023.[1] Due to increasing incidence and a persistently high mortality, and improving outcomes in other malignancies, it is estimated that PDAC will surpass colorectal cancer as the 2nd leading cause of cancer mortality by 2025.[2] The risk of PDAC increases with increasing age. However, recent trends show a worrisome and significant increase in the incidence of PDAC, together with several other obesity-associated malignancies, in young adults aged 25 to 49 years, with steeper rises in successively younger generations.[3] Additionally, racial disparities in this disease are becoming increasingly appreciated. Black versus white individuals have been found to have a higher incidence, a later stage at diagnosis and lower likelihood of surgical resection even when diagnosed at an early stage; these and other factors have resulted in shorter overall survival for black and Hispanic patients.[4] These trends and findings are the focus of much ongoing research, and highlight the need for an improved the understanding of disease biology and more effective therapies. The focus of this article will be on new and innovative treatments that have been and are currently in

Gastrointestinal Oncology Service, Cell Therapy Service, Memorial Sloan Kettering Cancer Center, 300 E 66th Street, New York, NY 10065, USA
E-mail address: yuk1@mskcc.org

Hematol Oncol Clin N Am 38 (2024) 617–627
https://doi.org/10.1016/j.hoc.2024.03.002
0889-8588/24/© 2024 Elsevier Inc. All rights reserved.

hemonc.theclinics.com

development, with a particular focus on biomarkers and genomically targeted therapeutics.

Ductal adenocarcinoma is the most common malignancy arising from the pancreas. PDAC tumors are thought to arise from one of the 2 precursor lesions. Most commonly, in 85% to 90% of tumors, the precursor lesion is defined as a pancreatic intraepithelial neoplasia (PanIN). Less commonly, tumors arise from precursor cystic lesions such as intraductal papillary mucinous neoplasms (IPMNs). The progression of normal ductal epithelium through PanIN or IPMN to invasive PDAC has been well defined at the molecular level. The initiating, oncogenic mutation is thought to occur in Kirsten Rat Sarcoma Viral Oncogene Homolog (*KRAS*). Activating mutations have been found in the earliest PanIN lesions, and are present in greater than 90% of PDAC tumors. Stepwise inactivation of tumor suppressors follows, most commonly in *TP53, SMAD4,* and *CDKN2A*. Looking at global patterns of gene expression, a number of efforts have been undertaken to classify PDAC tumors. A number of these studies have identified 2 overarching subtypes termed classical and basal.[5–7] The therapeutic and prognostic implications of tumor subtypes remains uncertain and an area of active investigation.[8,9] Mutation rate of cells present in human PDAC suggests a time interval of, on average, 11.7 years between the occurrence of the initiating mutation and the birth of the parental, nonmetastatic founder cell. On average, 6.8 more years are required for the acquisition of mutations conferring metastatic ability, suggesting an opportunity to intervene early in this disease.[10]

A substantial minority of patients with PDAC harbor a pathogenic germline gene variant associated with increased cancer risk, with estimates ranging from 3.8% to 9.7%. These variants occur most commonly in genes responsive to DNA damage repair, specifically *BRCA2, BRCA1,* and *ATM*.[11–13] Less commonly, germline variants in the mismatch repair genes *MLH1, MSH2, MSH6,* and *PMS2*, associated with Lynch syndrome, are present. While only 1% of patients with PDAC harbor a germline variant in mismatch repair genes, this can have important therapeutic implications.[14] Consequently, current National Comprehensive Cancer Network guidelines recommend the germline testing of all patients with newly diagnosed PDAC using a gene panel that includes *BRCA1, BRCA2, ATM, MLH1, MSH2, MSH6,* and *PMS2*.[15]

DISEASE STAGING

Traditionally, tumor staging has and continues to dictate the treatment modalities used for treating PDAC. In the absence of screening tools or symptoms capable of detecting tumors at an early stage, only 10% to 20% of tumors are detected early enough that surgical resection is possible. Localized tumors, without evident metastases, are deemed resectable based on the absence of vascular involvement. A combination of surgery and chemotherapy are typically used to treat these patients. PDAC is considered locally advanced and unresectable in the absence of distant metastasis and in the presence of vascular encasement, usually involving the superior mesenteric artery (SMA), superior mesenteric vein (SMV), celiac axis (CA) and/or portal vein. Chemotherapy and increasingly radiation therapy are typically used to treat these patients. In patients who experience a dramatic treatment response, surgery can be considered, however, this can only be achieved in a minority of patients. Of increased research interest are patients with borderline resectable PDAC. These tumors have a lesser degree of vascular involvement, typically defined as ≤ 180° involvement of key vascular structures such as the SMA, SMV, CA or PV.[16] Strategies combining chemotherapy and radiation therapy have been and continue to be studied, with a goal of rendering tumors eligible for surgical resection.

ADVANCES IN STANDARDS OF CARE: METASTASTIC DISEASE

The standard of care for treating all stages of PDAC has evolved dramatically since 2010, with major progress occurring by way of new developments in and innovative combinations of cytotoxic chemotherapeutic agents (**Table 1**). The PRODIGE 4/ ACCORD 11 trial demonstrated superior progression-free survival (PFS) and overall survival (OS) of a regimen consisting of 5-fluorouracil (5-FU), leucovorin (LV), oxaliplatin and irinotecan (FOLFIRINOX) compared with gemcitabine in patients with untreated, metastatic PDAC.[17] This 342 patient, randomized phase III trial found a median PFS of 6.4 months versus 3.3 months (hazard ratio (HR) 0.47; 95% confidence interval (CI), 0.37–0.59; $P < .001$) and median OS of 11.1 months versus 6.8 months (HR 0.57; 95% CI, 0.45–0.73; $P < .001$) for the FOLFIRINOX versus gemcitabine cohorts, respectively. Subsequently, the Metastatic Pancreatic Cancer Trial (MPACT) showed that the addition of albumin-bound (nab) paclitaxel to gemcitabine also improved median PFS and OS compared with gemcitabine alone in patients with untreated, metastatic PDAC.[18] This 861 patient, randomized phase III trial, found a median PFS of 5.5 months versus 3.7 months (HR 0.69; 95% CI, 0.58–0.82; $P < .001$) and

Table 1
Key endpoint from randomized clinical trials discussed

Experimental arm	Control arm	PFS	OS	Reference
Metastatic				
Frontline				
FOLFIRINOX	gemctabine	6.4 v 3.3 mo	11.1 v 6.8 mo	Conroy et al,[17] 2018
gemcitabine/ nab-paclitaxel	gemctabine	5.5 v 3.7 mo	8.5 v 6.7 mo	Von Hoff et al,[18] 2013
NALIRIFOX	gemcitabine/ nab-paclitaxel	7.4 v 5.6 mo	11.1 v 9.2 mo	Wainberg et al,[19] 2023
2nd line and beyond				
5-FU/LV/Nal-IRI	5-FU/LV	3.1 v 1.5 mo	6.1 v 4.2 mo	Wang-Gillam et al,[20] 2016
Maintenance, *BRCA* mutated				
Olaparib	placebo	7.4 v 3.8 mo	18.9 v 18.1 mo[a]	Golan et al,[25] 2014
Perioperative				
perioperative gemcitabine + radiation	adjuvant gemcitabine	8.1 v 7.7 mo	16.0 v 14.3 mo[a]	Versteijne et al,[36] 2020
mFOLFIRINOX	gemcitabine/ nab-paclitaxel	10.9 v 14.2 mo[a]	23.2 v 23.6 mo[a]	Ahmad et al,[37] 2020
Adjuvant				
FOLFIRINOX	gemcitabine	21.6 v 12.8 mo	54.4 v 35.0 mo	Conroy et al,[33] 2018
gemcitabine/ nab-paclitaxel	gemctabine	19.4 v 18.8 mo[a]	40.5 v 36.2 mo[a]	Tempero et al,[34] 2023
gemcitabine/ capecitabine	gemcitabine	13.9 v 13.1 mo[a]	28 v 25.5 mo	Neoptolemos et al,[35] 2017

[a] Difference is not statistically significant.

median OS of 8.5 months versus 6.7 months (HR 0.72; 95% confidence interval [CI], 0.62–0.83; $P < .001$) for the gemcitabine/nab-paclitaxel versus gemcitabine cohorts, respectively. Most recently, the NAPOLI-3 trial compared a novel, nanoliposomal formulation of irinotecan (Nal-IRI), combined with 5-FU, LV, irinotecan and oxaliplatin (NALIRIFOX) to gemcitabine/nab-paclitaxel in patients with untreated, metastatic PDAC. This 770 patient randomized phase III trial found a median PFS of 7.4 months versus 5.6 months (HR 0.69; 95% CI, 0.58–0.83; $P < .0001$) and median OS of 11.1 months versus 9.2 months (HR 0.83; 95% confidence interval [CI], 0.70–0.99; $P = .036$) for the NALIRIFOX versus gemcitabine/nab-paclitaxel cohorts, respectively.[19] These trials suggest superior survival for treatment with a triplet regimen combining infusional 5-FU, oxaliplatin and either irinotecan or Nal-IRI.

Beyond frontline treatment, the NAPOLI-1 trial demonstrated that Nal-IRI, together with 5-FU and LV, improved median PFS and OS compared with 5-FU/LV alone, in patients with metastatic PDAC after disease progression on gemcitabine-based treatment. This 417 patient, randomized phase III trial found a median PFS of 3.1 months versus 1.5 months (HR 0.57; 95% CI, 0.43–0.76; $P < .0001$) and a median OS of 6.1 months versus 4.2 months (HR 0.67; 95% CI, 0.49–0.92; $P = .012$) for the 5-FU/LV/Nal-IRI versus 5-FU/LV cohorts, respectively.[20]

Our group and others are actively studying biomarkers for selecting the optimal chemotherapy selection for individual patients. O'Kane and colleagues identified tumor GATA6 expression as a biomarker of PDAC subtyping, either basal (GATA6 low) or classical (GATA6 high), and intriguingly, this was associated with chemotherapy response.[8] GATA6 low and basal subtype tumors experienced significantly worse median OS compared with GATA6 high and classical subtype tumors when treated with FOLFIRINOX chemotherapy, but not gemcitabine/nab-paclitaxel. We participated in a large collaborative effort to develop and characterize patient-derived organoids (PDOs) as a model system for studying PDAC biology and therapeutics.[21] PDOs can be derived reliably from individual patients and grown in three-dimensional tissue culture indefinitely. Tiriac and colleagues found that the drug responses of PDOs paralleled patient outcomes. Furthermore, gene-expression signatures could be derived that correlated well with treatment response to gemcitabine and oxaliplatin.[22] Our group has also pioneered work profiling circulating tumor cells to predict chemotherapy response.[23] We have developed an innovative invasion assay to isolate circulating tumor and invasive cells from peripheral blood and perform expression profiling in these cells to predict treatment response to individual chemotherapeutic agents. Our most recent study enrolled 70 patients with newly diagnosed advanced PDAC prior to receiving either FOLFIRINOX or gemcitabine/nab-paclitaxel at a 1:1 ratio. Our drug profiling classified patients as "sensitive" if patients were treated with the regimen, either FOLFIRINOX or gemcitabine/nab-paclitaxel, containing the single, highest scoring drug, otherwise samples were classified as "resistant." Patients classified as sensitive experienced longer PFS (7.8 months vs 4.2 months; $P = .0002$) and OS (21.0 months vs 9.7 months; $P = .002$) compared with those who were resistant. There was no significant difference in survival based solely on the regimen received, and the Assay predicted survival regardless of the regimen administered. These and other predictive tools are being actively validated presently in an ongoing clinical trial.[9]

Developing targeted therapies effective for treatment PDAC has been challenging. Although the EGFR inhibitor erlotinib was shown by Moore and colleagues in 2007 to have modest efficacy in advanced PDAC, the benefit was not clinically meaningful, and was outweighed by associated toxicities.[24] Patients harboring pathogenic alterations in DNA damage repair genes such as *BRCA1* and *BRCA2* have been shown to have increased sensitivity to platinum-based chemotherapy[25] and the poly(adenosine diphosphate-ribose) polymerase (PARP) inhibitor olaparib.[26] The POLO trial enrolled patients with pathogenic germline *BRCA* mutations whose disease had not progressed after ≥ 16 weeks of frontline platinum-based chemotherapy. Patients were randomized to either olaparib or placebo. Patients in the olaparib arm experienced significantly longer time to progression compared with placebo (HR, 0.44; 95% CI, 0.30–0.66; $P < .0001$); however, median OS was not significantly different. Expanding these findings to patients with other DNA damage repair deficiencies, and developing more effective therapies, are currently under active investigation.

While therapies designed to stimulate the immune system have improved outcomes in many cancer types, the same cannot be said in PDAC. Several trials testing immune checkpoint inhibitors targeting programmed cell death protein 1 ligand (PD-L1)[27] and cytotoxic T-lymphocyte-associated antigen 4 (CTLA-4)[28] have shown these approaches to be entirely ineffective for the treatment of PDAC. A small subset of patients with PDAC (~1%) harbor pathogenic alterations in mismatch repair (MMR) genes, such as *MLH1, MSH2, PMS2,* and *MSH6.* The KEYNOTE-158 phase II trial treated patients with advanced PDAC, MSI-high/dMMR after progression on chemotherapy with the PD-1 inhibitor pembrolizumab.[14] Twenty-two patients were enrolled with an overall response rate (ORR) of 18.2% and a median duration of response of 13.4 months.

ADVANCES IN STANDARDS OF CARE: LOCALLY ADVANCED AND EARLY-STAGE DISEASE

Developments in the metastatic setting have informed studies and progress for treating locally advanced, unresectable, and borderline resectable disease. A number of studies have shown encouraging results from the administration of combination chemotherapy, particularly FOLFIRINOX, yielding high rates of surgical resection and survival.[29,30] Results from trials studying the role of radiation therapy have been disappointing, as typified by the LAP07 trial, a randomized phase III trial that did not show a benefit of standard dose and fraction chemoradiation after gemcitabine compared with gemcitabine alone in patients with locally advanced PDAC.[31] This study also included a randomization for erlotinib, which also did not show any benefit. Advancements in both chemotherapy and radiation have spurred interest in revisiting this approach. Our group has pioneered a hypofractionated ablative radiation approach, with promising results, both with regards to efficacy and safety.[32] These results stand in contrast to results from the multicenter AO21501 phase II trial, which did not show a benefit of adding stereotactic body radiotherapy to FOLFIRINOX chemotherapy in patients with borderline resectable PDAC. Further work to optimize the timing and dosing of chemotherapy and radiation are needed and are areas of active study.

Advancements in chemotherapy regimens have also translated to the adjuvant and perioperative setting. The pivotal randomized phase III trial conducted by the Canadian Cancer Trials and Unicancer-GI–PRODIGE Groups randomized 493 patients with resected PDAC to 24 weeks of either modified (m)FOLFIRINOX or gemcitabine adjuvant chemotherapy.[33] A significant benefit was seen in the mFOLFIRINOX cohort, with a median disease-free survival (mDFS) of 21.6 months versus 12.8 months (HR 0.58; 95% CI, 0.46–0.73; $P < .001$) and mOS of 54.4 months versus 35.0 months (HR0.64; 95% CI, 0.48–0.86; $P = .003$) in the gemcitabine cohort. A similar clinical benefit was not seen for gemcitabine/nab-paclitaxel in the adjuvant setting when compared with gemcitabine.[34] Not all patients are good candidates for mFOLFIRINOX chemotherapy in the adjuvant setting. The ESPAC-4[35] trial randomized 732 patients to a combination of gemcitabine and capecitabine compared with gemcitabine alone for 24 weeks after surgical resection. The mOS was 28.0 months compared with 25.5 months (HR 0.82; 95% CI, 0.68–0.98; P = .032) in the gemcitabine/capecitabine and gemcitabine alone cohorts, respectively.

There remains great interest in the utilization of chemotherapy in the perioperative and neoadjuvant settings for treating patients with resectable PDAC. The PREOPANC trial provided intriguing support for this approach.[36] This phase III trial randomized 246 patients to either gemcitabine-based preoperative chemoradiotherapy followed by surgical resection and adjuvant gemcitabine chemotherapy, or upfront surgery followed by adjuvant gemcitabine. The R0 resection rate was higher (71% vs 40%) in the preoperative chemoradiotherapy group compared with the adjuvant chemotherapy group. The mOS was favorable (16.0 months vs 14.3 months (HR 0.78; 95% CI, 0.58–1.05; P = .096) but not significantly improved in the preoperative compared with the adjuvant treatment group. Interestingly, in a subset of patients who ultimately underwent surgical resection, mOS was improved in the preoperative treatment group (35.2 months vs 19.8 months; HR, 0.58; 95% CI, 0.35–0.95; P = .029). The SWOG S1505 trial compared perioperative chemotherapy with mFOLFIRINOX to gemcitabine/nab-paclitaxel.[37] This randomized phase II trial enrolled 147 patients with resectable PDAC to one of these regimens administered more than 12 weeks before and 12 weeks after surgical resection. No significant difference was seen between the 2 cohorts with regards to mOS or mDFS. Further work is needed and is ongoing to determine the optimal treatment regimen and timing.

ADVANCES IN EXPERIMENTAL THERAPEUTICS

Although significant progress has focused on innovative combinations and formulations of cytotoxic chemotherapeutic agents, progress with regards to targeted agents and immune therapies have been more challenging. A number of promising approaches are currently being tested; selected examples are discussed.

TARGETING KIRSTEN RAT SARCOMA VIRAL ONCOGENE HOMOLOG

No target has held the promise and challenge of KRAS, due to the oncogenic role and near-universal presence in PDAC. Mutated *KRAS* has until recently proven difficult to drug due in part to its smooth protein surface, strong grip of the GTP-binding pocket to its substrate and complexity of both upstream and downstream signaling pathways.[38] Elegant medical chemistry has finally led to initial breakthroughs. The G12 C variant of *KRAS* was the first to be successfully targeted. AMG510 (sotorasib) and MRTX849 (adagrasib) were 2 of the lead candidates to enter clinical trial testing. AMG510 is a small molecule inhibitor that specifically inhibits *KRAS* G12 C by binding and locking KRAS in the inactive GDP binding state.[39,40] The G12 C variant is much more common in nonsmall-cell lung cancer (13%) and less common in colorectal cancer (1%–3%) PDAC (1%–2%). The phase I trial of sotorasib showed promising safety and efficacy results.[41] This study was enriched for patients with lung and colorectal cancer, all heavily pretreated and harboring a *KRAS* G12 C mutation. Notably, 32.2% of patients with lung cancer had an objective response, 88.1% with disease control and their mPFS was 6.3 months. Responses were also seen in patients with PDAC enrolled. A follow-up phase I/II study was conducted, enrolling 38 patients with metastatic and pretreated PDAC harboring *KRAS* G12 C mutation.[42] Promising objective response rate of 21%, an mPFS of 4.0 months, and an mOS of 6.9 months were seen, and treatment was generally safe. Adagrasib, similarly, shows promising early clinical results. In the phase II KRYSTAL-1 trial, 64 patients were accrued, including 21 with *KRAS* G12 C mutated PDAC. Adagrasib was found to be well tolerated and active, with a 33.3% objective response rate, mPFS of 5.4 months, and mOS of 8.0 in the PDAC cohort.

The development of inhibitors targeting the common pathogenic *KRAS* variants present in PDAC is perhaps an even more important recent advance. Medicinal chemistry was used to modify MRTX849 to specifically inhibit *KRAS* G12D, the most common PDAC variant.[43] The most promising compound, MRTX1133, is currently in clinical trial testing (ClinicalTrials.gov ID NCT05737706). Several other *KRAS* G12D inhibitors with high specificity and preclinical activity are currently in developments, including TH-Z827 and TH-Z835.[44] The tricomplex inhibitor, RMC-9805, binds covalently and specifically to KRAS G12D in the GTP-bound state, has promising preclinical activity, and is currently in early-phase clinical trial testing (ClinicalTrials.gov ID NCT06040541).[45] A number of other promising approaches to target *KRAS* are in clinical trial testing. One example involves the selective ubiquitination of target proteins, leading increased proteasome trafficking and degradation. ASP3082 selectively binds and induces the ubiquitination of KRAS G12D and is currently in early-phase clinical trial testing (ClinicalTrials.gov ID NCT05382559).

Effective strategies to target *KRAS* represent a major advance in treating PDAC. Despite promising early results, it is clear that these first generation of *KRAS* inhibitors are not capable of inducing cures or long-term remissions in the majority of patients treated. Further work to develop more effective inhibitors, as well as complimentary and synergistic approaches are underway and greatly needed.

IMMUNE THERAPY

The difficulty in leveraging the immune system to fight PDAC has been attributed to numerous factors, particularly an immunosuppressive tumor microenvironment and low mutation burden. Several promising efforts to overcome these obstacles are discussed.

As mentioned earlier, proof of principle has been established that for selected patients with DNA mismatch repair deficiency (dMMR) leading to microsatellite instability (MSI-H), checkpoint inhibition can be effective in PDAC.[14] Beyond the small cohort of patients with PDAC with these features (~1%), there is great interest in identifying other patients likely to benefit from immune therapy. Reiss and colleagues conducted a phase Ib/II study, using ongoing platinum chemotherapy response to select and randomize patients to treatment with a combination of the PARP inhibitor niraparib and either the CTLA-4 inhibitor ipilimumab or the PD-1 inhibitor nivolumab.[46] 91 patients were enrolled; interestingly, patients in the niraparib and ipilimumab cohort experienced a 6-month PFS of 59.6%, compared with 20.6% in the niraparib and nivolumab cohort. Validation of this study could yield a promising maintenance approach for patients following induction FOLFIRINOX chemotherapy. An ongoing study to further tease out genomic profiles and response to the PARP inhibitor olaparib with the PD-1 inhibitor pembrolizumab could help to validate and help select patients likely to benefit from this approach.[47]

While chimeric antigen receptor (CAR) T-cell therapy approaches have revolutionized the treatment of liquid tumors, translating these approaches to solid tumors, including PDAC, has been largely unsuccessful. Two small series show proof of principle. The first was a report on 2 patients with HLA-C*08:02 and *KRAS* G12D PDAC. Autologous T cells were engineered to target *KRAS* G12D and administered.[48] In one patient, metastatic lung lesions regressed, a partial response was achieved and was durable at 6 months of follow-up, with engineered T cells representing > 2% of circulating T cells. A second treated patient experienced significant cytokine release syndrome and only a transient tumor response. This approach is limited to patients with HLA-C*08:02, which is relatively rare, however, preliminary results are promising. Separately, scientists at the National Cancer Institute have identified KRAS neoantigens presented by HLA-A*11:01, an phase I/II clinical trial in ongoing (ClinicalTrials. gov ID NCT03745326).[49] A second proof of principle approach used CART cells engineered to target the Claudin18.2 tight junction isoform, often overexpressed in gastric cancer and PDAC. This CAR-CLDN18.2 product demonstrated activity in preclinical models and was tested in a phase I pilot study in 12 patients, 7 with advanced gastric cancer and 5 with advanced PDAC.[50] Treatment was well-tolerated and 1 PDAC patient had a partial response. Overall, the ORR was 33.3%, mPFS was 130 days.

Vaccine-based approaches have long been studied for treating PDAC with limited efficacy. One of the earliest and most promising vaccines developed was the GVAX vaccine, formulated from irradiated, granulocyte-macrophage colony-stimulating factor secreting allogeneic PDAC cell lines.[51] Initial promising results, however, were not validated in later phase clinical testing, even when combined with chemotherapy and other immune-stimulating agents.[52] More recently, the development of mRNA vaccine technology has allowed for the development of vaccines targeting patient-specific neoantigens. Balachandran and colleagues performed the DNA sequencing of resected tumors from 16 patients with early stage PDAC.[53] Neoantigens were computed, and individualized mRNA vaccines were manufactured for each patient. The autogene cevumeran vaccine was well-tolerated. Half of vaccinated patients (8/16) mounted a neoantigen-specific T cell response. Incredibly, median RFS was not reached in the 8 responders, compared with 13.4 months in the 8 nonresponders (HR 0.08; 95% CI, 0.01–0.4; $P = .003$). A randomized phase II trial to validate these promising results is currently underway (ClinicalTrials.gov ID NCT05968326).

SUMMARY

Significant progress has been made toward developing innovative therapies for PDAC. New and innovative combinations of cytotoxic chemotherapies have improved survival in perioperative and metastatic settings. Targeted and immune therapies have improved survival in the subset of patients with DDR deficiency and MSI-high/dMMR. New and innovative approaches targeting *KRAS* and immune therapies aim to have broad applicability.

REFERENCES

1. Siegel RL, Miller KD, Wagle NS, et al. Cancer statistics, 2023. CA Cancer J Clin 2023;73(1):17–48.

2. Rahib L, Wehner MR, Matrisian LM, et al. Estimated projection of US cancer incidence and death to 2040. JAMA Netw Open 2021;4(4):e214708.

3. Sung H, Siegel RL, Rosenberg PS, et al. Emerging cancer trends among young adults in the USA: analysis of a population-based cancer registry. Lancet Public Health 2019;4(3):e137–47.

4. Papageorge MV, Evans DB, Tseng JF. Health care disparities and the future of pancreatic cancer care. Surg Oncol Clin N Am 2021;30(4):759–71.

5. Bailey P, Chang DK, Nones K, et al. Genomic analyses identify molecular subtypes of pancreatic cancer. Nature 2016;531(7592):47–52.

6. Moffitt RA, Marayati R, Flate EL, et al. Virtual microdissection identifies distinct tumor- and stroma-specific subtypes of pancreatic ductal adenocarcinoma. Nat Genet 2015;47(10):1168–78.

7. Hayashi A, Fan J, Chen R, et al. A unifying paradigm for transcriptional heterogeneity and squamous features in pancreatic ductal adenocarcinoma. Nature Cancer 2020;1(1):59–74.

8. O'Kane GM, Grunwald BT, Jang GH, et al. GATA6 expression distinguishes classical and basal-like subtypes in advanced pancreatic cancer. Clin Cancer Res 2020;26(18):4901–10.

9. Knox JJ, Jaffee EM, O'Kane GM, et al. PASS-01: Pancreatic adenocarcinoma signature stratification for treatment–01. J Clin Oncol 2022;40(4_suppl):TPS635.

10. Yachida S, Jones S, Bozic I, et al. Distant metastasis occurs late during the genetic evolution of pancreatic cancer. Nature 2010;467(7319):1114–7.

11. Shindo K, Yu J, Suenaga M, et al. Deleterious germline mutations in patients with apparently sporadic pancreatic adenocarcinoma. J Clin Oncol 2017;35(30): 3382–90.

12. Hu C, Hart SN, Polley EC, et al. Association between inherited germline mutations in cancer predisposition genes and risk of pancreatic cancer. JAMA 2018; 319(23):2401–9.

13. Golan T, Kindler HL, Park JO, et al. Geographic and ethnic heterogeneity of germline BRCA1 or BRCA2 mutation prevalence among patients with metastatic pancreatic cancer screened for entry into the POLO trial. J Clin Oncol 2020; 38(13):1442–54.

14. Marabelle A, Le DT, Ascierto PA, et al. Efficacy of pembrolizumab in patients with noncolorectal high microsatellite instability/mismatch repair-deficient cancer: results from the phase II KEYNOTE-158 study. J Clin Oncol 2020;38(1):1–10.

15. Rainone M, Singh I, Salo-Mullen EE, et al. An emerging paradigm for germline testing in pancreatic ductal adenocarcinoma and immediate implications for clinical practice: a review. JAMA Oncol 2020;6(5):764–71.

16. Sabater L, Munoz E, Rosello S, et al. Borderline resectable pancreatic cancer. Challenges and controversies. Cancer Treat Rev 2018;68:124–35.

17. Conroy T, Desseigne F, Ychou M, et al. FOLFIRINOX versus gemcitabine for metastatic pancreatic cancer. N Engl J Med 2011;364(19):1817–25.

18. Von Hoff DD, Ervin T, Arena FP, et al. Increased survival in pancreatic cancer with nab-paclitaxel plus gemcitabine. N Engl J Med 2013;369(18):1691–703.

19. Wainberg ZA, Melisi D, Macarulla T, et al. NALIRIFOX versus nab-paclitaxel and gemcitabine in treatment-naive patients with metastatic pancreatic ductal adenocarcinoma (NAPOLI 3): a randomised, open-label, phase 3 trial. Lancet 2023; 402(10409):1272–81.

20. Wang-Gillam A, Li CP, Bodoky G, et al. Nanoliposomal irinotecan with fluorouracil and folinic acid in metastatic pancreatic cancer after previous gemcitabine-based therapy (NAPOLI-1): a global, randomised, open-label, phase 3 trial. Lancet 2016;387(10018):545–57.

21. Boj SF, Hwang C-I, Baker LA, et al. Organoid models of human and mouse ductal pancreatic cancer. Cell 2015;160:1–15.

22. Tiriac H, Belleau P, Engle DD, et al. Organoid profiling identifies common responders to chemotherapy in pancreatic cancer. Cancer Discov 2018;8(9): 1112–29.

23. Yu KH, Ricigliano M, Hidalgo M, et al. Pharmacogenomic modeling of circulating tumor and invasive cells for prediction of chemotherapy response and resistance in pancreatic cancer. Clin Cancer Res 2014;20(20):5281–9.

24. Moore MJ, Goldstein D, Hamm J, et al. Erlotinib plus gemcitabine compared with gemcitabine alone in patients with advanced pancreatic cancer: a phase III trial of the National Cancer Institute of Canada Clinical Trials Group. J Clin Oncol 2007;25(15):1960–6.

25. Golan T, Kanji ZS, Epelbaum R, et al. Overall survival and clinical characteristics of pancreatic cancer in BRCA mutation carriers. Br J Cancer 2014;111(6): 1132–8.

26. Kindler HL, Hammel P, Reni M, et al. Overall survival results from the POLO trial: a phase III study of active maintenance olaparib versus placebo for germline BRCA-mutated metastatic pancreatic cancer. J Clin Oncol 2022;40(34):3929–39.

27. Brahmer JR, Tykodi SS, Chow LQ, et al. Safety and activity of anti-PD-L1 antibody in patients with advanced cancer. N Engl J Med 2012;366(26):2455–65.

28. Royal RE, Levy C, Turner K, et al. Phase 2 trial of single agent Ipilimumab (anti-CTLA-4) for locally advanced or metastatic pancreatic adenocarcinoma. J Immunother 2010;33(8):828–33.

29. Hackert T, Sachsenmaier M, Hinz U, et al. Locally advanced pancreatic cancer: neoadjuvant therapy with folfirinox results in resectability in 60% of the patients. Ann Surg 2016;264(3):457–63.

30. Ferrone CR, Marchegiani G, Hong TS, et al. Radiological and surgical implications of neoadjuvant treatment with FOLFIRINOX for locally advanced and borderline resectable pancreatic cancer. Ann Surg 2015;261(1):12–7.

31. Hammel P, Huguet F, van Laethem JL, et al. Effect of chemoradiotherapy vs chemotherapy on survival in patients with locally advanced pancreatic cancer controlled after 4 months of gemcitabine with or without erlotinib: the LAP07 randomized clinical trial. JAMA 2016;315(17):1844–53.

32. Reyngold M, O'Reilly EM, Varghese AM, et al. Association of ablative radiation therapy with survival among patients with inoperable pancreatic cancer. JAMA Oncol 2021;7(5):735–8.

33. Conroy T, Hammel P, Hebbar M, et al. FOLFIRINOX or gemcitabine as adjuvant therapy for pancreatic cancer. N Engl J Med 2018;379(25):2395–406.

34. Tempero MA, Pelzer U, O'Reilly EM, et al. Adjuvant nab-paclitaxel + gemcitabine in resected pancreatic ductal adenocarcinoma: results from a randomized, open-label, phase III trial. J Clin Oncol 2023;41(11):2007–19.

35. Neoptolemos JP, Palmer DH, Ghaneh P, et al. Comparison of adjuvant gemcitabine and capecitabine with gemcitabine monotherapy in patients with resected pancreatic cancer (ESPAC-4): a multicentre, open-label, randomised, phase 3 trial. Lancet 2017;389(10073):1011–24.

36. Versteijne E, Suker M, Groothuis K, et al. Preoperative chemoradiotherapy versus immediate surgery for resectable and borderline resectable pancreatic cancer: results of the dutch randomized phase III PREOPANC trial. J Clin Oncol 2020; 38(16):1763–73.

37. Ahmad SA, Duong M, Sohal DPS, et al. Surgical outcome results from SWOG S1505: a randomized clinical trial of mFOLFIRINOX versus gemcitabine/nab-paclitaxel for perioperative treatment of resectable pancreatic ductal adenocarcinoma. Ann Surg 2020;272(3):481–6.

38. Mullard A. Cracking KRAS. Nat Rev Drug Discov 2019;18(12):887–91.

39. Zhu C, Guan X, Zhang X, et al. Targeting KRAS mutant cancers: from druggable therapy to drug resistance. Mol Cancer 2022;21(1):159.

40. Canon J, Rex K, Saiki AY, et al. The clinical KRAS(G12C) inhibitor AMG 510 drives anti-tumour immunity. Nature 2019;575(7781):217–23.

41. Hong DS, Fakih MG, Strickler JH, et al. KRAS(G12C) inhibition with Sotorasib in advanced solid tumors. N Engl J Med 2020;383(13):1207–17.

42. Strickler JH, Satake H, George TJ, et al. Sotorasib in KRAS p.G12C-mutated advanced pancreatic cancer. N Engl J Med 2023;388(1):33–43.

43. Wei D, Wang L, Zuo X, et al. A Small molecule with big impact: MRTX1133 targets the KRASG12D mutation in pancreatic cancer. Clin Cancer Res 2024;30(4): 655–62.

44. Li L, Liu J, Yang Z, et al. Discovery of Thieno[2,3-d]pyrimidine-based KRAS G12D inhibitors as potential anticancer agents via combinatorial virtual screening. Eur J Med Chem 2022;233:114243.

45. Knox JE, Jiang J, Burnett GL, et al. Abstract 3596: RM-036, a first-in-class, orally-bioavailable, tri-complex covalent KRASG12D(ON) inhibitor, drives profound anti-tumor activity in KRASG12D mutant tumor models. Cancer Res 2022; 82(12_Supplement):3596.

46. Reiss KA, Mick R, Teitelbaum U, et al. Niraparib plus nivolumab or niraparib plus ipilimumab in patients with platinum-sensitive advanced pancreatic cancer: a randomised, phase 1b/2 trial. Lancet Oncol 2022;23(8):1009–20.

47. Park W, O'Connor C, Chou JF, et al. Phase 2 trial of pembrolizumab and olaparib (POLAR) maintenance for patients (pts) with metastatic pancreatic cancer (mPDAC): Two cohorts B non-core homologous recombination deficiency (HRD) and C exceptional response to platinum-therapy. J Clin Oncol 2023; 41(16_suppl):4140.

48. Leidner R, Sanjuan Silva N, Huang H, et al. Neoantigen T-cell receptor gene therapy in pancreatic cancer. N Engl J Med 2022;386(22):2112–9.

49. Wang QJ, Yu Z, Griffith K, et al. Identification of T-cell receptors targeting KRAS-mutated human tumors. Cancer Immunol Res 2016;4(3):204–14.

50. Zhan X, Wang B, Li Z, et al. Phase I trial of Claudin 18.2-specific chimeric antigen receptor T cells for advanced gastric and pancreatic adenocarcinoma. J Clin Oncol 2019;37(15_suppl):2509.

51. Laheru D, Lutz E, Burke J, et al. Allogeneic granulocyte macrophage colony-stimulating factor-secreting tumor immunotherapy alone or in sequence with cyclophosphamide for metastatic pancreatic cancer: a pilot study of safety, feasibility, and immune activation. Clin Cancer Res 2008;14(5):1455–63.

52. Le DT, Picozzi VJ, Ko AH, et al. Results from a Phase IIb, randomized, multicenter study of GVAX Pancreas and CRS-207 compared with chemotherapy in adults with previously treated metastatic pancreatic adenocarcinoma (ECLIPSE Study). Clin Cancer Res 2019;25(18):5493–502.

53. Rojas LA, Sethna Z, Soares KC, et al. Personalized RNA neoantigen vaccines stimulate T cells in pancreatic cancer. Nature 2023;618(7963):144–50.

Advances in Surgery and (Neo) Adjuvant Therapy in the Management of Pancreatic Cancer

Mengyuan Liu, MD, Alice C. Wei, MD, MSc*

KEYWORDS

- Pancreatic cancer • Resectability • Pancreatectomy • Borderline-resectable
- Locally-advanced • Neoadjuvant therapy • Adjuvant therapy

KEY POINTS

- Surgical resection remains the curative therapy for pancreatic adenocarcinoma; thus, resectability should be evaluated at diagnosis. Patients with localized disease who receive systemic therapy as initial treatment should have regular multidisciplinary reevaluation.
- The role of neoadjuvant chemotherapy for upfront resectable tumors has not been established.
- Induction chemotherapy for borderline resectable tumors is the current standard of care but the role of radiation is not clear.
- Patients with locally advanced tumors should receive induction chemotherapy followed by chemoradiation dependent on response.
- Pancreas surgery at high-volume centers is associated with higher survival and better perioperative and oncologic outcomes.

INTRODUCTION

Death from pancreatic adenocarcinoma (PDAC) is predicted to surpass colorectal cancer to become the second leading cause of cancer-related death by 2030.[1] The incidence of PDAC is expected to increase to 88,000 cases annually, emphasizing the need for more effective treatments. To date, surgical resection as part of a multimodal treatment approach provides the best chance of cure. However, only ~15% of patients present with upfront resectable disease, whereas the remaining will have borderline resectable/locally advanced (BR/LA) PDAC due to vascular involvement (35%) or metastatic disease (50%), precluding surgery.[2] Despite modern chemotherapy, only a

Department of Surgery, Memorial Sloan Kettering Cancer Center, 1275 York Avenue, New York, NY 10065, USA
* Corresponding author. 1275 York Avenue, C-886A, New York, NY 10065.
E-mail address: weia@mskcc.org

Hematol Oncol Clin N Am 38 (2024) 629–642
https://doi.org/10.1016/j.hoc.2024.01.004
0889-8588/24/© 2024 Elsevier Inc. All rights reserved.

minority of patients with BR/LA PDAC will be suitable for resection after induction therapy.[3]

This review will discuss the advances and challenges in treating the increasing pool of patients for whom surgery may be an option, highlighting the importance of multi-modality therapy.

SURGICAL APPROACH
Defining Resectability

Surgical assessment of PDAC begins with technical evaluation of resectability based on anatomic definitions. This requires high-quality cross-sectional pancreatic imaging that includes noncontrast, arterial, portal-venous, and venous phases. Generally, tumors are categorized as upfront resectable, BR PDAC, and LA PDAC based on the relationship with the portal vein (PV)/superior mesenteric vein (SMV) and the celiac axis (CA)/superior mesenteric artery (SMA; **Table 1**).

The National Comprehensive Cancer Network (NCCN) guidelines define resectable as no tumor contact with CA, common hepatic artery (CHA), or SMA and less than 180° contact with PV or SMV; BR PDAC as less than 180° arterial contact and venous involvement suitable for reconstruction; and LA PDAC include those with 180° or greater arterial involvement and nonreconstructable venous involvement.[4] The Americas Hepato-Pancreato-Biliary Association (AHPBA), Society of Surgical Oncology (SSO), and Society for Surgery of the Alimentary Tract (SSAT) have similar definitions for venous involvement but add a hierarchical breakdown of arterial involvement.[5] Finally, the International Association of Pancreatology (IAP) further stratifies the definition of venous involvement by discriminating between unilateral versus bilateral SMV/PV narrowing and whether the tumor extent is caudal to the inferior border of the duodenum.[6] Although these guidelines each illustrate that vascular contact limits PDAC resectability, anatomic resectability is a spectrum, which limits the interpretation and application of the studies that use these definitions.

Interobserver agreement among radiologists and surgeons on PDAC resectability is low.[7] For example, in the SWOG S1505 trial of neoadjuvant chemotherapy for resectable PDAC, 30% of patients enrolled with resectable tumors were found to be ineligible after centralized review highlighting the difficulty of characterizing resectability.[8] As a result, modern day randomized trials that include surgical resection as an intervention have mandated centralized review of resectability.[9,10]

In addition to anatomic suitability, there are biologic considerations in determining resectability. Because patients with elevated cancer antigen (CA) 19-9 may have occult metastatic disease that portends poor biology, the IAP contends that CA 19-9 greater than 500 U/mL should be included in the definition of BR PDAC.[6] Finally, patients should have an adequate physiologic reserve to tolerate pancreatectomy, which has a postoperative morbidity rate of up to 50%.[11] Determining which medical comorbidities can be optimized and which are fixed conditions that preclude surgery requires a collaborative effort across multiple subspecialties.

The Trans-Atlantic Pancreatic Surgery Consortium reported that the anatomic, biologic, and conditional (ABC) criteria are independently prognostic for PDAC in patients who received induction fluorouracil, leucovorin, irinotecan, oxaliplatin (FOLFIRINOX).[12] This is a 4-point scale in which BR PDAC is 1 point, LA PDAC is 2 points, CA 19-9 greater than 500 U/mL is 1 point, and performance status greater than 0 is 1 point. A patient without any of these features has a favorable 5-year overall survival (OS) of 47% but each additional point halves the survival. Thus, incorporating the ABC staging criteria into surgical assessment may help determine which patients may benefit from surgery.

Table 1
Anatomic resectability definitions

	NCCN		AHPBA/SSO/SSAT		IAP	
	Arterial	Venous	Arterial	Venous	Arterial	Venous
Resectable	No contact with CA, CHA, and SMA	<180 contact with SMV, PV without vein irregularity	No abutment or encasement of CA, SMA, and CHA	No abutment, encasement or occlusion of SMV/PV	No contact with CA, CHA, and SMA	No tumor contact or unilateral narrowing SMV/PV
Borderline	<180 contact with SMA, CA; Contact with CHA allows for reconstruction; Contact with variant anatomy	>180 contact with SMV, PV, or <180 with thrombus but with suitable reconstruction	No abutment of CA; Abutment of SMA or CHA; Short segment encasement of CHA, amenable for reconstruction	Abutment, encasement, or occlusion of SMV/PV	<180 contact of SMA, CA without deformity or stenosis; Tumor contact of CHA without PHA and/or CA	>180 contact SMV/PV or bilateral narrowing, not past the inferior border of duodenum
Locally advanced unresectable	>180 SMA or CA; Contact with aorta	Unreconstructable SMV/PV	Abutment of CA; Encasement of SMA; Unreconstructable CHA	Unreconstructable SMV/PV	>180 contact of SMA, CA without deformity or stenosis; Tumor contact of CHA with PHA and/or CA	Bilateral narrowing of SMV/PV past the inferior border of duodenum

Abbreviations: AHPBA, Americas Hepato-Pancreato-Biliary Association; CA, celiac axis; CHA, common hepatic artery; IAP, International Association of Pancreatology; NCCN, National Comprehensive Cancer Network; PV, portal vein; SMA, superior mesenteric artery; SMV, superior mesenteric vein; SSAT, Society for Surgery of the Alimentary Tract; SSO, Society of Surgical Oncology.

Surgery for Resectable Tumors: Pancreatic Adenocarcinoma Without Vascular Involvement

For patients with resectable PDAC, upfront surgery followed by adjuvant chemotherapy is the current standard of care. In the case of a solid pancreatic mass and very high radiologic or clinical suspicion of malignancy, preoperative endoscopic biopsy and/or endoscopic retrograde cholangiography is not essential because the results do not usually influence the need for surgery. Routine preoperative biliary drainage is also not necessary[13] but may be considered based on the intensity of jaundice symptoms, need for induction chemotherapy, diagnostic uncertainty, or logistics of surgical planning.

For PDAC in the pancreatic head, a pancreaticoduodenectomy or Whipple procedure is performed. This involves removing the head of the pancreas, duodenum, and extrahepatic bile duct and reconstructing with a loop of jejunum for the pancreaticojejunostomy, hepatico-jejunostomy, and gastro-jejunostomy.[14] Regional lymphadenectomy, with goal to harvest 15 or greater lymph nodes, is necessary for accurate staging and has been shown to predict better stage-for-stage survival compared with inadequate lymphadenectomy.[15] Extended lymphadenectomy to include more proximal lymph node basins (ie, CA and SMA) does not improve outcomes and is associated with increased perioperative morbidity.[16]

For PDAC of the pancreatic body/tail (ie, to the left of the PV), a distal pancreatectomy and splenectomy is the standard operation. In 2003, Strasberg described the radical antegrade modular pancreatosplenectomy procedure, which involves lymphadenectomy around the CA and the retroperitoneal fat encasing the adrenal gland and the kidney.[17] This radicality is associated with increased R0 resection rates and lymph node harvest but does not improve recurrence or survival outcomes compared to a standard surgical approach.[18]

Rarely, for patients with multifocal PDAC, a total pancreatectomy is required but this procedure results in complete endocrine and exocrine pancreatic insufficiency and is reserved for patients with excellent performance status.

Exploratory Laparoscopy

Despite high-quality staging and upfront chemotherapy, up to 25% of patients will have unresectable disease[5,19] found at the time of surgery. Thus, some surgeons perform exploratory laparoscopy either as a separate procedure or at the time of planned resection to rule out occult metastatic disease. At this time, exploratory laparoscopy is not mandatory, but may be considered selectively in high-risk patients with anatomically extensive tumors or significant clinical symptoms (pain and weight loss).[15] The pretest probability of finding metastases increases with elevated CA 19-9 levels (>100 U/mL) and equivocal radiology,[5] and these patients may benefit from exploratory laparoscopy.

If tumors are unresectable at surgery, palliative procedures may be considered to alleviate biliary and/or gastric obstruction on a case-by-case basis, depending on endoscopic drainage options and the anticipated life span. These procedures are well tolerated but are unlikely to alter the number of future interventions or length of hospital stay.[20] When resection is aborted, minimizing postoperative recovery time is an important surgical principle to allow timely start of next treatment (usually chemotherapy).

RECENT SURGICAL ADVANCES
Minimally Invasive Pancreas Surgery

Minimally invasive surgery (MIS), either laparoscopic or robotic, can be safely performed for both pancreaticoduodenectomy and distal pancreatectomy.[21,22] There is slow but steady adoption of MIS pancreatectomy globally as more surgeons overcome the steep learning curve for these complex procedures.[23–25] The Miami International Guidelines on MIS pancreatectomy reinforced that these technically challenging procedures should be performed at high-volume centers.[26] Multiple retrospective studies have shown equivalent oncologic outcomes to open surgery with a slightly shorter length of stay and less blood loss.[27,28] Several randomized controlled trials (RCTs) are underway to assess whether there are oncologic benefits to minimally invasive techniques, such as time to adjuvant chemotherapy.[29]

Surgery for Pancreatic Adenocarcinoma with Vessel Involvement

Localized tumors with vascular involvement pose specific surgical challenges. In addition to pancreatectomy, resection/reconstruction of portovenous (PV) and arterial involvement may be required for surgical extirpation with negative margins. Management of these patients requires iterative multidisciplinary assessment to optimize whether surgical resection is appropriate and determine the sequence of chemotherapy, surgery, and/or radiotherapy (RT).

For patients with limited PV involvement (resectable and BR PDAC), pancreatectomy with venous resection should be considered standard of care. In a modern hepatopancreaticobiliary (HPB) surgical practice, up to 25% of resectable PDAC[30] and up to 75% of BR PDAC after induction therapy[31] will require PV resection. The morbidity of PV resection is similar to standard pancreaticoduodenectomy in high-volume centers and does not affect operative mortality.[32,33]

In contrast, tumor arterial involvement of the CA, CHA, and SMA has traditionally been contraindications to surgery because arterial resection is associated with prohibitively high perioperative morbidity (30%–100%) and mortality (0%–17%).[32,33] In the era of more effective chemotherapy/chemoradiotherapy, however, there is growing experience in arterial resection in highly selected patients.[34] In addition, aggressive local tumor clearance around the mesenteric arteries may be possible with meticulous dissection or divestment, not necessarily arterial resection.[35] Such arterial approaches represent surgical advances that are not yet standard practice and should be performed selectively in high-volume centers with experience in vascular reconstruction to minimize morbidity.

Surgery in High-Volume Centers

Despite the complexities of pancreatectomy, mortality is low in high-volume centers due to early recognition of complications and interventions to mitigate severe consequences.[11] Studies to quantify the impact of volume have found the failure-to-rescue rate is almost 2 times higher in low-volume centers as compared with high-volume centers (12% vs 6.4%, $P < .001$).[36]

Regionalized care is one proposed solution to minimize the outcomes disparity between high-volume and low-volume centers. Since 2000, the number of hospitals performing pancreas resections has decreased by 13%, and this centralization may account for the observed temporal decreases in failure-to-rescue rates and mortality across all hospital volumes.[36] Furthermore, it is estimated that if the quality of care at low-volume centers and high-volume centers were equivalent, 491 deaths from pancreas surgery might be avoided annually in the United States.[37] Thus, regionalization of care may contribute the most to improved pancreas surgery outcomes.

TIMING AND SEQUENCE OF CHEMOTHERAPY
Adjuvant Chemotherapy

The standard of care following surgery is adjuvant chemotherapy for 6 months. Triplet modified FOLFIRINOXHPB-hepatopancreaticobiliary (mFOLFIRINOX) is the preferred regimen based on data from PRODIGE-24, which showed mFOLFIRINOX improved OS compared with gemcitabine (54.4 vs 35 months, $P = .003$) in patients with resected PDAC.[30] mFOLFIRINOX, however, is associated with more grade 3 adverse events than gemcitabine (76% vs 53%) and may not be tolerated. Alternate regimens, including gemcitabine/nab-paclitaxel[38] and gemcitabine/capecitabine,[39] are suitable for patients who do not tolerate mFOLFIRINOX (**Table 2**). Although gemcitabine/nab-paclitaxel did not meet its primary endpoint of improved disease-free survival (DFS) by independent assessment in the adjuvant APACT trial, it improved OS compared with gemcitabine (40.5 vs 36.2 months, $P = .045$). The selection of optimal chemotherapy regimen continues to evolve, and there is evidence that molecular biomarkers may predict sensitivity to chemotherapy regimens. For example, *SMAD4* mutation is associated with progressive metastatic disease in patients receiving induction FOLFIRINOX but not gemcitabine/nab-paclitaxel.[40] In addition, GATA6 expression associated with classic PDAC phenotype is shown to have improved outcomes and chemotherapy responses compared with basal PDAC.[41]

Induction Chemotherapy

Interest in induction (eg, neoadjuvant) chemotherapy for all patients with PDAC is increasing, with advocates highlighting several theoretic benefits. First, a higher proportion of patients would get chemotherapy and treatment response can be determined after resection. Pancreatectomy is a complex oncologic procedure with high morbidity, and poor postoperative functional status may delay or defer chemotherapy. In adjuvant chemotherapy trials, up to 20% of patients have a delay in the start of allocated treatment and 50% of patients will require dose reductions.[42] Finally, because a fraction of patients (14%–36%) will develop metastatic disease on chemotherapy, induction chemotherapy can help avoid futile surgery.[10,19]

Neoadjuvant Chemotherapy for Resectable Pancreatic Adenocarcinoma

Several retrospective studies suggest a potential benefit of neoadjuvant therapy in patients with resectable PDAC.[43] However, RCTs have failed to find a survival advantage for a neoadjuvant strategy (**Table 3**). In the PREOPANC-1 trial, which compared perioperative chemoradiation with gemcitabine to resection alone,[19] there was no difference in OS or DFS with neoadjuvant therapy in the predefined subgroup of resectable PDAC. Using modern regimens, SWOG S1505 randomized patients with resectable PDAC to preoperative mFOLFIRINOX versus gemcitabine/nab-paclitaxel[10]; neither regimen met the predetermined threshold of improvement over the historic 2-year OS of 40% without preoperative therapy. Most recently, the benefit of neoadjuvant therapy for resectable disease was called into question with the results of the NORPACT-1 trial comparing short-course neoadjuvant mFOLFIRINOX (8 weeks) to upfront surgery.[44] In intention-to-treat and per-protocol analysis, there was no difference in OS between the neoadjuvant and upfront surgery arms (25.1 vs 38.5 months, $P = .09$). Interestingly, the neoadjuvant arm had a significantly higher R0 resection rate than upfront surgery (56% vs 39%, $P = .01$) but OS was unaffected.

The role of neoadjuvant chemotherapy in resectable PDAC continues to be addressed in several ongoing trials, including Alliance 021806 (neoadjuvant vs adjuvant mFOLFIRINOX[45]), PANCHE1/PRODIGE 48 (neoadjuvant FOLFOX/mFOLFIRINOX[46]), PREOPANC II (total neoadjuvant mFOLFIRINOX vs neoadjuvant gemcitabine/radiotherapy (RT) with adjuvant gemcitabine[47]), and PREOPANC III (neoadjuvant/adjuvant FOLFIRINOX vs adjuvant FOLFIRINOX[48]).

Table 2
Adjuvant chemotherapy randomized controlled trials after resection of pancreas cancer

Trial Name, Year	Size	Arms	DFS (mo)	P-Value	OS (mo)	P-Value
APACT, 2023[38]	N = 866	Gemcitabine/nab-P vs gemcitabine	19.4 vs 18.8	.184	40.5 vs 36.2	.045
PRODIGE-24, 2018[30]	N = 493	mFOLFIRINOX vs gemcitabine	21.6 vs 12.8	<.001	54.4 vs 35.0	.003
ESPAC-4, 2017[39]	N = 730	Gemcitabine/capecitabine vs gemcitabine	13.9 vs 13.1	.082	28.0 vs 25.5	.032
CONKO-001, 2013[61]	N = 368	Gemcitabine vs observation	13.4 vs 6.7	<.001	22.1 vs 20.2	.01

Abbreviation: nab-P, nab-paclitaxel.

Induction Chemotherapy for Borderline Resectable Pancreatic Adenocarcinoma

Unlike resectable tumors, data support the role of preoperative induction chemotherapy for BR PDAC (**Table 4**). In the PREOPANC-1 trial, the BR PDAC subgroup benefited from induction therapy, with significant improvements in median OS for neoadjuvant therapy versus upfront surgery (17.6 vs 13.2 months, $P = .029$) and R0 resection rate (79% vs 13%, $P = .001$).[19]

The optimal regimen and duration of induction chemotherapy is unknown. Given the success of adjuvant FOLFIRINOX in the PRODIGE-24 trial,[30] the Nupat-01 trial compared induction mFOLFIRINOX to gemcitabine/nab-paclitaxel and found no significant difference in OS, resection rate, or R0 resection rate between the regimens.[31] A 4-arm randomized trial compared combinations of gemcitabine and FOLFIRINOX regimens (ESPAC 5) but it did not meet its accrual target of 100 patients.[49] The results of efficacy are difficult to interpret because it reported low R0 resection rates (14%–38%), which may reflect differences in the stringency of pathology assessment. For

Table 3
Neoadjuvant chemotherapy/chemoradiotherapy randomized controlled trials for resectable pancreas cancer

Trial Name, Year	Size	Arms	OS (mo)	Resection Rate	R0 Resection Rate
NORPACT-1, 2023[44]	N = 140, intention to treat	Neoadjuvant mFOLFIRINOX vs upfront surgery	25.1 vs 38.5	82% vs 89%	56% vs 39%
SWOG S1505, 2021[10]	N = 102, pick the winner	Neoadjuvant mFOLFIRINOX and gem/nab-P	22.4 and 23.6	73% and 70%	85% and 85%
PREOPANC-1, 2020[19] (resectable only)	N = 133 intention to treat	Neoadjuvant gem/RT then surgery vs upfront surgery	14.6 vs 15.6	68% vs 79%	66% vs 59%

Abbreviations: Gem, gemcitabine; nab-p, nab-paclitaxel; RT, radiotherapy.

Table 4
Induction chemotherapy/chemoradiotherapy randomized controlled trials for borderline resectable pancreas cancer

Trial Name, Year	Size	Arms	OS (mo Unless Noted)	Resection Rate	R0 Resection Rate
ESPAC 5, 2023[49]	N = 90, intention to treat	1. Upfront surgery vs 2. Neoadjuvant gem/cape vs 3. Neoadjuvant FOLFIRINOX vs 4. Neoadjuvant cape/RT	1-y OS: 1. 39% 2. 78% 3. 84% 4. 60%	1. 68% 2. 58% 3. 55% 4. 50%	1. 14% 2. 18% 3. 18% 4. 38%
Alliance A021501, 2022[45]	N = 110, pick the winner	Neoadjuvant mFOLFIRINOX and mFOLFIRINOX/RT	29.8 and 17.1	58% and 51%	88% and 78%
Nupat-01, 2022[31]	N = 51, intention to treat	Neoadjuvant FOLFIRINOX vs gem nab-P	38.6 (combined)	89% vs 80%	73% vs 56%
PREOPANC-1, 2020[19] (BR only)	N = 113, intention to treat	Neoadjuvant gem/RT then surgery vs upfront surgery	17.6 vs 13.2[a]	52% vs 64%	79% vs 13%[a]

Abbreviations: cape, capecitabine; Gem, gemcitabine; nab-P, nab-paclitaxel; OS, overall survival; RT, radiotherapy.
[a] Denotes statistical significance.

example, the Leeds protocol, which examines the anterior, posterior, and SMV groove margins along radial slices, was shown to detect a higher proportion of R1 resections compared with nonstandard pathology protocols (85% vs 53%).[50] More research is needed to determine optimal induction therapy, which in the future will likely include tailored approaches that consider molecular features of the tumor.

RADIOTHERAPY

The role of perioperative RT in PDAC treatment is controversial. The early ESPAC-1 trial showed the worst survival outcomes after PDAC resection in the chemoradiotherapy group compared with either resection alone or adjuvant chemotherapy only groups. In contrast, retrospective studies from large institutional databases found a survival benefit with the addition of radiation, even when adjusted for competing risks.[51] Currently, RT is currently not part of standard adjuvant therapy after PDAC resection.

The benefit of RT in the preoperative setting is still uncertain. The Alliance A021501 trial compared mFOLFIRINOX ± RT in BR PDAC[9] but the RT group was terminated early after failing to meet R0 resection thresholds. In addition, the 47% 18-month median OS in the RT group failed to surpass the historic control rate of 50%. Final results from the CONKO-007 trial comparing chemotherapy against chemoradiotherapy in the locally advanced setting are pending but preliminarily show no differences in resection rate or OS with radiation.[52]

For patients who are not surgical candidates, RT can be used for local control, as short-course stereotactic body radiotherapy, long-course external beam, or high-dose ablative radiation. The latter modality delivers high biologically effective doses (>98 Gy) to the tumor bed, and achieves durable local control, with 2-year local progression rate of only 32.8%.[53] Our group has reported that ablative radiation had similar rates of locoregional control compared to pancreatectomy (16% vs 21%, $P = .252$).[54] In the correct setting, ablative radiation offers substantial disease control for patients with locally advanced unresectable PDAC.

EMERGING THERAPIES

The response rate to current immunotherapies is marginal in PDAC.[55] The discovery of immunologically "hot tumors" in exceptional survivors[56] led to phase-1 trial testing of adjuvant personalized mRNA neoantigen vaccines in patients with resected PDAC.[57] This approach was safe and feasible, and half of the patients developed a durable immune response after vaccination. Currently, a multicenter RCT of mRNA neoantigen vaccines + mFOLFIRINOX versus mFOLFIRINOX alone is underway (NCT05968326).

All patients with PDAC should undergo next-generation sequencing to determine the presence of targetable mutations. About 19% of patients will have mutations in homologous recombination deficiency genes[58] and benefit from platinum-based chemotherapy or the poly (ADP-ribose)-polymerase (PARP) inhibitor olaparib.[59] Although greater than 90% of PDAC carry an activating mutation in *KRAS*, targeting downstream *KRAS*-pathways have largely been unsuccessful. Of those, 1% to 2% contains *KRAS* G12 C mutation and can be targeted with the small molecule inhibitor sotorasib.[60] There is ongoing research to curb *KRAS* signaling in PDAC through either direct inhibition or its downstream pathways.

DISCUSSION

Surgery remains center stage in the treatment of PDAC because it is the only intervention that offers the possibility of cure. Currently, tumors are defined as resectable, BR, or LA based on anatomic criteria but there is no consensus definition. The best evidence supports upfront surgery for resectable tumors and induction chemotherapy for the BR/LA tumors. For patients who are not surgical candidates (for anatomic or biologic reasons), ablative radiation may provide adequate local control and extend survival, although this remains an area of investigation.

Pancreatectomy is complex oncologic surgery, associated with high perioperative morbidity; the ability to manage complications of surgery is important. High-volume pancreas centers have better perioperative and oncologic outcomes. These centers also can safely offer advanced surgical techniques, such as venous resection, which are considered standard of care for pancreas surgery.

Ultimately, pancreatic cancer is a challenging cancer to treat, with high recurrence rates, even when pancreatectomy is possible. Advances in multimodal therapy strive to increase the proportion of patients who will most likely benefit from surgical resection while preventing progression of systemic disease.

SUMMARY

The optimal management of pancreas cancer is multimodal and requires determination of the appropriateness of surgery, chemotherapy, and radiation, which is best accomplished in high-volume centers experienced with the nuances of each intervention.

CLINICS CARE POINTS

- Surgical resectability of PDAC is a spectrum based on anatomic, biologic, and conditional criteria and spans upfront resectable, BR, and locally advanced unresectable disease. As resectability can change after induction chemotherapy, it requires reevaluation.
- Upfront resectable tumors should proceed to surgery based on current evidence but randomized trials are underway to assess the benefit of neoadjuvant chemotherapy.
- BR tumors should be considered for induction chemotherapy, although the choice of regimen and duration of treatment remain under investigation.
- Locally advanced tumors that remain unresectable after induction chemotherapy should receive chemoradiation depending on response. Ablative radiation offers durable local control.

DISCLOSURE

A.C. Wei received institutional clinical trial funding from IPSEN pharmaceuticals. M. Liu has no relevant conflicts of interest to report. Memorial Sloan Kettering has institutional financial interests relative BioNTech, Epistem Prognostics, Clarity Pharmaceuticals.

REFERENCES

1. Rahib L, Smith BD, Aizenberg R, et al. Projecting cancer incidence and deaths to 2030: the unexpected burden of thyroid, liver, and pancreas cancers in the United States. Cancer Res 2014;74(11):2913–21.
2. Suker M, Beumer BR, Sadot E, et al. FOLFIRINOX for locally advanced pancreatic cancer: a systematic review and patient-level meta-analysis. Lancet Oncol 2016;17(6):801–10.
3. Springfeld C, Ferrone CR, Katz MHG, et al. Neoadjuvant therapy for pancreatic cancer. Nat Rev Clin Oncol 2023;20(5):318–37.

4. Tempero MA, Malafa MP, Al-Hawary M, et al. Pancreatic Adenocarcinoma, Version 2.2021, NCCN Clinical Practice Guidelines in Oncology. J Natl Compr Cancer Netw 2021;19(4):439–57.

5. Callery MP, Chang KJ, Fishman EK, et al. Pretreatment assessment of resectable and borderline resectable pancreatic cancer: expert consensus statement. Ann Surg Oncol 2009;16(7):1727–33.

6. Isaji S, Mizuno S, Windsor JA, et al. International consensus on definition and criteria of borderline resectable pancreatic ductal adenocarcinoma 2017. Pancreatology 2018;18(1):2–11.

7. Badgery HE, Muhlen-Schulte T, Zalcberg JR, et al. Determination of "borderline resectable" pancreatic cancer - a global assessment of 30 shades of grey. Oxford: HPB; 2023. https://doi.org/10.1016/j.hpb.2023.07.883.

8. Ahmad SA, Duong M, Sohal DPS, et al. Surgical Outcome Results From SWOG S1505: A Randomized Clinical Trial of mFOLFIRINOX Versus Gemcitabine/Nab-paclitaxel for Perioperative Treatment of Resectable Pancreatic Ductal Adenocarcinoma. Ann Surg 2020;272(3):481–6.

9. Katz MHG, Shi Q, Meyers J, et al. Efficacy of Preoperative mFOLFIRINOX vs mFOLFIRINOX Plus Hypofractionated Radiotherapy for Borderline Resectable Adenocarcinoma of the Pancreas: The A021501 Phase 2 Randomized Clinical Trial. JAMA Oncol 2022;8(9):1263–70.

10. Sohal DPS, Duong M, Ahmad SA, et al. Efficacy of Perioperative Chemotherapy for Resectable Pancreatic Adenocarcinoma: A Phase 2 Randomized Clinical Trial. JAMA Oncol 2021;7(3):421–7.

11. Ratnayake B, Pendharkar SA, Connor S, et al. Patient volume and clinical outcome after pancreatic cancer resection: A contemporary systematic review and meta-analysis. Surgery 2022;172(1):273–83.

12. Dekker EN, van Dam JL, Janssen QP, et al. Improved Clinical Staging System for Localized Pancreatic Cancer Using the ABC Factors: A TAPS Consortium Study. J Clin Oncol 2024;JCO2301311. https://doi.org/10.1200/JCO.23.01311.

13. van der Gaag NA, Rauws EA, van Eijck CH, et al. Preoperative biliary drainage for cancer of the head of the pancreas. N Engl J Med 2010;362(2):129–37.

14. Whipple AO, Parsons WB, Mullins CR. Treatment of Carcinoma of the Ampulla of Vater. Ann Surg 1935;102(4):763–79.

15. American College of Surgeons, Alliance for clinical trials in Oncology. Operative standards for cancer surgery. Wolters Kluwer Health; 2015. 1-3 volumes.

16. Dasari BV, Pasquali S, Vohra RS, et al. Extended Versus Standard Lymphadenectomy for Pancreatic Head Cancer: Meta-Analysis of Randomized Controlled Trials. J Gastrointest Surg 2015;19(9):1725–32.

17. Strasberg SM, Drebin JA, Linehan D. Radical antegrade modular pancreatosplenectomy. Surgery 2003;133(5):521–7.

18. Cao F, Li J, Li A, et al. Radical antegrade modular pancreatosplenectomy versus standard procedure in the treatment of left-sided pancreatic cancer: A systemic review and meta-analysis. BMC Surg 2017;17(1):67.

19. Versteijne E, Suker M, Groothuis K, et al. Preoperative Chemoradiotherapy Versus Immediate Surgery for Resectable and Borderline Resectable Pancreatic Cancer: Results of the Dutch Randomized Phase III PREOPANC Trial. J Clin Oncol 2020;38(16):1763–73.

20. Lyons JM, Karkar A, Correa-Gallego CC, et al. Operative procedures for unresectable pancreatic cancer: does operative bypass decrease requirements for postoperative procedures and in-hospital days? HPB (Oxford) 2012;14(7):469–75.

21. Chen K, Pan Y, Liu XL, et al. Minimally invasive pancreaticoduodenectomy for periampullary disease: a comprehensive review of literature and meta-analysis of outcomes compared with open surgery. BMC Gastroenterol 2017;17(1):120.

22. Pfister M, Probst P, Muller PC, et al. Minimally invasive versus open pancreatic surgery: meta-analysis of randomized clinical trials. BJS Open 2023;7(2). https://doi.org/10.1093/bjsopen/zrad007.

23. van Ramshorst TME, van Hilst J, Bannone E, et al. International survey on opinions and use of robot-assisted and laparoscopic minimally invasive pancreatic surgery: 5-year follow up. Oxford: HPB; 2023. https://doi.org/10.1016/j.hpb.2023.09.004.

24. Zwart MJW, van den Broek B, de Graaf N, et al. The Feasibility, Proficiency, and Mastery Learning Curves in 635 Robotic Pancreatoduodenectomies Following A Multicenter Training Program: 'Standing on the Shoulders of Giants'. Ann Surg 2023. https://doi.org/10.1097/SLA.0000000000005928.

25. Liu Q, Zhao Z, Zhang X, et al. Perioperative and Oncological Outcomes of Robotic Versus Open Pancreaticoduodenectomy in Low-Risk Surgical Candidates: A Multicenter Propensity Score-Matched Study. Ann Surg 2023;277(4):e864–71.

26. Asbun HJ, Moekotte AL, Vissers FL, et al. The Miami International Evidence-based Guidelines on Minimally Invasive Pancreas Resection. Ann Surg 2020; 271(1):1–14.

27. Torphy RJ, Friedman C, Halpern A, et al. Comparing Short-term and Oncologic Outcomes of Minimally Invasive Versus Open Pancreaticoduodenectomy Across Low and High Volume Centers. Ann Surg 2019;270(6):1147–55.

28. Sweigert PJ, Wang X, Eguia E, et al. Does minimally invasive pancreaticoduodenectomy increase the chance of a textbook oncologic outcome? Surgery 2021; 170(3):880–8.

29. Jin J, Shi Y, Chen M, et al. Robotic versus Open Pancreatoduodenectomy for Pancreatic and Periampullary Tumors (PORTAL): a study protocol for a multicenter phase III non-inferiority randomized controlled trial. Trials 2021;22(1):954.

30. Conroy T, Hammel P, Hebbar M, et al. FOLFIRINOX or Gemcitabine as Adjuvant Therapy for Pancreatic Cancer. N Engl J Med 2018;379(25):2395–406.

31. Yamaguchi J, Yokoyama Y, Fujii T, et al. Results of a Phase II Study on the Use of Neoadjuvant Chemotherapy (FOLFIRINOX or GEM/nab-PTX) for Borderline-resectable Pancreatic Cancer (NUPAT-01). Ann Surg 2022;275(6):1043–9.

32. Kasumova GG, Conway WC, Tseng JF. The Role of Venous and Arterial Resection in Pancreatic Cancer Surgery. Ann Surg Oncol 2018;25(1):51–8.

33. Younan G, Tsai S, Evans DB, et al. Techniques of Vascular Resection and Reconstruction in Pancreatic Cancer. Surg Clin North Am 2016;96(6):1351–70.

34. Tee MC, Krajewski AC, Groeschl RT, et al. Indications and Perioperative Outcomes for Pancreatectomy with Arterial Resection. J Am Coll Surg 2018;227(2): 255–69.

35. Diener MK, Mihaljevic AL, Strobel O, et al. Periarterial divestment in pancreatic cancer surgery. Surgery 2021;169(5):1019–25.

36. Amini N, Spolverato G, Kim Y, et al. Trends in Hospital Volume and Failure to Rescue for Pancreatic Surgery. J Gastrointest Surg 2015;19(9):1581–92.

37. Bilimoria KY, Bentrem DJ, Feinglass JM, et al. Directing surgical quality improvement initiatives: comparison of perioperative mortality and long-term survival for cancer surgery. J Clin Oncol 2008;26(28):4626–33.

38. Tempero MA, Pelzer U, O'Reilly EM, et al. Adjuvant nab-Paclitaxel + Gemcitabine in Resected Pancreatic Ductal Adenocarcinoma: Results From a Randomized, Open-Label, Phase III Trial. J Clin Oncol 2023;41(11):2007–19.

39. Neoptolemos JP, Palmer DH, Ghaneh P, et al. Comparison of adjuvant gemcitabine and capecitabine with gemcitabine monotherapy in patients with resected pancreatic cancer (ESPAC-4): a multicentre, open-label, randomised, phase 3 trial. Lancet 2017;389(10073):1011–24.
40. Ecker BL, Tao AJ, Janssen QP, et al. Genomic Biomarkers Associated with Response to Induction Chemotherapy in Patients with Localized Pancreatic Ductal Adenocarcinoma. Clin Cancer Res 2023;29(7):1368–74.
41. O'Kane GM, Grunwald BT, Jang GH, et al. GATA6 Expression Distinguishes Classical and Basal-like Subtypes in Advanced Pancreatic Cancer. Clin Cancer Res 2020;26(18):4901–10.
42. Valle JW, Palmer D, Jackson R, et al. Optimal duration and timing of adjuvant chemotherapy after definitive surgery for ductal adenocarcinoma of the pancreas: ongoing lessons from the ESPAC-3 study. J Clin Oncol 2014;32(6):504–12.
43. Versteijne E, Vogel JA, Besselink MG, et al. Meta-analysis comparing upfront surgery with neoadjuvant treatment in patients with resectable or borderline resectable pancreatic cancer. Br J Surg 2018;105(8):946–58.
44. Labori KJ, Bratlie SO, Andersson B, et al. Neoadjuvant FOLFIRINOX versus upfront surgery for resectable pancreatic head cancer (NORPACT-1): a multicentre, randomised, phase 2 trial. Lancet Gastroenterol Hepatol 2024. https://doi.org/10.1016/S2468-1253(23)00405-3.
45. Chawla A, Shi Q, Ko AH, et al. Alliance A021806: A phase III trial evaluating perioperative versus adjuvant therapy for resectable pancreatic cancer. J Clin Oncol 2023;41(16_suppl):TPS4204.
46. Schwarz L, Vernerey D, Bachet JB, et al. Resectable pancreatic adenocarcinoma neo-adjuvant FOLF(IRIN)OX-based chemotherapy - a multicenter, non-comparative, randomized, phase II trial (PANACHE01-PRODIGE48 study). BMC Cancer 2018;18(1):762.
47. Janssen QP, van Dam JL, Bonsing BA, et al. Total neoadjuvant FOLFIRINOX versus neoadjuvant gemcitabine-based chemoradiotherapy and adjuvant gemcitabine for resectable and borderline resectable pancreatic cancer (PREOPANC-2 trial): study protocol for a nationwide multicenter randomized controlled trial. BMC Cancer 2021;21(1):300.
48. van Dam JL, Verkolf EMM, Dekker EN, et al. Perioperative or adjuvant mFOLFIRINOX for resectable pancreatic cancer (PREOPANC-3): study protocol for a multicenter randomized controlled trial. BMC Cancer 2023;23(1):728.
49. Ghaneh P, Palmer D, Cicconi S, et al. Immediate surgery compared with short-course neoadjuvant gemcitabine plus capecitabine, FOLFIRINOX, or chemoradiotherapy in patients with borderline resectable pancreatic cancer (ESPAC5): a four-arm, multicentre, randomised, phase 2 trial. Lancet Gastroenterol Hepatol 2023;8(2):157–68.
50. Verbeke CS, Leitch D, Menon KV, et al. Redefining the R1 resection in pancreatic cancer. Br J Surg 2006;93(10):1232–7.
51. Herman JM, Swartz MJ, Hsu CC, et al. Analysis of fluorouracil-based adjuvant chemotherapy and radiation after pancreaticoduodenectomy for ductal adenocarcinoma of the pancreas: results of a large, prospectively collected database at the Johns Hopkins Hospital. J Clin Oncol 2008;26(21):3503–10.
52. Fietkau R, Ghadimi M, Grützmann R, et al. Randomized phase III trial of induction chemotherapy followed by chemoradiotherapy or chemotherapy alone for nonresectable locally advanced pancreatic cancer: First results of the CONKO-007 trial. J Clin Oncol 2022;40(16 suppl):4008.

53. Reyngold M, O'Reilly EM, Varghese AM, et al. Association of Ablative Radiation Therapy With Survival Among Patients With Inoperable Pancreatic Cancer. JAMA Oncol 2021;7(5):735–8.

54. Jolissaint JS, Reyngold M, Bassmann J, et al. Local Control and Survival After Induction Chemotherapy and Ablative Radiation Versus Resection for Pancreatic Ductal Adenocarcinoma With Vascular Involvement. Ann Surg 2021;274(6): 894–901.

55. Royal RE, Levy C, Turner K, et al. Phase 2 trial of single agent Ipilimumab (anti-CTLA-4) for locally advanced or metastatic pancreatic adenocarcinoma. J Immunother 2010;33(8):828–33.

56. Balachandran VP, Luksza M, Zhao JN, et al. Identification of unique neoantigen qualities in long-term survivors of pancreatic cancer. Nature 2017;551(7681): 512–6.

57. Rojas LA, Sethna Z, Soares KC, et al. Personalized RNA neoantigen vaccines stimulate T cells in pancreatic cancer. Nature 2023;618(7963):144–50.

58. Park W, Chen J, Chou JF, et al. Genomic methods identify homologous recombination deficiency in pancreas adenocarcinoma and optimize treatment selection. Clin Cancer Res 2020;26(13):3239–47.

59. Golan T, Hammel P, Reni M, et al. Maintenance olaparib for germline BRCA-mutated metastatic pancreatic cancer. N Engl J Med 2019;381(4):317–27.

60. Strickler JH, Satake H, George TJ, et al. Sotorasib in KRAS p.G12C-Mutated Advanced Pancreatic Cancer. N Engl J Med 2023;388(1):33–43.

61. Oettle H, Neuhaus P, Hochhaus A, et al. Adjuvant chemotherapy with gemcitabine and long-term outcomes among patients with resected pancreatic cancer: the CONKO-001 randomized trial. JAMA 2013;310(14):1473–81.

Immunotherapy

A Sharp Curve Turn at the Corner of Targeted Therapy in the Treatment of Biliary Tract Cancers

Layal Al Mahmasani, MD[a], James J. Harding, MD[a,b],
Ghassan Abou-Alfa, MD, MBA[a,b,c],*

KEYWORDS

- Biliary tract cancers • Cholangiocarcinoma • Gallbladder cancer
- Cytotoxic chemotherapy • Immune checkpoint inhibitors • Targeted therapy
- Precision medicine

KEY POINTS

- The combination of chemotherapy and immune checkpoint inhibitors has become the standard of care in advanced biliary tract cancer.
- Advances in precision medicine have led to the discovery of multiple targets in addition to drugs directed toward these targets.
- Second-line treatment is based on genomic alterations, if present. In the absence of alterations, chemotherapy remains the standard of care.
- Several investigational therapeutic approaches are emerging with promising results.

INTRODUCTION

Biliary tract cancers (BTCs) incidence is increasing in incidence and has a high mortality rate. BTCs include cholangiocarcinoma (CCA), both intrahepatic CCA (iCCA) and extrahepatic CCA (eCCA), and gallbladder (GB) carcinomas. For early-stage disease, surgical resection remains the only potentially curative treatment option.[1] There is continued evaluation of liver transplant for perihilar CCA,[2] with a high rate of recurrence is noted.[3,4] In the last decade, numerous systemic therapies have demonstrated efficacy in advanced disease, which are described herein.

[a] Memorial Sloan Kettering Cancer Center, 300 East 66th Street, New York, NY, USA; [b] Weill Medical College at Cornell University, New York, NY, USA; [c] Trinity College Dublin, Dublin, Ireland
* Corresponding author. Memorial Sloan Kettering Cancer Center, 300 East 66th Street, New York, NY 10065, USA
E-mail address: abou-alg@MSKCC.ORG

Hematol Oncol Clin N Am 38 (2024) 643–657
https://doi.org/10.1016/j.hoc.2024.01.005
0889-8588/24/© 2024 Elsevier Inc. All rights reserved.

NEW DEVELOPMENTS IN SYSTEMIC THERAPY FOR ADVANCED DISEASE
Chemoimmunotherapy

Gemcitabine plus cisplatin demonstrated a survival advantage over gemcitabine alone and has remained the standard of care in the first-line setting for over a decade.[5] Combining immune checkpoint inhibitors (ICIs) with chemotherapy has now been demonstrated to improve overall survival (OS). The pivotal TOPAZ-1 trial was a multi-center, double-blind, randomized phase III clinical trial evaluating and the anti-PDL-1 antibody durvalumab versus placebo in combination with gemcitabine plus cisplatin[6] (**Table 1**). Systemic therapy was stopped at 6 months and patients continued durva-lumab or placebo. Improved survival was observed in all prespecified subgroups. KETNOTE-996, a randomized phase III trial evaluated the addition of the anti-PD-1 antibody pembrolizumab to gemcitabine plus cisplatin versus placebo also in the first-line setting.[7] In contrast to TOPAZ-1, a greater proportion of patients were accrued in non-Asia and cytotoxic chemotherapy could continue beyond 6 months. The results showed the addition of pembrolizumab to improve median OS and progression-free survival (PFS). The data from these trials have prompted several questions: Who are the long-term responders? can tumor or patient-specific factors function as biomarkers of response and resistance?[8] is there a role for continuation of chemotherapy or intensification of treatment during maintenance therapy? and should ICI be continued beyond progression?

Cytotoxic Chemotherapy

In tandem with the development chemoimmunotherapy, several studies assessed chemotherapy intensification in the first-line setting (see **Table 1**). The PRODIGE38-AMEBICA phase III clinical trial compared oxaliplatin, irinotecan, and 5-fluorouracil to gemcitabine/cisplatin. The study did not meet the primary endpoint for 6 month PFS.[9] SWOG-1815 investigated triplet combination, adding nab-paclitaxel to gemci-tabine/cisplatin, and failed to show a survival benefit.[10] Ad hoc analysis suggested a benefit in patients with GB cancer or locally advanced disease; however, the data are hypothesis generating and require prospective confirmation. A multicenter phase III study evaluated the addition of S1 to gemcitabine/cisplatin. Combination therapy demonstrated survival benefits and higher objective response rate (ORR) at the expense of a higher incidence of diarrhea, stomatitis, and rash.[11] In summary, triplet-based chemotherapy does not necessarily lead to superior outcomes, and toxicity seems to increase with additional agents. Early enthusiasm for the phase II data led to the addition of triplet regimen gemcitabine, cisplatin plus nab-paclitaxel to the National Comprehensive Cancer Network (NCCN) guidelines[12]

Clinical equipoise, a "state of genuine uncertainty" in the community of providers regarding superior treatment for a given clinical scenario, has been described in BTC.[13] Defining the boundaries between investigative work and clinical practice, and ensuring patients receive proven, standard-of-care treatment until sufficient evi-dence exists, need to be emphasized to avoid harm from the dependence on encour-aging early phase II data. This also implies the need for new strategies to reduce clinical trial size and duration[13] to answer questions in a more expeditious fashion.

In the second-line setting, combination regimens have demonstrated modest effi-cacy. The ABC-06 clinical trial showed that FOLFOX compared with active symptom control modestly improved median OS.[14,15] A pivotal study is the phase IIb NIFTY trial which showed improvement in PFS and OS with the use 5-fluorouracil/leucovorin and liposomal irinotecan.[16] An investigator-initiated, retrospective analysis across 3 study sites of contemporary second-line outcomes showed that 5-fluorouracil was used in

Table 1
Phase II/III studies in the first-line and second-line setting in advanced biliary tract cancer

Trial Names	Phase	Population	Treatment Arms	ORR	Median PFS (mo)	Median OS (mo)
First line						
TOPAZ-1[8]	III	Previously untreated unresectable or metastatic BTC or recurrent disease N = 685	Gemcitabine/cisplatin ± durvalumab, followed by durvalumab vs placebo	26.7% vs 18.7%	7.2 vs 5.7 HR 0.75 (95% CI 0.63–0.89), P = 0.001	12.8 vs 11.5 HR 0.76 (95% CI 0.64–0.91), P = 0.021
Keynote-966[9]	III	Previously untreated, unresectable, locally advanced or metastatic BTC N = 1069	Gemcitabine/cisplatin ± pembrolizumab vs placebo	29% both arms	6.5 vs 5.6 HR 0.86 (95% CI 0.75–1.00), P = 0.023	12.7 vs 10.9 HR 0.83 (95% CI 0.72–0.95), P = 0·0034
PRODIGE38-AMEBICA[11]	II–III	Locally advanced or metastatic BTC N = 191	mFOLFIRINOX vs gemcitabine/cisplatin (GemCis)	25.0% vs 19.4%	5.4 vs 6.8	11.7 vs 13.8
SWOG 1815[12]	III	Advanced BTC N = 441	Gemcitabine/cisplatin ± nab-paclitaxel (GAP) vs placebo (GC)	34% vs 25%	8.2 vs 6.4 HR 0.92 (95% CI 0.72–1.16), P = 0.47	14 vs 2.7 HR 0.93 (95% CI 0.74–1.19), P = 0.58
KHBO1401-MITSUBA[13]	III	Advanced BTC N = 246	Gemcitabine/cisplatin ± S1 (GPCS) vs placebo (GC)	41.5% vs 15.0%	7.4 vs 5.5 HR 0.75 (95% CI 0.577–0.970), P = 0.015	13.5 vs 12.6 HR 0.79 (95% CI 0.628–0.996), P = 0.046
Second line						
ABC-06[16]	III	Advanced BTC, progression to first-line cisplatin and gemcitabine N = 162	FOLFOX vs active symptom control (ACS)	-	-	6·2 vs 5.3 HR 0.69 (95% CI 0.50–0.97), P = 0.031
NIFTY[18]	IIb	Advanced BTC, progression on gemcitabine plus cisplatin N = 174	LV/FU/nal-IRI vs LV/FU	12.5% vs 3.5% P = 0.04	4.2 vs 1.7 HR 0.61, P = 0.004	8.6 vs 5.3 HR 0.68 (95% CI 0.48–0.95), P = 0.02

Abbreviations: FU, 5-flurouracil; GAP, Gemcitabine, cisplatin plus nab-paclitaxel; GC, Gemcitabine plus cisplatin; GPCS, Gemcitabine,cisplatin plus S-1 versus placebo; IRI, Irinotecan; LV, Leucovorin.

more than 60% of the patients in regimens such as 5-fluorouracil/irinotecan [FOLFIRI] or oxaliplatin [FOLFOX], whereas 18% received gemcitabine.[17] As such, fluoropyridine doublets have become acceptable regimens after failure of a front-line gemcitabine containing regimen—specifically in the absence of a gene alteration amenable to precision medicine.

Precision Medicine

It is estimated that up to 30% to 40% of patients with BTC harbor at least one actionable or potentially actionable genetic alteration (**Fig. 1**).[18–20] Based on observations from real-world experience, the prevalence of alterations seems much lower. Data show that the incidence of isocitrate dehydrogenese (IDH)1/2 mutation ranges from 15% to 20% in iCCA, 3% to 4% in eCCA and approaches 0% in GB cancer. The incidence for fibroblas growth factor receptor (FGFR) gene fusions ranges from 11% to 12% in iCCA, 0% in eCCA, and 1% in GB cancer.[21] Molecular profiles differ by anatomic sites, IDH1/2, FGFR2, and BRAF, are predominantly drivers in iCCA, whereas MDM2 loss and ERBB2 alterations are more frequent in eCCA and GB cancer.[22] Some genomic alterations seem to be mutually exclusive, suggesting that such alterations identify biologically distinct molecular subtypes and potentially clinical behavior.[19]

IDH Inhibitors

In the presence of IDH1/2 mutation, the mutant protein results in the production of a "neo"- or "onco"-metabolite, 2-hydroxyglutarate, whose accumulation impairs cellular differentiation by direct effects on DNA methylation and chromatin structure.[22] Ivosidenib, a selective inhibitor of mutant IDH1, was found to be safe and tolerable with cytostatic antitumor activity.[23] These data prompted the ClarIDHy study, a double-blind, placebo-controlled, phase III trial which confirmed its activity.[24] The trial permitted crossover on progression based on input from patient advocacy groups and clinicians. Crossover could have had a confounding effect on treatment effect estimation. When adjusting for crossover, the median OS was 5.1 months for placebo compared with 10.3 months for ivosidenib.[25] The final analysis showed that ivosidenib improved OS, despite a high rate of crossover from the placebo group (70%).[25] Correlative studies have identified isoform switching and second site mutations as potential resistance mechanisms to IDH1 inhibition.[26,27] Second-generation molecules blocking IDH1/2 and second-site mutations are under investigation.[28] The role of combination therapies with IDH1 inhibition or combinations of IDH1 inhibition and ICI, such as the phase II trial investigating ivosidenib in combination with nivolumab (NCT04056910), is ongoing.[29,30]

FGFR2 Inhibitors

Selective FGFR inhibitors have gained accelerated US FDA approval for previously treated FGFR2-fusion-positive CCAs. Infigratinib, one of the first FGFR1-4 inhibitors studied, demonstrated modest antitumor efficacy.[31] Although the confirmatory phase III trial (PROOF301) studying infigratinib as a first-line setting compared with the gemcitabine/cisplatin therapy was launched,[32] the study closed after the accrual of 48 of a planned 300 patients due to poor accrual.[33,34] Issues were also related to the need to perform broad genomic profiling early in the disease course and the need for a realistic expectation of the frequency of genomic alteration.

Pemigatinib, a non-covalent FGFR inhibitor, received approval based on the FIGHT-202 study, which confirmed antitumor activity.[35] The results of the phase II FOENIX-CA2 trial with futibatinib, a covalent FGFR1-4 inhibitor, demonstrated similar results.[36]

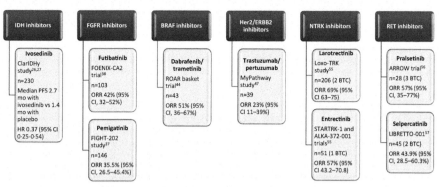

Fig. 1. Currently FDA-approved precision medicines and gene targets.

Both agents, conditionally approved by the FDA, moved into front-line randomized phase 3 studies; however, the phase 3 of futibatinib was resigned to a smaller randomized phase 2 study, whereas the study of pemigatinib is currently ongoing. The experience indicates that in these uncommon alterations in an uncommon disease, novel clinical trial design (ie, randomized phase 2), surrogates (ie, ciculating free DNA (cfDNA) or short-term time-to-event analysis), as well as real-world data are critical for feasibility and to confirm efficacy. Enrolling patients to phase III trials might take decades, making evidence-based medicine options not available for years.

For future drug development, nontarget FGFR alterations may be candidates for FGFR-targeted strategies in addition to the activating fusions.[37] Secondary mutations in the kinase domain of FGFR2, which prevent the inhibitors from binding, may represent a significant resistance mechanism.[38] Other mutations result in the abolition of molecular interactions or conformational changes in the receptor that destabilize a strong inhibitor–receptor interaction or stabilize a weak inhibitor–receptor interaction.[39] Novel inhibitors designed to overcome resistance are in active clinical development,[22] and more potent and selective inhibitors such as gunagratinib and RLY-4008 are in early-stage testing. Reported results are promising with improvements in ORR and disease control rate (DCR).[40,41]

Other Alterations

BRAF mutations are found in approximately 1% to 5% of BTC.[39] In the Rare Oncology Agnostic Research basket trial, treatment with dabrafenib and trametinib targeted BRAF V600 E mutations and resulted in an ORR of 51%.[42] Accordingly, dabrafenib in combination with trametinib received a tumor agnostic accelerated approval for non-colorectal cancers harboring BRAF V600 E mutations. Newer classes of RAF inhibitors, referred to as "paradox breakers," are currently in phase 1 studies; these drugs inhibit signaling by disrupting BRAF-containing dimers with a greater potency.[43] For patients whose tolerance to cytotoxic chemotherapy is concerning, the use of BRAF inhibitors in the first-line setting might be a reasonable because BRAF inhibitors are generally well tolerated. This approach is to be confirmed in clinical trials.

HER2 overexpression or pathway activation is present in 5% to 20% of CCAs and 15% to 30% of GB cancer.[18,44] Several human epithelian growth factor 2 (Her2) targeting agents have been tested including tyrosine kinase inhibitors, monoclonal antibodies, antibody-drug conjugates (ADCs), and combination therapies. Response rates range from 22% to 46.7%.[45–51] Next-generation molecules and novel combinations have offered the highest ORR, especially in Her2 immunohistochemistry 3+

cases, with a manageable safety profile. Targeting the activating HER2 single-nucleotide variant with neratinib resulted in ORR of 16%.[52] It remains unclear if this unique subset is targetable with monoclonal antibodies and next-generation ADCs. More data on the mechanism of resistance and predictors of response are yet to be identified.

Other rare genomic drivers include the neurotrophic tyrosine receptor kinase genes (NTRK1-3). Two selective inhibitors, larotrectinib and entrectinib, have showed activity in early clinical trials; a grouped analysis of the clinical trials reported an ORR of 57%.[53] RET inhibitors, pralsetinib and selpercatinib, improved ORR according to AR-ROW[54] and LIBRETTO-001[55] studies, respectively. Inactivation in mismatch repair enzymes occurs in less than 2% of BTC; pembrolizumab is approved in the deficient mismatch repair/MSI-high setting, with a phase 2 study showing an ORR of 41%. Multiple randomized controlled trials are ongoing to expand the role of ICI in advanced BTC.[56] Whether patients with MSI-high disease will benefit from treatment de-escalation remains to be answered.

EMERGING INVESTIGATIONAL THERAPIES

Newer targets have emerged including the MDM2 protein, an E3 ubiquitin ligase that targets the tumor suppressor p53.[57] MDM2 inhibitors block the MDM2-p53 protein–protein interaction leading to restoration of TP53 function. Early studies have shown a signal and are currently in late-stage clinical development.[58–60] Other targets include activating mutations in RAS which occur in up to 40% of BTC with a higher frequency in eCCA.[22] Targeting RAS through KRAS G12 C, which occurs in less than 1% of BTC, may have a future treatment role. The phase II KRYSTAL-1 trial of adagrasib has shown partial responses in 4 of 8 participants to date.[4] This and other advances have ushered in the study of selective and nonselective KRAS inhibitors and molecular degraders aimed at making the previously undruggable KRAS, a druggable target.[39]

Targeting multiple immunosuppressive pathways simultaneously is a field of interest aimed at achieving additional benefit over single pathway targeting. The use of two molecules which have inhibit independent, yet overlapping, pathways (TIGIT:CD155, programmed call death 1 [PD-1]/programmed cell death ligand 1 [PD-L1], and trans-formign growth factor beta [TGFβ]) is one example.[61] Another approach is through the combination of ICI and targeted therapies. Results from LEAP-005 study combining lenvatinib and pembrolizumab showed an ORR of 9.7% and DCR of 68%.[62] The use of anti-ascular endothelial growth factor (VEGF) therapy is also being investigated. IMBRAVE 151 is a phase 2 randomized double-blind placebo-controlled trial of first-line treatment in patients with advanced BTC, adding bevacizumab to atezolizumab/cisplatin/gemcitabine. Preliminary results showed a higher 6 month PFS rate.[63] Follow-up on this trial, including OS, is required to confirm efficacy.

Cellular Therapy and Cancer Vaccine

Chimeric antigen receptor (CAR) T-cell therapy, an innovative form of immunotherapy that involves genetically modified T cells to express CARs and enable them to recognize and target specific cancer cells, leads to a highly targeted anticancer response. CAR T-cell therapy has shown promising efficacy for hematologic malignancies.[64] Currently, CAR T-cell therapy does not work well in solid tumors due to challenges posed by several characteristics of solid tumors and the toxicity of the treatment itself.[65] However, there is a growing interest in the role of CAR T-cell therapy in solid tumors.[66] One clinical study used a combination of CAR-T therapies in patients with terminal CCA with the sequential infusion of EGFR-specific and CD133-specific

Table 2
Key clinical trials on adjuvant therapy in biliary tract cancer

Trial Names	Phase	Treatment Arms	Population	Results	Impression
European Study Group for Pancreatic Cancer (ESPAC)-3 periampullary[73]	III	Observation group or treatment group 1: folinic acid/fluorouracil, or treatment group 2: gemcitabine for 6 mo	428 patients (297 had ampullary, 96 had bile duct, and 35 had other cancers)	Median survival: Observation group 35.2 mo Chemotherapy group: 43.1 HR 0.86 (95% CI, 0.66–1.11), $P = 0.25$	No significant survival benefit
PRODIGE12-ACCORD18[74]	III	Observation (arm A) or chemotherapy GEMOX (gemcitabine/oxaliplatin) (arm B)	193 patients	Median RFS: Arm A 30.4 mo Arm B 18.5 mo HR 0.88 (95% CI, 0.62–1.25), $P = 0.48$	No benefit of adjuvant GEMOX
BCAT[75]	III	Observation or adjuvant gemcitabine for 6 cycles	225 patients	Median OS: Observation arm: 62.3 mo Gemcitabine: 63.8 mo HR 1·01 (95% CI 0·70–1·45), $P = 0.964$ Median RFS: Observation arm: 36.0 Gemcitabine: 39.9 HR 0·93 (95% CI 0·66–1·32), $P = 0.693$	No significant differences in overall survival
BILCAP[77]	III	8 cycles of adjuvant capecitabine or surveillance	447 patients	Median OS intention-to-treat analysis Control arm: 36.4 mo Capecitabine arm: 51.1 mo HR 0·81 (95% CI 0·63–1·04), $P = 0.097$ Protocol-specified sensitivity analysis: OS HR 0.71 (95% CI 0.55–0.92)	First positive study in the adjuvant setting

(continued on next page)

Table 2
(continued)

Trial Names	Phase	Treatment Arms	Population	Results	Impression
ASCOT[78]	III	Observation or S-1 for 4 cycles	440 patients	3 y OS: Observation arm: 67.6% S1 arm: 77.1% HR 0.69 (95% CI 0.51–0.94), p0.0080 3 y RFS Observation arm: 50.9% S1 arm: 62.4% HR 0.80 (95% CI 0.61–1.04), $P = 0.088$	Suggested improvement in survival
SWOG S0809[80]	II	4 cycles of gemcitabine/ capecitabine followed by concurrent capecitabine/ radiotherapy	79 patients with GB cancer or eCCA, stage pT2-4 or N+ or positive resection margins	Median OS 35 mo (R0, 34 mo; R1, 35 mo)	Promising efficacy for non-iCCA patients

Abbreviations: CI, confidence interval; HR, hazard ratio.

CAR-T cells. Results showed that treatment is feasible and safe without overt evidence of off-tumor on-target toxicity against normal tissues.[67] The data are promising yet premature, and more studies are needed. Peptide-derived vaccines and dendritic cell vaccines have emerged with positive clinical outcomes in case reports and early phase clinical trials.[68] This remains an active area of investigation with promising data from in vitro studies.[69] A key for success of these therapies is finding personalized neoantigens to tailor personalized therapy to potentially achieve better outcomes.

SYSTEMIC THERAPIES MOVEMENT TO EARLY STAGES OF DISEASE

Prospective phase 3 studies have assessed chemotherapy as an adjuvant therapy (**Table 2**).[70–73] Although most studies were negative, two trials suggest a benefit for fluoropyrimidine adjuvant therapy including the BILCAP[74] and ASCOT trials.[75,76] Further studies of adjuvant therapy are ongoing, and it is likely that immunotherapeutics will move into this space. The role of adjuvant radiotherapy has yet to be fully clarified. SWOG S0809 trial favored the use of radiation therapy in node positive or margin positive disease in patients diagnosed with GB cancer or eCCA after radical resection.[73,77] Critiques about this study include grouping different diseases with disparate biology, differences of resectability definitions, and treatment interruption.[78] Without a control group, this study is of limited application and the efficacy of radiotherapy remains debatable.

Perioperative therapy has potential advantages over adjuvant therapy including early treatment of micro-metastatic disease, increasing the R0 resection rate and N0 rate, assessment of antitumor activity in situ, and assessment of tumor biology. If immunotherapy is applied, there are theoretic benefits in early-stage disease.[79,80] At present, perioperative therapy remains under investigation with ongoing studies including the Optimal Perioperative Therapy for Incidental Gallbladder Cancer.[81] Small prospective studies such as NEO-GAP phase II study of neoadjuvant gemcitabine/cisplatin/nab-paclitaxel demonstrate feasibility and safety, but we await RFS and OS data.[82]

SUMMARY

BTCs are diverse cancers with unique biological and clinical behavior. In advanced disease, the first-line treatment includes combination of chemotherapy and ICI. For second-line and beyond, targeting genomic alterations, if present, is recommended. If no genomic alterations exist, chemotherapy is the choice of treatment. The role of perioperative therapy remains to be investigated. Despite the advances in molecular profiling and targeted therapies, studies on BTC remain challenging due to the small number of patients. We need better drugs and drug combinations to enhance disease control, improve survival, and overcome drug resistance.

CLINICS CARE POINTS

- Biliary tract cancer (BTC) is a rare subset of gastrointestinal tumors that are subclassified as intrahepatic cholangiocarcinoma (CCA), extrahepatic CCA, and gallbladder cancer.
- In advanced disease, chemotherapy in combination with immune checkpoint inhibitors is a standard of care in the first-line setting.
- For the second-line treatment, BTC should be assessed for genomic alterations to identify an appropriate use of targeted therapies.

- In patients with no known driver alteration or targetable mutations or unavailable genomic analysis, cytotoxic chemotherapy remains the second-line choice.
- There are ongoing studies with newer drugs and drug combinations, as well as cellular therapy.
- For localized and resectable disease, surgery remains the only curative intervention.
- Adjuvant chemotherapy reduces recurrence risk after surgical intervention.
- No current trials support the use of perioperative therapy.

DISCLOSURE

J.J. Harding reports research from Bristol-Myers Squibb, United States, Pfizer, United States, Lilly, United States, Novartis, Switzerland, Incyte, United States, Calithera Biosciences, United States, Polaris, Yiviva, Debiopharm Group, Zymeworks, Boehringer Ingelheim, United States, Loxo, Genoscience Pharma, Codiak Biosciences, and a consulting role from Bristol Myers Squibb, CytomX Therapeutics, Lilly, Eisai, Imvax, Merck, Exelixis, Zymeworks, Adaptimmune, QED Therapeutics, Hepion Pharmaceuticals, Medivir, and Elevar Therapeutics and G. Abou-Alfa reports research from Agenus, Arcus, AstraZeneca, United Kingdom, BioNTech, BMS, United States, Elicio, Genentech/Roche, Helsinn, Switzerland, Parker Institute, United States, Pertzye, Puma, QED, Yiviva, and consulting support from Astra Zeneca, Autem, Berry Genomics, BioNtech, Boehringer Ingelheim, BMS, Eisai, Exelixis, Genentech/Roche, Incyte, Ipsen, Merck, Merus, Neogene, Novartis, Servier, Tempus, Vector, Yiviva.

REFERENCES

1. Dickson PV, Behrman SW. Distal cholangiocarcinoma. Surgical Clinics 2014; 94(2):325–42.
2. Zamora-Valdes D, Heimbach JK. Liver Transplant for Cholangiocarcinoma. Gastroenterol Clin North Am 2018;47(2):267–80.
3. Fairweather M, Balachandran VP, D'Angelica MI. Surgical management of biliary tract cancers. Chin Clin Oncol 2016;5(5):63.
4. Bekaii-Saab TS, Yaeger R, Spira AI, et al. Adagrasib in Advanced Solid Tumors Harboring a KRAS(G12C) Mutation. J Clin Oncol 2023;41(25):4097–106.
5. Valle J, Wasan H, Palmer DH, et al. Cisplatin plus gemcitabine versus gemcitabine for biliary tract cancer. N Engl J Med 2010;362(14):1273–81.
6. Oh D-Y, Ruth He A, Qin S, et al. Durvalumab plus gemcitabine and cisplatin in advanced biliary tract cancer. NEJM evidence 2022;1(8). EVIDoa2200015.
7. Kelley RK, Ueno M, Yoo C, et al. Pembrolizumab in combination with gemcitabine and cisplatin compared with gemcitabine and cisplatin alone for patients with advanced biliary tract cancer (KEYNOTE-966): a randomised, double-blind, placebo-controlled, phase 3 trial. Lancet 2023;401(10391):1853–65.
8. Frega G, Cossio FP, Banales JM, et al. Lacking Immunotherapy Biomarkers for Biliary Tract Cancer: A Comprehensive Systematic Literature Review and Meta-Analysis. Cells 2023;12(16). https://doi.org/10.3390/cells12162098.
9. Phelip J-M, Edeline J, Blanc J-F, et al. Modified FOLFIRINOX versus CisGem first-line chemotherapy for locally advanced non resectable or metastatic biliary tract cancer (AMEBICA)-PRODIGE 38: Study protocol for a randomized controlled multicenter phase II/III study. Dig Liver Dis 2019;51(2):318–20.

10. Shroff RT, Guthrie KA, Scott AJ, et al. SWOG 1815: A phase III randomized trial of gemcitabine, cisplatin, and nab-paclitaxel versus gemcitabine and cisplatin in newly diagnosed, advanced biliary tract cancers, J Clin Oncol, 41, 2023 (suppl 4, abstr LBA490).

11. Ioka T, Kanai M, Kobayashi S, et al. Randomized phase III study of gemcitabine, cisplatin plus S-1 versus gemcitabine, cisplatin for advanced biliary tract cancer (KHBO1401- MITSUBA). J Hepatobiliary Pancreat Sci 2023;30(1):102–10.

12. NCCN guidelines on management of Biliary tract cancers. V. 3 2023.

13. Lee TY, Bates SE, Abou-Alfa GK. Equipoise, drug development, and biliary cancer. Cancer 2022;128(5):944–9.

14. Lamarca A, Palmer DH, Wasan HS, et al. Second-line FOLFOX chemotherapy versus active symptom control for advanced biliary tract cancer (ABC-06): a phase 3, open-label, randomised, controlled trial. Lancet Oncol 2021;22(5): 690–701.

15. Choi IS, Kim KH, Lee JH, et al. A randomised phase II study of oxaliplatin/5-FU (mFOLFOX) versus irinotecan/5-FU (mFOLFIRI) chemotherapy in locally advanced or metastatic biliary tract cancer refractory to first-line gemcitabine/cisplatin chemotherapy. Eur J Cancer 2021;154:288–95.

16. Yoo C, Kim K-P, Jeong JH, et al. Liposomal irinotecan plus fluorouracil and leucovorin versus fluorouracil and leucovorin for metastatic biliary tract cancer after progression on gemcitabine plus cisplatin (NIFTY): a multicentre, open-label, randomised, phase 2b study. Lancet Oncol 2021;22(11):1560–72.

17. Lowery MA, Goff LW, Keenan BP, et al. Second-line chemotherapy in advanced biliary cancers: A retrospective, multicenter analysis of outcomes. Cancer 2019;125(24):4426–34.

18. Javle M, Bekaii-Saab T, Jain A, et al. Biliary cancer: utility of next-generation sequencing for clinical management. Cancer 2016;122(24):3838–47.

19. Lowery MA, Ptashkin R, Jordan E, et al. Comprehensive molecular profiling of intrahepatic and extrahepatic cholangiocarcinomas: potential targets for intervention. Clin Cancer Res 2018;24(17):4154–61.

20. Mody K, Jain P, El-Refai SM, et al. Clinical, genomic, and transcriptomic data profiling of biliary tract cancer reveals subtype-specific immune signatures. JCO Precision Oncology 2022;6:e2100510.

21. Bridgewater JA, Goodman KA, Kalyan A, et al. Biliary tract cancer: epidemiology, radiotherapy, and molecular profiling. American Society of Clinical Oncology Educational Book 2016;36:e194–203.

22. Harding JJ, Khalil DN, Fabris L, et al. Rational development of combination therapies for biliary tract cancers. J Hepatol 2023;78(1):217–28.

23. Lowery MA, Burris HA, Janku F, et al. Safety and activity of ivosidenib in patients with IDH1-mutant advanced cholangiocarcinoma: a phase 1 study. Lancet Gastroenterology & Hepatology 2019;4(9):711–20.

24. Abou-Alfa GK, Macarulla T, Javle MM, et al. Ivosidenib in IDH1-mutant, chemotherapy-refractory cholangiocarcinoma (ClarIDHy): a multicentre, randomised, double-blind, placebo-controlled, phase 3 study. Lancet Oncol 2020;21(6): 796–807.

25. Zhu AX, Macarulla T, Javle MM, et al. Final overall survival efficacy results of ivosidenib for patients with advanced cholangiocarcinoma with IDH1 mutation: the phase 3 randomized clinical claridhy trial. JAMA Oncol 2021;7(11):1669–77.

26. Harding JJ, Lowery MA, Shih AH, et al. Isoform switching as a mechanism of acquired resistance to mutant isocitrate dehydrogenase inhibition. Cancer Discov 2018;8(12):1540–7.

27. Cleary JM, Rouaisnel B, Daina A, et al. Secondary IDH1 resistance mutations and oncogenic IDH2 mutations cause acquired resistance to ivosidenib in cholangiocarcinoma. npj Precis Oncol 2022;6(1):61.

28. Rodon J, Goyal L, Mercade TM, et al. Abstract CT098: A first-in-human phase 1 study of LY3410738, a covalent inhibitor of mutant IDH, in advanced IDH-mutant cholangiocarcinoma and other solid tumors. Cancer Res 2023;83(8_Supplement): CT098.

29. Clinicaltrials.gov. 2023. clinicaltrial.gov/study/NCT04056910.

30. Lo JH, Agarwal R, Goff LW, et al. Immunotherapy in Biliary Tract Cancers: Current Standard-of-Care and Emerging Strategies. Cancers 2023;15(13):3312.

31. Javle M, Lowery M, Shroff RT, et al. Phase II Study of BGJ398 in Patients With FGFR-Altered Advanced Cholangiocarcinoma. J Clin Oncol 2018;36(3):276–82.

32. Makawita S, Abou-Alfa GK, Roychowdhury S, et al. Infigratinib in patients with advanced cholangiocarcinoma with FGFR2 gene fusions/translocations: the PROOF 301 trial. Future Oncol 2020;16(30):2375–84.

33. https://www.biospace.com/article/bridgebio-takes-hit-as-partner-ends-2-4b-partnership-for-liver-cancer-candidate/. 2023.

34. Abou-Alfa GK, Borbath I, Goyal L, et al. Proof 301: a multicenter, open-label, randomized, phase 3 trial of infigratinib versus gemcitabine plus cisplatin in patients with advanced cholangiocarcinoma with an FGFR2 gene fusion/rearrangement, 2022, *J Clini Oncol*, 40, 16 (TSP4171).

35. Abou-Alfa GK, Sahai V, Hollebecque A, et al. Pemigatinib for previously treated, locally advanced or metastatic cholangiocarcinoma: a multicentre, open-label, phase 2 study. Lancet Oncol 2020;21(5):671–84.

36. Goyal L, Meric-Bernstam F, Hollebecque A, et al. Futibatinib for FGFR2-rearranged intrahepatic cholangiocarcinoma. N Engl J Med 2023;388(3):228–39.

37. Choudhury NJ, Harada G, Whiting K, et al. Genomic characterization of FGFR-altered solid tumors using a clinically annotated pan-cancer repository. J Clin Oncol 2023;41(16_suppl):3074.

38. Facchinetti F, Hollebecque A, Bahleda R, et al. Facts and new hopes on selective FGFR inhibitors in solid tumors. Clin Cancer Res 2020;26(4):764–74.

39. Valery M, Vasseur D, Fachinetti F, et al. Targetable Molecular Alterations in the Treatment of Biliary Tract Cancers: An Overview of the Available Treatments. Cancers 2023;15(18):4446.

40. Hollebecque A, Borad M, Goyal L, et al. LBA12 Efficacy of RLY-4008, a highly selective FGFR2 inhibitor in patients (pts) with an FGFR2-fusion or rearrangement (f/r), FGFR inhibitor (FGFRi)-naïve cholangiocarcinoma (CCA): ReFocus trial. Ann Oncol 2022;33:S1381.

41. Guo Y, Yuan C, Ding W, et al. Gunagratinib, a highly selective irreversible FGFR inhibitor, in patients with previously treated locally advanced or metastatic cholangiocarcinoma harboring FGFR pathway alterations: a phase IIa dose-expansion study. American Society of Clinical Oncology; 2023.

42. Salama AKS, Li S, Macrae ER, et al. Dabrafenib and trametinib in patients with tumors with BRAF V600E/K mutations: Results from the molecular analysis for therapy choice (MATCH) Arm H. J Clin Oncol 2019;37(15_suppl):3002.

43. Yaeger R, Corcoran RB. Targeting Alterations in the RAF-MEK Pathway. Cancer Discov 2019;9(3):329–41.

44. Hwajeong L, Kai W, Adrienne J, et al. Comprehensive genomic profiling of extrahepatic cholangiocarcinoma reveals a long tail of therapeutic targets. J Clin Pathol 2016;69(5):403.

45. Javle M, Borad MJ, Azad NS, et al. Pertuzumab and trastuzumab for HER2-positive, metastatic biliary tract cancer (MyPathway): a multicentre, open-label, phase 2a, multiple basket study. Lancet Oncol 2021;22(9):1290–300.

46. Ohba A, Morizane C, Ueno M, et al. Multicenter phase II trial of trastuzumab deruxtecan for HER2-positive unresectable or recurrent biliary tract cancer: HERB trial. Future Oncol 2022;18(19):2351–60.

47. Meric-Bernstam F, Makker V, Oaknin A, et al. Efficacy and safety of trastuzumab deruxtecan (T-DXd) in patients (pts) with HER2-expressing solid tumors: DESTINY-PanTumor02 (DP-02) interim results, 2023, J Clin Oncol, 41, 17 (LBA3000).

48. Pant S, Fan J, Oh D-Y, et al. Results from the pivotal phase (Ph) 2b HERIZON-BTC-01 study: Zanidatamab in previously-treated HER2-amplified biliary tract cancer (BTC). J Clin Oncol 2023;41(16_suppl):4008.

49. Harding JJ, Fan J, Oh DY, et al. Zanidatamab for HER2-amplified, unresectable, locally advanced or metastatic biliary tract cancer (HERIZON-BTC-01): a multicentre, single-arm, phase 2b study. Lancet Oncol 2023;24(7):772–82.

50. Bekaii-Saab T, Jin F, Ramos J, et al. P-74 SGNTUC-019: Phase 2 basket study of tucatinib and trastuzumab in previously treated solid tumors with HER2 alterations: Biliary tract cancer cohort (trial in progress). Ann Oncol 2022;33:S273–4.

51. Nakamura Y, Mizuno N, Sunakawa Y, et al. Tucatinib and trastuzumab for previously treated HER2-positive metastatic biliary tract cancer (SGNTUC-019): A phase 2 basket study. J Clin Oncol 2023;41(16_suppl):4007.

52. Harding JJ, Piha-Paul SA, Shah RH, et al. Antitumour activity of neratinib in patients with HER2-mutant advanced biliary tract cancers. Nat Commun 2023; 14(1):630.

53. Doebele RC, Drilon A, Paz-Ares L, et al. Entrectinib in patients with advanced or metastatic NTRK fusion-positive solid tumours: integrated analysis of three phase 1-2 trials. Lancet Oncol 2020;21(2):271–82.

54. Subbiah V, Cassier PA, Siena S, et al. Pan-cancer efficacy of pralsetinib in patients with RET fusion-positive solid tumors from the phase 1/2 ARROW trial. Nat Med 2022;28(8):1640–5.

55. Subbiah V, Wolf J, Konda B, et al. Tumour-agnostic efficacy and safety of selpercatinib in patients with RET fusion-positive solid tumours other than lung or thyroid tumours (LIBRETTO-001): a phase 1/2, open-label, basket trial. Lancet Oncol 2022;23(10):1261–73.

56. Kang S, El-Rayes BF, Akce M. Evolving Role of Immunotherapy in Advanced Biliary Tract Cancers. Cancers (Basel) 2022;14(7). https://doi.org/10.3390/cancers14071748.

57. Bond GL, Hu W, Levine AJ. MDM2 is a central node in the p53 pathway: 12 years and counting. Curr Cancer Drug Targets 2005;5(1):3–8.

58. Aguilar A, Thomas JE, Wang S. Targeting MDM2 for the development of a new cancer therapy: progress and challenges. Med Chem Res 2023;32(7):1334–44.

59. Goyal L, Harding JJ, Ueno M, et al. A phase IIa/IIb, open-label trial of BI 907828, an MDM2–p53 antagonist, in patients with locally advanced/metastatic biliary tract carcinoma or pancreatic ductal adenocarcinoma: Brightline-2. J Clin Oncol 2023;41(16_suppl):TPS4179.

60. LoRusso P, Yamamoto N, Patel MR, et al. The MDM2-p53 Antagonist Brigimadlin (BI 907828) in Patients with Advanced or Metastatic Solid Tumors: Results of a Phase Ia, First-in-Human, Dose-Escalation Study. Cancer Discov 2023;13(8): 1802–13.

61. Franks SE, Fabian KP, Santiago-Sánchez G, et al. Immune targeting of three independent suppressive pathways (TIGIT, PD-L1, TGFβ) provides significant

antitumor efficacy in immune checkpoint resistant models. OncoImmunology 2022;11(1):2124666.

62. Villanueva L, Lwin Z, Chung HC, et al. Lenvatinib plus pembrolizumab for patients with previously treated biliary tract cancers in the multicohort phase II LEAP-005 study. American Society of Clinical Oncology; 2021.

63. Hack SP, Verret W, Mulla S, et al. IMbrave 151: a randomized phase II trial of atezolizumab combined with bevacizumab and chemotherapy in patients with advanced biliary tract cancer. Therapeutic Advances in Medical Oncology 2021;13. 17588359211036544.

64. Ali S, Kjeken R, Niederlaender C, et al. The European Medicines Agency Review of Kymriah (Tisagenlecleucel) for the Treatment of Acute Lymphoblastic Leukemia and Diffuse Large B-Cell Lymphoma. Oncologist 2020;25(2):e321–7.

65. Feng Q, Sun B, Xue T, et al. Advances in CAR T-cell therapy in bile duct, pancreatic, and gastric cancers. Front Immunol 2022;13:1025608.

66. Sangsuwannukul T, Supimon K, Sujjitjoon J, et al. Anti-tumour effect of the fourth-generation chimeric antigen receptor T cells targeting CD133 against cholangiocarcinoma cells. Int Immunopharm 2020;89:107069.

67. Beatty GL, Haas AR, Maus MV, et al. Mesothelin-specific chimeric antigen receptor mRNA-engineered T cells induce anti-tumor activity in solid malignancies. Cancer Immunol Res 2014;2(2):112–20.

68. Han S, Lee SY, Wang WW, et al. A Perspective on Cell Therapy and Cancer Vaccine in Biliary Tract Cancers (BTCs). Cancers (Basel) 2020;12(11). https://doi.org/10.3390/cancers12113404.

69. Rojas-Sepúlveda D, Tittarelli A, Gleisner MA, et al. Tumor lysate-based vaccines: on the road to immunotherapy for gallbladder cancer. Cancer Immunol Immunother 2018;67(12):1897–910.

70. Neoptolemos JP, Moore MJ, Cox TF, et al. Effect of adjuvant chemotherapy with fluorouracil plus folinic acid or gemcitabine vs observation on survival in patients with resected periampullary adenocarcinoma: the ESPAC-3 periampullary cancer randomized trial. JAMA 2012;308(2):147–56.

71. Edeline J, Benabdelghani M, Bertaut A, et al. Gemcitabine and oxaliplatin chemotherapy or surveillance in resected biliary tract cancer (PRODIGE 12-ACCORD 18-UNICANCER GI): a randomized phase III study. J Clin Oncol 2019;37(8):658–67.

72. Ebata T, Hirano S, Konishi M, et al. Randomized clinical trial of adjuvant gemcitabine chemotherapy versus observation in resected bile duct cancer. Journal of British Surgery 2018;105(3):192–202.

73. Ben-Josef E, Guthrie KA, El-Khoueiry AB, et al. SWOG S0809: a phase II intergroup trial of adjuvant capecitabine and gemcitabine followed by radiotherapy and concurrent capecitabine in extrahepatic cholangiocarcinoma and gallbladder carcinoma. J Clin Oncol 2015;33(24):2617.

74. Primrose JN, Fox RP, Palmer DH, et al. Capecitabine compared with observation in resected biliary tract cancer (BILCAP): a randomised, controlled, multicentre, phase 3 study. Lancet Oncol 2019;20(5):663–73.

75. Nakachi K, Ikeda M, Konishi M, et al. Adjuvant S-1 compared with observation in resected biliary tract cancer (JCOG1202, ASCOT): a multicentre, open-label, randomised, controlled, phase 3 trial. Lancet 2023;401(10372):195–203.

76. Kefas J, Bridgewater J, Vogel A, et al. Adjuvant therapy of biliary tract cancers. Ther Adv Med Oncol 2023;15. https://doi.org/10.1177/17588359231163785. 17588359231163785.

77. Gholami S, Colby S, Horowitz DP, et al. Adjuvant chemoradiation in patients with lymph node-positive biliary tract cancers: secondary analysis of a single-arm clinical trial (Swog 0809). Ann Surg Oncol 2023;30(3):1354–63.

78. Warner SG, Starlinger P. Comparing Apples to Oranges: Commentary on a Secondary Analysis of SWOG 0809. Ann Surg Oncol 2023;30(3):1285–6.

79. Yoo C, Shin SH, Park JO, et al. Current Status and Future Perspectives of Perioperative Therapy for Resectable Biliary Tract Cancer: A Multidisciplinary Review. Cancers (Basel) 2021;13(7). https://doi.org/10.3390/cancers13071647.

80. Moris D, Palta M, Kim C, et al. Advances in the treatment of intrahepatic cholangiocarcinoma: An overview of the current and future therapeutic landscape for clinicians. CA A Cancer J Clin 2023;73(2):198–222.

81. Maithel SK, Hong SC, Ethun CG, et al. Optimal perioperative therapy for incidental gallbladder cancer (OPT-IN): A randomized phase II/III trial—ECOG-ACRIN EA2197. J Clin Oncol 2023;41(4_suppl):TPS620.

82. Maithel SK, Javle MM, Mahipal A, et al. NEO-GAP: A phase II single-arm prospective feasibility study of neoadjuvant gemcitabine/cisplatin/nab-paclitaxel for resectable high-risk intrahepatic cholangiocarcinoma. J Clin Oncol 2022; 40(16_suppl):4097.

Targeted Agents in Esophagogastric Cancer Beyond Human Epidermal Growth Factor Receptor-2

Eric Mehlhaff, MD[a,1], Devon Miller, MD[a,1],
Johnathan D. Ebben, MD, PhD[a], Oleksii Dobrzhanskyi, MD[b,2],
Nataliya V. Uboha, MD, PhD[a,c],*

KEYWORDS

- Esophageal cancer • Gastric cancer • Gastroesophageal junction adenocarcinoma
- Biomarker • CLDN18.2 • FGFR2b • DKN-01 • Receptor tyrosine kinases

KEY POINTS

- Tumor biomarker testing is essential for optimal treatment selection.
- CLDN18.2 is the newest established biomarker with associated therapies in advanced upper GI cancers.
- There are multiple targeted agents in development.
- Biomarker overlap and tumor heterogeneity must be considered during targeted drug development.

INTRODUCTION

Gastroesophageal cancer is a significant global health challenge, and the identification and validation of reliable biomarkers have become increasingly important for early diagnosis, prognosis, and personalized treatment strategies. Esophageal cancer is currently ranked seventh and gastric cancer fifth in cancer-related causes of death.[1] In 2020, there were more than 26,000 new cases of gastric cancer and 18,309 new cases of esophageal cancer in the United States.[1] Approximately half of upper

[a] Division of Hematology, Medical Oncology and Palliative Care, Department of Medicine, University of Wisconsin School of Medicine and Public Health, University of Wisconsin, 600 Highland Avenue, Madison, WI 53792, USA; [b] Upper Gastrointestinal Tumors Department, National Cancer Institute, Kyiv, Ukraine; [c] University of Wisconsin, Carbone Cancer Center, Madison, WI, USA
[1] These authors contributed equally.
[2] Present address: Julii Zdanovskoji Street 33/34, Kyiv 03022, Ukraine.
* Corresponding author. 600 Highland Avenue, K4/518, Madison, WI 53792.
E-mail address: nvuboha@medicine.wisc.edu

Hematol Oncol Clin N Am 38 (2024) 659–675
https://doi.org/10.1016/j.hoc.2024.02.006
0889-8588/24/© 2024 Elsevier Inc. All rights reserved.

gastrointestinal (GI) cancers are detected in advanced stages, and a notable portion of individuals with early stage disease experience recurrences following definitive treatments.[2,3] Overall survival (OS) for patients with advanced disease remains less than 2 years with current treatments.[4] There remains a significant unmet need to improve outcomes for patients with this disease.

Across cancer types, incorporation of biomarker-based therapies results in better patient outcomes. Biomarker-based treatments not only offer better efficacy but also spare patient toxicities when treatments are unlikely to work. There are several clinically relevant biomarkers and associated therapies that are part of standard care for patients with upper GI cancers. However, gastroesophageal tumors are a group of heterogeneous malignancies, anatomically and molecularly.[5,6] This extensive tumor heterogeneity has posed challenges for effective drug development, especially when studies enroll patients without appropriate selection measures. Over the last decade, there have been significant advances in the understanding of molecular characteristics of gastric and esophageal cancers. The Cancer Genome Atlas network has grouped these tumors into four subclasses, the incidence of which varies depending on the primary tumor location, gene copy alteration, point mutations, patterns of gene expression, and changes in DNA methylation.[5] Currently, there is a growing number of biomarker-based therapies in development for upper GI cancers. Here we review ongoing research efforts focusing on novel biomarker-based therapies for patients with gastroesophageal cancers. We highlight relevant clinical studies and discuss existing questions regarding incorporation of these emerging therapies into current treatment paradigms.

CURRENT BIOMARKERS

Upper GI malignancies are increasingly managed using biomarker-based approaches. In advanced disease, treatment selection based on human epidermal growth factor receptor-2 (HER2), programmed death receptor ligand 1 (PD-L1), or microsatellite instability (MSI) status or mismatch repair (MMR) protein expression has become standard practice.

Human Epidermal Growth Factor Receptor-2

HER2 family receptors are known to play a critical role in tumorigenesis.[7] HER2 overexpression is seen in up to 20% of esophageal and gastric adenocarcinoma. HER2 status is typically assessed using immunohistochemistry (IHC) and in situ hybridization method. Trastuzumab, a monoclonal antibody (mAb) that binds to the extracellular domain of the HER2 receptor, has been approved for the treatment of advanced gastroesophageal adenocarcinoma (GEA) based on randomized phase 3 TOGA trial.[8] Recently, trastuzumab deruxtecan (HER2 directed antibody drug conjugate [ADC]) received approval in the late-line setting after progression on trastuzumab-containing systemic therapy.[9]

Programmed Death Ligand-1

PD-L1 is a biomarker used to select patients with advanced GEA that are likely to benefit from checkpoint inhibitors. Although higher PD-L1 expression in tumor and immune cells predicts immunotherapy (IO) therapy response, its applicability in upper GI cancers is evolving and its use is complicated by differing scoring systems, antibodies, and thresholds of detection in various studies.[10–12] Nevertheless, presently all advanced-stage tumors should undergo evaluation for PD-L1 expression via IHC to determine combined positive score (CPS) that helps guide therapy selection.

DNA Mismatch Repair/Microsatellite Instability

Microsatellites are short and repetitive DNA sequences randomly widespread throughout the genome. The MMR system deficiency (dMMR) is caused by germline mutations or sporadic epigenetic silencing and result in aberrant presence of microsatellite regions in the DNA defined as MSI.[13] Evaluation for MSI of dMMR should be performed on all tumors, regardless of stage, because they predict response to immunotherapy and are associated with longer progression-free survival (PFS) and OS in patients who receive immunotherapy.[14] Incorporation of immune checkpoint inhibitors should be considered across disease stages for patients with MSI-H/dMMR tumors.[15]

TARGETED AGENTS IN DEVELOPMENT
Claudin 18.2–Directed Therapies

Claudin 18.2 function

Within the biomarker-driven therapy development for GEA, claudin 18.2 (CLDN18.2) has emerged as an attractive target because of significant expression in upper GI malignancies, and restricted expression in normal tissues. CLDN18.2 is a member of CLDN family of proteins.[16] CLDNs are 20- to 27-kDa transmembrane proteins that consist of four transmembrane domains and two extracellular loops.[17] CLDNs have a crucial role in maintaining the integrity and selective permeability of epithelial cell barriers.[17,18] CLDN18.2 is primarily expressed in normal gastric mucosa.[16] When present as component of protein scaffolding in tight junctions, CLDN18.2 extracellular regions are typically inaccessible for antibody targeting. However, its expression can be dysregulated in multiple cancers. During carcinogenesis, CLDN18.2 can relocalize over the cellular membrane resulting in loss of cellular polarity and accessibility of CLDN18.2 extracellular domains for antibody binding (**Fig. 1**). Such dysfunctionality of tight junction proteins results in abnormal cellular cytoskeletal organization that underlies epithelial-mesenchymal transition, which in turn results in increased cellular migration, proliferation, and invasion.[19]

More than a third of advanced GEA have upregulated CLDN18.2 expression.[20,21] Multiple definitions for CLDN18.2 positivity via IHC have been used across studies, and standardizing staining and scoring is critical for unified classifications during ongoing drug development. On a molecular level, CLDN18.2 gene fusions have been detected in gastric cancer. The incidence of fusions is low (1.3%–4%), but they are seen at higher frequency (up to 15%) in genomically stable tumors as defined per Cancer Genome Atlas Research Network Classification.[5,22]

Several different therapeutics targeting CLDN18.2 are in development, including CLDN18.2-directed mAbs, bispecific antibodies and T-cell engagers, ADCs, and cell therapies involving chimeric antigen receptor (CAR) T cells (see **Fig. 1**). Within these different therapeutic classes, there is ongoing work to explore rational combinations, such as the addition of immunotherapy to CLDN18.2 targeting. Sections discussed next describe select therapeutic agents within each of these classes, their established efficacy, associated toxicities, and ongoing development efforts.

Anticlaudin monoclonal antibody: zolbetuximab

Zolbetuximab is a chimeric IgG1 mAb that binds to the extracellular loop of CLDN18.2 on tumor cell surface. This antibody is engineered to involve antibody-dependent cellular cytotoxicity (ADCC) and complement-dependent cytotoxicity tumor killing.[23] Zolbetuximab demonstrated promising activity in early phase studies, alone and in combination with chemotherapy.[24,25] More recently, zolbetuximab activity was confirmed in two randomized phase 3 studies (SPOTLIGHT and GLOW).[21,26]

A Claudin 18.2: A Novel Tumor-Associated Target

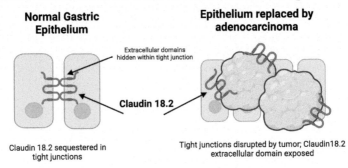

B   Therapeutic Strategies Targeting Claudin18.2

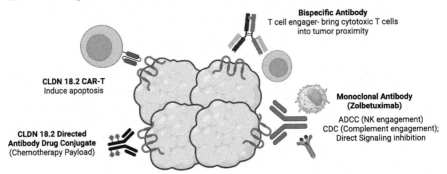

Fig. 1. (*A*) CLDN18.2 expression in normal and cancer cells. (*B*) Methods for targeting CLDN18.2 during drug development. (Created with BioRender.com.)

In the phase 3 SPOTLIGHT trial, patients with locally advanced, previously untreated, HER2-negative gastric and gastroesophageal junction (G/GEJ) adenocarcinoma were randomized to either modified 5-fluorouracil, leucovorin, and oxaliplatin chemotherapy (mFOLFOX6) plus zolbetuximab or mFOLFOX6 plus placebo.[27] Eligible patients had CLDN18.2-positive tumors, which was defined as greater than or equal to 75% of tumor cells with moderate-to-strong membranous CLDN18 staining. The study met its primary end point of median PFS improvement with zolbetuximab addition (10.61 vs 8.67 months; hazard ratio [HR], 0.75).[21] Median OS was also significantly improved with zolbetuximab addition (18.23 vs 15.54 months; HR, 0.75). The objective response rate (ORR) was similar between the two groups. The randomized phase 3 GLOW study had similar design but used capecitabine and oxaliplatin (CAPOX) as a chemotherapy backbone.[26] Similar to the SPOTLIGHT trial, PFS (8.21 vs 6.80 months; HR, 0.687) and OS (14.39 vs 12.16 months; HR, 0.771) were improved with zolbetuximab addition to chemotherapy in a biomarker-select patient population. There were no differences in ORR (42.5% in the zolbetuximab arm vs 40.3% in the control arm) in the GLOW trial as well. In both studies, zolbetuximab demonstrated a similar safety profile, with nausea and vomiting being the only adverse events (AEs) with more than 10% difference between the treatment arms. These toxicities are likely caused by on-target effects of zolbetuximab related to normal expression of CLDN18.2 in gastric mucosa. In both studies, these GI toxicities were more prominent during the first treatment cycle and decreased with subsequent treatments.

Both SPOTLIGHT and GLOW trials used chemotherapy alone as a control arm, which was appropriate at the time these studies launched. However, more recently nivolumab plus chemotherapy has become standard first-line treatment of advanced HER2-negative GEA per CheckMate 649.[4] Despite broad Food and Drug Administration approval of nivolumab for all patients with advanced GEA regardless of PD-L1 expression, activity of anti-PD1 agents seems to be restricted to patients whose tumors have higher PD-L1 CPS.[28] The recent updates in the standard of care should be incorporated in the design of future studies. Nevertheless, given positive results from two global phase 3 studies, CLDN18.2 has now been established as a clinically relevant biomarker for GEA, and zolbetuximab has emerged as a new targeted agent for this disease and is currently awaiting Food and Drug Administration approval.

Combination strategies

There are ongoing efforts to better characterize CLDN18.2 expression in the context of existing biomarkers that currently drive clinical decision making. In particular, overlap between CLDN18.2 and PD-L1 expression has been evaluated in several prior investigations. In SPOTLIGHT and GLOW trials, 13% and 21.9% of assessed patients, respectively, had tumors with PD-L1 CPS greater than or equal to five, respectively.[21,26] In a retrospective analysis of single-institution archival tissue samples from 408 patients, CLDN18.2 positivity (defined similarly to the SPOTLIGHT and GLOW trial definitions as moderate-to-strong expression in $\geq$75% of tumor cells) was evenly distributed across various molecular (dMMR, Epstein-Barr virus–positive, HER2-positive and -negative) and histologic (diffuse or intestinal) subtypes.[29] In this study, there was significant overlap in tumors expressing both CLDN18.2 and PD-L1, with 41.9% in CLDN18.2-positive tumors having PD-L1 CPS greater than or equal to five.[29] When HER2-positive, Epstein-Barr virus–positive, and dMMR tumors were excluded from the latter analysis, only 20% of PD-L1 CPS greater than or equal to five tumors were also positive for CLDN18.2. In another single-institution study, coexpression between PD-L1 CPS greater than or equal to five and CLDN18.2 was seen in 30% of tumors.[20] These results indicate that there will be patients who qualify for treatments with either anti-PD1 or anti-CLDN antibodies, warranting studying combination of these agents in a biomarker-select patient population. Evaluation of zolbetuximab in combination with immunotherapy is further supported by the preclinical data demonstrating increased T-cell infiltration in CLDN18.2-positive tumors, suggesting that strategies that augment the immune response may have synergistic value with CLDN18.2-directed therapies.[30]

The ongoing multicohort phase 2 ILUSTRO trial is evaluating novel combinations with zolbetuximab, including anti-PD-L1 antibodies, given this significant biomarker overlap and strong preclinical rationale (NCT03505320). In one of the completed cohorts, the study enrolled heavily pretreated patients for treatment with zolbetuximab and pembrolizumab in the third-line setting.[31] Although anticancer activity of this combination was limited, the study did not reveal any new safety signals when an anti-PD-L1 agent and zolbetuximab were combined. Two new groups, 4A (designated as the safety cohort) and 4B, are scheduled to enroll approximately 12 and 50 patients, respectively. Their primary objective is to evaluate the safety and efficacy of the combination of zolbetuximab, mFOLFOX6, and nivolumab for G/GEJ adenocarcinomas in the first-line setting. These cohorts are specifically seeking patients whose tumors do not express HER2, but show notable levels of CLDN18.2 as indicated by moderate-to-strong IHC staining intensity in at least 75% of tumor cells (considered as high) or in at least 50% but less than 75% of tumor cells (considered as intermediate).[27] If clinically relevant signal is seen with this combination regimen, further evaluation in a randomized phase 3 trial would be warranted.

Claudin-directed bispecific antibodies

Bispecific antibodies harness the capabilities of mAbs with an additional therapeutic enhancement of targeting multiple epitopes or pathways.[32,33] The bulk of the bispecific CLDN18.2-directed antibodies either directly engage T cells or bind targets that have a potential to enhance intrinsic immune responses. Two of the most advanced bispecific antibodies fall into this later class, with CLDN18.2 × 4-1BB bispecific antibody (also known as Givastomig or ABL111) representing a prototypical molecule that binds to CLDN18.2, and 4-1BB, a surface marker present on activated T cells.[34] The therapeutic goal is to tether activated T cells in close proximity to CLDN18.2-expressing tumor cells, with the underlying concept being an ability to reengage activated T cells within the tumor microenvironment, without driving systemic immune-related toxicities. This agent is currently in phase 1 clinical trial (NCT04900818). PT886 is another bispecific antibody that targets CD47 in addition to CLDN18.2.[35] CD47 protein is frequently overexpressed on the tumor cell surface and it can inhibit phagocytosis by binding SIRPα on an immune cell. The dual targeting of these two cell surface proteins is thought to potentially better illuminate CLDN-expressing tumor cells to the immune system (ADCC), while also increasing capacity for clearance through negation of CD47 signaling.

Claudin-directed antibody drug conjugates

ADCs combine the specificity of an antibody therapeutic with a tethered chemotherapeutic payload to increase tumor-directed chemotherapy concentration, while limiting off-target toxicities.[36] Numerous CLDN18.2-directed ADCs are currently in development and in early phase clinical trials.[37] Early activity seen thus far is promising and warrants investigation in larger studies. For instance, phase 1 study with CMG901 ADC with monomethyl auristatin E demonstrated acceptable safety profile and an ORR of 75% in patients' gastric, GEJ, and pancreas adenocarcinomas with a median of two prior treatment lines.[38] A similar compound SYSA1801, also with monomethyl auristatin E payload, demonstrated an ORR of 47% among 17 patients with gastric cancer,[39] and further trials with this compound are now under investigation in the United States.

Claudin 18.2 chimeric antigen receptor T cells

This class of cellular therapy is defined by the artificial introduction of a CAR, which directly binds to and stimulates T-cell activation in response to CLDN18.2. CT041 is a second-generation CAR-T (CD28 costimulatory domain) that targets CLDN18.2.[40] In a phase 1 study, this agent demonstrated an overall favorable safety profile, with anticipated AEs related to preconditioning before CAR-T infusion, and low-grade cytokine release syndrome. Nearly all participants experienced grade 1 or grade 2 cytokine release syndrome, with no grade 3 events observed. Promising efficacy data were seen with ORR of 57.1% in heavily pretreated patient population. Although 6-month OS rate of 81.2% was clinically meaningful, duration of response was short at 6.4 months, given the complexity and expense of this treatment.[40] It is possible that better efficacy signals can be seen if CAR-T therapy is used in earlier lines of treatment and with further modifications of the CAR-T constructs.

Fibroblast Growth Factor Receptor–Directed Therapies

Fibroblast growth factor receptor 2 signaling

Fibroblast growth factor receptor 2 (FGFR2) is a receptor tyrosine kinase that is predominantly expressed in epithelial and mesenchymal tissues.[41–43] Activation of the receptor occurs after binding with ligand fibroblast growth factors leading to cross-phosphorylation and further cytosolic signaling.[44] On formation of the FGF-FGFR complex, several downstream signaling pathways are activated, including the Ras-dependent MAPK (RAS-MAPK) pathway, Ras-independent phosphoinositide 3-kinase (PI3K-Akt) pathway, PLCγ-Ca2+-PKC pathway, and Janus kinase-signal transducers and activators of transcription (JAK-STAT) pathway.[45] In normal cells, these pathways orchestrate critical cellular functions, such as proliferation, survival, and transformation. In cancer cells, FGFR2 signaling can become dysregulated. FGFR2b is one of the isoforms of FGFR2. It is primarily expressed in epithelial tissues and is involved in cell proliferation and tissue repair. *FGFR2* gene amplification is one of the most common gene aberrations in gastric cancer, which leads to FGFR2 over-expression and constitutive signaling of the FGFR pathway.[45]

Anti–fibroblast growth factor receptor 2b antibody: bemarituzumab

Bemarituzumab, formerly known as FPA144, is an mAb designed to target the extra-cellular domain of FGFR2b. It is a recombinant humanized IgG1 kappa mAb.[46,47] Bemarituzumab binds to the extracellular domain of FGFR2b, preventing the binding of its natural ligands. This inhibits the activation of FGFR2b and disrupts the down-stream signaling pathways involved in cell growth and survival.[46,48] Bemarituzumab has also been engineered to prevent fucosylation, which leads to the activation of FcγRIIIa (CD16a) and increased binding affinity for natural killer cells (NK) cells, enhancing their ability to recognize and destroy cancer cells expressing FGFR2b through ADCC.[49]

The FIGHT trial (NCT03694522) was a randomized, double-blind, placebo-controlled phase 2 study assessing the efficacy and safety of bemarituzumab in com-bination with mFOLFOX6 during first-line treatment of patients with FGFR2b-positive unresectable or metastatic G/GEJ.[50] The trial included patients whose tumors had FGFR2b overexpression determined by IHC and/or *FGFR2* amplification detected through plasma next-generation sequencing of cell-free circulating tumor DNA. Pos-itive FGFR2b overexpression by IHC was defined as moderate (2+) or strong (3+) membranous staining of more than 0% of tumor cells.

Of 910 patients assessed, 274 patients (30%) had a positive result for FGFR2b over-expression or *FGFR2* amplification. Most patients eligible for this study were selected based on FGFR2b overexpression (29% of screened patients), whereas only 4% of screened patients had *FGFR2* amplification on genetic testing. The trial initially was designed as a phase 3 study with a planned sample size of 540 patients, which was based on the assumption that most FGFR2b-positive tumors would have overexpres-sion of the FGFR2b protein and amplification of the *FGFR2* gene. During the study conduct it was found that patients predominantly had overexpression of FGFR2b without concurrent amplification of *FGFR2*. This finding prompted a pause in enroll-ment, and study design was updated to a phase 2 trial.

The primary end point of improved PFS was not reached in this study, although numerically patients in the bemarituzumab cohort had better PFS outcomes (9.5 vs 7.4 months; HR, 0.68; $P = .073$).[50] OS also favored the bemarituzumab group, with a median OS not reached in the bemarituzumab group versus 12.9 months in the placebo group at the time of the initial analysis with 10.9 months of median follow-up. During post hoc analysis with longer follow-up time of 12.5 months, me-dian OS in the bemarituzumab group was 19.2 months versus 13.5 months in the pla-cebo group (HR, 0.60).[50] Bemarituzumab treatment also resulted in higher ORR compared with placebo group (47% vs 33%) and longer duration of response (12.2 vs 7.1 months).

Importantly, the level of FGFR2b expression correlated with outcomes. Prespecified exploratory analyses were conducted on predefined subgroups of patients exhibiting FGFR2b overexpression in at least 5% of tumor cells and in at least 10% of tumor cells. OS in these cohorts was longer than in the control arm (25.4 vs 12.5 months and HR of 0.49 in tumors with at least 5% cells with FGFR2b overexpression; NR vs 11.1 months and HR of 0.41 in tumors with at least 10% of cells with FGFR2b overexpression).

Several drug-specific adverse effects were associated with the bemarituzumab treatment group, including stomatitis and corneal events. Corneal toxicities are of particular importance given that 20 (26%) patients in the bemarituzumab group discontinued treatment because of corneal AEs. Aggressive supportive measures and risk identification are warranted because this agent is undergoing further investigations in phase 3 trials. FORTITUDE-101 trial (NCT05052801) is a global phase 3 study exploring the use of bemarituzumab in combination with mFOLFOX6 in patients with FGFR2b-positive advanced G/GEJ adenocarcinoma. FORTITUDE-102 trial (NCT05111626) is a global phase 3 trial of bemarituzumab versus placebo in combination with mFOLFOX6 and nivolumab for patients with FGFR2b overexpression and unresectable advanced G/GEJ adenocarcinoma.

Fibroblast growth factor receptor tyrosine inhibitors

Several tyrosine kinase inhibitors (TKI) targeting FGFR have also been evaluated in patients with G/GEJ adenocarcinoma with aberrant FGFR2 signaling. Both selective and nonselective TKIs (those targeting multiple other receptor tyrosine kinases) have been assessed in this setting. Derazantinib, a competitive pan-FGFR inhibitor predominantly targeting FGFR1-3, is currently under investigation as second-line therapy alone or in combination with paclitaxel and ramucirumab, and/or atezolizumab, in G/GEJ adenocarcinoma with FGFR2 amplifications or translocations in three substudies of a phase I/II trial (NCT04604132). Futibatinib is an irreversible FGFR1-4 inhibitor being investigated in the second line for advanced G/GEJ cancers with FGFR2 amplifications in a phase 2 clinical trial where ORR is the primary end point (NCT04189445). Erdafitinib, a reversible pan-FGFR inhibitor being investigated in a phase 2 clinical trial examining ORR across multiple cancers including upper GI cancers with FGFR alterations (NCT02699606). If a signal of activity is seen in these early studies, further investigations in larger trials will be warranted. However, based on the low incidence of FGFR2 gene alterations in upper GI cancers, and molecular heterogeneity frequently observed, feasibility may pose challenges for the conduct of larger and randomized studies.

Dickkopf-1 Targeting

Dickkopf-1 signaling

Aberrancy within the Wnt/β-catenin cascade, which is an integral part of cellular proliferation and tissue homeostasis, has been described in a variety of cancer types, including G/GEJ adenocarcinoma.[51] Dickkopf-1 (DKK1) is a secreted protein that plays a crucial role in regulating the Wnt signaling pathway.[52–54] DKK1 functions as an inhibitor of the Wnt pathway by binding to and blocking the Wnt coreceptor LRP5/6, preventing the activation of the pathway. DKK1 has also been found to interact with cytoskeleton-associated protein 4 (CKAP4) on macrophage surfaces leading to downstream activation of PI3K-AKT signaling, modulation of tumor microenvironment, and dampening of immune response through myeloid-derived suppressor cells and downregulation of NK cells.[55–57] In cancer cells, DKK1 overexpression has been associated with aggressive tumor growth and worse clinical outcomes.[57]

The mechanisms underlying DKK1 dysregulation in cancer are not fully understood and can vary depending on the cancer type. Both genetic and epigenetic changes, such as gene amplification and promoter hypermethylation, can contribute to the overexpression of DKK1 in cancer cells. An emerging therapeutic strategy is aimed at DKK1 inhibition to promote antitumor response and improve immune-mediated surveillance.

DKN-01

DKN-01 is a humanized IgG4 mAb targeting DKK1. Preclinical data have shown DKN-01 to stimulate NK cells, downregulate Akt activity, and upregulate PD-L1 expression.[58] As a result, synergistic combination with checkpoint inhibitors is a promising treatment strategy that is being explored. One of the newer anti-PD-1 inhibitors, tislelizumab, has demonstrated encouraging antitumor activity in patients with G/GEJ adenocarcinoma in several studies.[59,60] It is structurally unique with decreased PD-1 and FC-gamma receptor (FcγR) interaction, which thereby decreases antibody-dependent macrophage-mediated destruction of effector T cells to overcome potential resistance.[61–63]

DisTinGuish is an ongoing phase 2a trial (NCT04363801) investigating DKN-01 in combination with tislelizumab with or without chemotherapy in the treatment of advanced G/GEJ adenocarcinoma. The study has multiple parts that enroll patients in different lines of treatment. Part A has now completed enrollment of 25 patients with HER2-negative tumors that have received no prior therapies in advanced setting.[64] Patients in this cohort received DKN-01, tislelizumab, and CAPOX. The primary efficacy end point of ORR was 73% in the modified intention-to-treat population (n = 22). Efficacy signals were explored in the prespecified subgroup analysis based on DKK1 mRNA levels. Tumoral DKK1 mRNA expression was evaluated by a chromogenic in situ hybridization RNAscope assay and assigned an H-score of 0 to 300 (high defined ≥35). Between DKK1-high (n = 10) and DKK1-low (n = 9) patients, the ORR was 90% and 67%, respectively. Durable responses were notably observed in patients with PD-L1-low (CPS <5) tumors. With follow-up time of 2 years, median OS was 19.5 months and median PFS was 11.3 months in the Part A cohort. Most treatment-related AEs were low-grade (76%) with the most frequent ones being fatigue, nausea, diarrhea. Six patients had serious DKN-01-related events, and one discontinued treatment because of DKN-01-related toxicity. With these promising results in Part A of the study, the ongoing Part C is a randomized phase 2 study evaluating DKN-01 in combination with tislelizumab and chemotherapy (CAPOX or mFOLFOX6) versus tislelizumab plus chemotherapy in patients with advanced GEA in the first-line setting (NCT04363801).[65] Part B evaluated the efficacy of DKN-01 and tislelizumab in 30 patients with high tumoral DKK1 expression in the second-line setting. Out of 26 evaluable patients, five (19%) achieved partial response.[66] Based on the ongoing DisTinGuish trial, high DKK1 expression was seen in 57% of treatment-naive patients and 33% of patients enrolled in second-line. This suggests that a significant portion of patients may qualify for DKK1-targeted therapies based on the positive biomarker status. Given early efficacy signals with DKN01 and favorable safety profile, there are ongoing efforts to further characterize DKK1 as a predictive biomarker and therapeutic target.

Epidermal Growth Factor Receptor–Directed Therapies

The overexpression of the epidermal growth factor receptor (EGFR) occurs in nearly 50% of patients, whereas approximately 6% exhibit EGFR gene amplification in GEA.[67,68] Increased EGFR expression in gastric cancer has been shown to correlate with worse prognosis.[69,70] Multiple trials to date (EXPAND, REAL3, and COG) have investigated the efficacy of EGFR inhibitors in unselected cohorts with disappointing results.[71-73] EXPAND study investigated the efficacy of cetuximab, an anti-EGFR antibody, in combination with chemotherapy for advanced G/GEJ cancer.[72] The study found that the addition of cetuximab to chemotherapy improved PFS, but did not significantly impact OS. In the REAL3 phase 3 trial, addition of panitumumab to the first-line systemic chemotherapy did not improve OS in unselect patient population.[71] In phase 3 COG trial, gefitinib (small molecule EGFR inhibitor) did not improve outcomes in late lines.[73] However, subsequent analyses suggest that patients with EGFR-amplified tumors may represent a unique cohort of patients with potential benefit from EGFR-directed therapy.[74,75] A retrospective, pooled analysis found that 43% of these patients were able to achieve an objective response when treated with EGFR-directed therapy alone or in combination with chemotherapy.[76] These results highlight the importance of appropriate selection of patients for the use of targeted therapies based on the biomarker characteristics of their tumors. Additional research efforts are warranted to further investigate EGFR-directed therapies, including bispecific antibodies and EGFR-targeted ADCs, and appropriately defined patient population to address intrinsic and acquired resistance patterns and tumor heterogeneity.

Multitarget Receptor Tyrosine Kinase Inhibitors

Several multitarget TKIs have been explored in the treatment of upper GI cancers. These types of agents lack kinase selectivity and target multiple signaling pathways, including VEGFR, KIT, FGFR, and RET. Recently, the activity of some of these agents have been investigated in randomized clinical trials. Regorafenib is an oral multitarget TKI that is actively being studied in this disease.[77] In the phase 3 INTEGRATE IIa study, regorafenib was compared with placebo in the third-line setting. Although statistically significant improvement in OS was observed, the median improvement of OS of less than 1 month may not be clinically relevant.[78] It is hoped that the ongoing INTEGRATE IIb study, which compares combination of regorafenib and nivolumab to investigator choice chemotherapy in a similar setting, will yield more positive results. Lenvatinib is another TKI under active investigation in this disease. Similar to regorafenib, lenvatinib in combination with immunotherapy demonstrated promising results in early phase studies.[79,80] The ongoing phase 3 LEAP-015 study is currently evaluating lenvatinib, pembrolizumab, and chemotherapy in the first-line setting (NCT04662710).

SUMMARY

There have been significant efforts to develop biomarker-based therapies for patients with upper GI cancers. Improved subclassification of these diseases and application of targeted therapies and immunotherapy when appropriate has resulted in significant survival gains for patients.

Currently, there are several biomarkers that have an established role in treatment selection. There are also several novel biomarkers and associated targeted agents that are under active investigation, with promising results in ongoing and completed clinical trials. CLDN18.2 has emerged as the newest biomarker with an established activity anti-CLDN18.2 antibody zolbetuximab in two phase 3 clinical trials. Several other targets (eg, as FGFR2b, DKK1) and associated therapeutic agents (bemarituzumab and DKN-01) are being evaluated in ongoing clinical trials. There exists a potential for overlap in biomarker expression within the same tumor. Moreover, variable expressions of these biomarkers may be seen across different metastatic sites and throughout the course of treatment. We have learned from HER2-positive upper GI cancers that tumor heterogeneity has been a challenge for precision oncology in these diseases. Nevertheless, it is exciting to see that management of patients with upper GI cancers is evolving and becoming more nuanced based on tumor unique characteristics. As clinicians start to incorporate novel targeted agents into practice, particular attention should be focused on safety profiles. Treatment-related toxicities will also be of paramount importance as clinicians start combining these agents in future studies. In summary, there are several promising targeted therapeutics in development for upper GI cancers. The advancement of future treatments should prioritize integration of the distinctive characteristics of each patient and their specific tumors to enhance overall outcomes.

FUNDING

Supported by University of Wisconsin, Carbone Cancer Center (P30 CA014520).

REFERENCES

1. Sung H, Ferlay J, Siegel RL, et al. Global cancer statistics 2020: GLOBOCAN Estimates of incidence and mortality worldwide for 36 cancers in 185 countries. CA Cancer J Clin 2021;71(3):209–49. https://doi.org/10.3322/caac.21660.

2. Kelly RJ, Ajani JA, Kuzdzal J, et al. Adjuvant nivolumab in resected esophageal or gastroesophageal junction cancer. N Engl J Med 2021;384(13):1191–203. https://doi.org/10.1056/NEJMoa2032125.

3. Al-Batran SE, Homann N, Pauligk C, et al. Perioperative chemotherapy with fluorouracil plus leucovorin, oxaliplatin, and docetaxel versus fluorouracil or capecitabine plus cisplatin and epirubicin for locally advanced, resectable gastric or gastro-oesophageal junction adenocarcinoma (FLOT4): a randomised, phase 2/3 trial. Lancet 2019;393(10184):1948–57. https://doi.org/10.1016/s0140-6736(18)32557-1.

4. Janjigian YY, Shitara K, Moehler M, et al. First-line nivolumab plus chemotherapy versus chemotherapy alone for advanced gastric, gastro-oesophageal junction, and oesophageal adenocarcinoma (CheckMate 649): a randomised, open-label, phase 3 trial. Lancet 2021. https://doi.org/10.1016/S0140-6736(21)00797-2.

5. Cancer Genome Atlas Research N. Comprehensive molecular characterization of gastric adenocarcinoma. Nature 2014;513(7517):202–9. https://doi.org/10.1038/nature13480.

6. Integrated genomic characterization of oesophageal carcinoma. Nature 2017;541(7636):169–75. https://doi.org/10.1038/nature20805.

7. Iqbal N, Iqbal N. Human epidermal growth factor receptor 2 (HER2) in cancers: overexpression and therapeutic implications. Molecular biology international 2014;2014:852748. https://doi.org/10.1155/2014/852748.

8. Bang YJ, Van Cutsem E, Feyereislova A, et al. Trastuzumab in combination with chemotherapy versus chemotherapy alone for treatment of HER2-positive advanced gastric or gastro-oesophageal junction cancer (ToGA): a phase 3, open-label, randomised controlled trial. Lancet 2010;376(9742):687–97. https://doi.org/10.1016/S0140-6736(10)61121-X.

9. Shitara K, Bang YJ, Iwasa S, et al. Trastuzumab deruxtecan in previously treated HER2-positive gastric cancer. N Engl J Med 2020;382(25):2419–30. https://doi.org/10.1056/NEJMoa2004413.

10. Janjigian YY, Shitara K, Moehler MH, et al. Nivolumab (NIVO) plus chemotherapy (chemo) vs chemo as first-line (1L) treatment for advanced gastric cancer/gastroesophageal junction cancer/esophageal adenocarcinoma (GC/GEJC/EAC): 3-year

follow-up from CheckMate 649. J Clin Oncol 2023;41(4_suppl):291. https://doi.org/10.1200/JCO.2023.41.4_suppl.291.

11. Patel MA, Kratz JD, Lubner SJ, et al. Esophagogastric cancers: integrating immunotherapy therapy into current practice. J Clin Oncol 2022;40(24):2751–62. https://doi.org/10.1200/jco.21.02500.

12. Shah MA, Kennedy EB, Alarcon-Rozas AE, et al. Immunotherapy and targeted therapy for advanced gastroesophageal cancer: ASCO Guideline. J Clin Oncol 2023;41(7):1470–91. https://doi.org/10.1200/jco.22.02331.

13. Hudler P. Genetic aspects of gastric cancer instability. TheScientificWorldJOURNAL 2012;2012:761909. https://doi.org/10.1100/2012/761909.

14. Lemery S, Keegan P, Pazdur R. First FDA approval agnostic of cancer site: when a biomarker defines the indication. N Engl J Med 2017;377(15):1409–12. https://doi.org/10.1056/NEJMp1709968.

15. Andre T, Tougeron D, Piessen G, et al. Neoadjuvant nivolumab plus ipilimumab and adjuvant nivolumab in patients (pts) with localized microsatellite instability-high (MSI)/mismatch repair deficient (dMMR) oeso-gastric adenocarcinoma (OGA): The GERCOR NEONIPIGA phase II study. J Clin Oncol 2022; 40(4_suppl):244. https://doi.org/10.1200/JCO.2022.40.4_suppl.244.

16. Sahin U, Koslowski M, Dhaene K, et al. Claudin-18 splice variant 2 is a pancancer target suitable for therapeutic antibody development. Clin Cancer Res 2008;14(23):7624–34. https://doi.org/10.1158/1078-0432.Ccr-08-1547.

17. Tabariès S, Siegel PM. The role of claudins in cancer metastasis. Oncogene 2017;36(9):1176–90. https://doi.org/10.1038/onc.2016.289.

18. Tsukita S, Furuse M, Itoh M. Multifunctional strands in tight junctions. Nat Rev Mol Cell Biol 2001;2(4):285–93. https://doi.org/10.1038/35067088.

19. Kyuno D, Takasawa A, Kikuchi S, et al. Role of tight junctions in the epithelial-to-mesenchymal transition of cancer cells. Biochim Biophys Acta Biomembr 2021; 1863(3):183503.

20. Pellino A, Brignola S, Riello E, et al. Association of CLDN18 protein expression with clinicopathological features and prognosis in advanced gastric and gastro-esophageal junction adenocarcinomas. J Personalized Med 2021;(11):11. https://doi.org/10.3390/jpm11111095.

21. Shitara K, Lordick F, Bang YJ, et al. Zolbetuximab plus mFOLFOX6 in patients with CLDN18.2-positive, HER2-negative, untreated, locally advanced unresectable or metastatic gastric or gastro-oesophageal junction adenocarcinoma (SPOTLIGHT): a multicentre, randomised, double-blind, phase 3 trial. Lancet 2023;401(10389):1655–68. https://doi.org/10.1016/S0140-6736(23)00620-7.

22. Kato K, Cho BC, Takahashi M, et al. Nivolumab versus chemotherapy in patients with advanced oesophageal squamous cell carcinoma refractory or intolerant to previous chemotherapy (ATTRACTION-3): a multicentre, randomised, open-label, phase 3 trial. Lancet Oncol 2019;20(11):1506–17. https://doi.org/10.1016/S1470-2045(19)30626-6.

23. Sahin U, Schuler M, Richly H, et al. A phase I dose-escalation study of IMAB362 (zolbetuximab) in patients with advanced gastric and gastro-oesophageal junction cancer. Eur J Cancer 2018;100:17–26.

24. Sahin U, Türeci Ö, Manikhas G, et al. FAST: a randomised phase II study of zolbetuximab (IMAB362) plus EOX versus EOX alone for first-line treatment of advanced CLDN18.2-positive gastric and gastro-oesophageal adenocarcinoma. Ann Oncol 2021;32(5):609–19. https://doi.org/10.1016/j.annonc.2021.02.005.

25. Türeci O, Sahin U, Schulze-Bergkamen H, et al. A multicentre, phase IIa study of zolbetuximab as a single agent in patients with recurrent or refractory advanced

adenocarcinoma of the stomach or lower oesophagus: the MONO study. Ann Oncol 2019;30(9):1487–95. https://doi.org/10.1093/annonc/mdz199.

26. Shah MA, Shitara K, Ajani JA, et al. Zolbetuximab plus CAPOX in CLDN18.2-positive gastric or gastroesophageal junction adenocarcinoma: the randomized, phase 3 GLOW trial. Nat Med 2023;29(8):2133–41. https://doi.org/10.1038/s41591-023-02465-7.

27. Shitara K, Yamaguchi K, Shoji H, et al. Phase 2 trial of zolbetuximab in combination with mFOLFOX6 and nivolumab in patients with advanced or metastatic claudin 18.2-positive, HER2-negative gastric or gastroesophageal junction adenocarcinomas. J Clin Oncol 2023;41(16_suppl):TPS4173. https://doi.org/10.1200/JCO.2023.41.16_suppl.TPS4173.

28. Zhao JJ, Yap DWT, Chan YH, et al. Low programmed death-ligand 1–expressing subgroup outcomes of first-line immune checkpoint inhibitors in gastric or esophageal adenocarcinoma. J Clin Oncol 2022. https://doi.org/10.1200/jco.21.01862. 0(0):JCO.21.01862.

29. Kubota Y, Kawazoe A, Mishima S, et al. Comprehensive clinical and molecular characterization of claudin 18.2 expression in advanced gastric or gastroesophageal junction cancer. ESMO Open 2023;8(1):100762. https://doi.org/10.1016/j.esmoop.2022.100762.

30. Jia K, Chen Y, Sun Y, et al. Multiplex immunohistochemistry defines the tumor immune microenvironment and immunotherapeutic outcome in CLDN18.2-positive gastric cancer. BMC Med 2022;20(1):223. https://doi.org/10.1186/s12916-022-02421-1.

31. Klempner SJ, Lee KW, Shitara K, et al. ILUSTRO: phase II multicohort trial of zolbetuximab in patients with advanced or metastatic claudin 18.2-positive gastric or gastroesophageal junction adenocarcinoma. Clin Cancer Res 2023;29(19): 3882–91. https://doi.org/10.1158/1078-0432.CCR-23-0204.

32. Labrijn AF, Janmaat ML, Reichert JM, et al. Bispecific antibodies: a mechanistic review of the pipeline. Nat Rev Drug Discov 2019;18(8):585–608. https://doi.org/10.1038/s41573-019-0028-1.

33. Liguori L, Polcaro G, Nigro A, et al. Bispecific antibodies: a novel approach for the treatment of solid tumors. Pharmaceutics 2022;14(11):2442.

34. Gao J, Wang Z, Jiang W, et al. CLDN18.2 and 4-1BB bispecific antibody givastomig exerts antitumor activity through CLDN18.2-expressing tumor-directed T-cell activation. Journal for ImmunoTherapy of Cancer 2023;11(6):e006704. https://doi.org/10.1136/jitc-2023-006704.

35. Overman MJ, Melhem R, Blum-Murphy MA, et al. A phase I, first-in-human, open-label, dose escalation and expansion study of PT886 in adult patients with advanced gastric, gastroesophageal junction, and pancreatic adenocarcinomas. J Clin Oncol 2023;41(4_suppl):TPS765. https://doi.org/10.1200/JCO.2023.41.4_suppl.TPS765.

36. Dumontet C, Reichert JM, Senter PD, et al. Antibody–drug conjugates come of age in oncology. Nat Rev Drug Discov 2023;22(8):641–61. https://doi.org/10.1038/s41573-023-00709-2.

37. Mullard A. Claudin-18.2 attracts the cancer crowd. Nat Rev Drug Discov 2023; 22(9):683–6. https://doi.org/10.1038/d41573-023-00120-x.

38. Xu R-h, Wei X, Zhang D, et al. A phase 1a dose-escalation, multicenter trial of anti-claudin 18.2 antibody drug conjugate CMG901 in patients with resistant/refractory solid tumors. J Clin Oncol 2023;41(4_suppl):352. https://doi.org/10.1200/JCO.2023.41.4_suppl.352.

39. Wang Y, Gong J, Lin R, et al. First-in-human dose escalation and expansion study of SYSA1801, an antibody-drug conjugate targeting claudin 18.2 in patients with resistant/refractory solid tumors. J Clin Oncol 2023;41(16_suppl):3016. https://doi.org/10.1200/JCO.2023.41.16_suppl.3016.

40. Qi C, Gong J, Li J, et al. Claudin18.2-specific CAR T cells in gastrointestinal cancers: phase 1 trial interim results. Nat Med 2022;28(6):1189–98. https://doi.org/10.1038/s41591-022-01800-8.

41. Peters KG, Werner S, Chen G, et al. Two FGF receptor genes are differentially expressed in epithelial and mesenchymal tissues during limb formation and organogenesis in the mouse. Development 1992;114(1):233–43. https://doi.org/10.1242/dev.114.1.233.

42. Orr-Urtreger A, Bedford MT, Burakova T, et al. Developmental localization of the splicing alternatives of fibroblast growth factor receptor-2 (FGFR2). Dev Biol 1993;158(2):475–86. https://doi.org/10.1006/dbio.1993.1205.

43. Eswarakumar VP, Monsonego-Ornan E, Pines M, et al. The IIIc alternative of Fgfr2 is a positive regulator of bone formation. Development 2002;129(16):3783–93. https://doi.org/10.1242/dev.129.16.3783.

44. Ghedini GC, Ronca R, Presta M, et al. Future applications of FGF/FGFR inhibitors in cancer. Expert Rev Anticancer Ther 2018;18(9):861–72. https://doi.org/10.1080/14737140.2018.1491795.

45. Turner N, Grose R. Fibroblast growth factor signalling: from development to cancer. Nature reviews Cancer 2010;10(2):116–29. https://doi.org/10.1038/nrc2780.

46. Gemo AT, Deshpande AM, Palencia S, et al. FPA144: a therapeutic antibody for treating patients with gastric cancers bearing FGFR2 gene amplification. Cancer Res 2014;74(19_Supplement):5446.

47. Catenacci DVT, Rasco D, Lee J, et al. Phase I escalation and expansion study of bemarituzumab (FPA144) in patients with advanced solid tumors and FGFR2b-selected gastroesophageal adenocarcinoma. J Clin Oncol 20 2020;38(21):2418–26. https://doi.org/10.1200/jco.19.01834.

48. Powers J, Palencia S, Foy S, et al. Abstract 1407: FPA144, a therapeutic monoclonal antibody targeting the FGFR2b receptor, promotes antibody dependent cell-mediated cytotoxicity and stimulates sensitivity to PD-1 in the 4T1 syngeneic tumor model. Cancer Res 2016;76:1407. https://doi.org/10.1158/1538-7445.AM2016-1407.

49. Xiang H, Chan AG, Ahene A, et al. Preclinical characterization of bemarituzumab, an anti-FGFR2b antibody for the treatment of cancer. mAbs 2021;13(1):1981202. https://doi.org/10.1080/19420862.2021.1981202.

50. Wainberg ZA, Enzinger PC, Kang YK, et al. Bemarituzumab in patients with FGFR2b-selected gastric or gastro-oesophageal junction adenocarcinoma (FIGHT): a randomised, double-blind, placebo-controlled, phase 2 study. Lancet Oncol 2022;23(11):1430–40. https://doi.org/10.1016/S1470-2045(22)00603-9.

51. Kagey MH, He X. Rationale for targeting the Wnt signalling modulator Dickkopf-1 for oncology. Br J Pharmacol 2017;174(24):4637–50. https://doi.org/10.1111/bph.13894.

52. Logan CY, Nusse R. The Wnt signaling pathway in development and disease. Annu Rev Cell Dev Biol 2004;20:781–810. https://doi.org/10.1146/annurev.cellbio.20.010403.113126.

53. Clevers H, Nusse R. Wnt/β-catenin signaling and disease. Cell 2012;149(6):1192–205. https://doi.org/10.1016/j.cell.2012.05.012.

54. Sedgwick AE, D'Souza-Schorey C. Wnt signaling in cell motility and invasion: drawing parallels between development and cancer. Cancers 2016;8(9). https://doi.org/10.3390/cancers8090080.

55. Wang S, Zhang S. Dickkopf-1 is frequently overexpressed in ovarian serous carcinoma and involved in tumor invasion. Clin Exp Metastasis 2011;28(6):581–91. https://doi.org/10.1007/s10585-011-9393-9.

56. Kimura H, Fumoto K, Shojima K, et al. CKAP4 is a Dickkopf1 receptor and is involved in tumor progression. J Clin Invest 2016;126(7):2689–705. https://doi.org/10.1172/jci84658.

57. Shi T, Zhang Y, Wang Y, et al. DKK1 promotes tumor immune evasion and impedes anti-PD-1 treatment by inducing immunosuppressive macrophages in gastric cancer. Cancer Immunol Res 2022;10(12):1506–24. https://doi.org/10.1158/2326-6066.Cir-22-0218.

58. Haas MS, Kagey MH, Heath H, et al. mDKN-01, a novel anti-DKK1 mAb, enhances innate immune responses in the tumor microenvironment. Mol Cancer Res 2021;19(4):717–25. https://doi.org/10.1158/1541-7786.Mcr-20-0799.

59. Moehler MH, Kato K, Arkenau H-T, et al. Rationale 305: phase 3 study of tislelizumab plus chemotherapy vs placebo plus chemotherapy as first-line treatment (1L) of advanced gastric or gastroesophageal junction adenocarcinoma (GC/GEJC). J Clin Oncol 2023;41(4_suppl):286. https://doi.org/10.1200/JCO.2023.41.4_suppl.286.

60. Xu J, Bai Y, Xu N, et al. Tislelizumab plus chemotherapy as first-line treatment for advanced esophageal squamous cell carcinoma and gastric/gastroesophageal junction adenocarcinoma. Clin Cancer Res 2020;26(17):4542–50. https://doi.org/10.1158/1078-0432.Ccr-19-3561.

61. Zhang T, Song X, Xu L, et al. The binding of an anti-PD-1 antibody to FcγRI has a profound impact on its biological functions. Cancer Immunol Immunother 2018;67(7):1079–90. https://doi.org/10.1007/s00262-018-2160-x.

62. Gül N, van Egmond M. Antibody-dependent phagocytosis of tumor cells by macrophages: a potent effector mechanism of monoclonal antibody therapy of cancer. Cancer Res 2015;75(23):5008–13. https://doi.org/10.1158/0008-5472.Can-15-1330.

63. Dahan R, Sega E, Engelhardt J, et al. FcγRs modulate the anti-tumor activity of antibodies targeting the PD-1/PD-L1 axis. Cancer Cell 2015;28(3):285–95. https://doi.org/10.1016/j.ccell.2015.08.004.

64. Klempner SJ, Sonbol BB, Wainberg ZA, et al. A phase 2 study (DisTinGuish) of DKN-01 in combination with tislelizumab + chemotherapy as first-line (1L) therapy in patients with advanced gastric or GEJ adenocarcinoma (GEA). J Clin Oncol 2023;41(16_suppl):4027. https://doi.org/10.1200/JCO.2023.41.16_suppl.4027.

65. Lee K-W, Moehler MH, Cunningham D, et al. Trial in progress: a phase 2, multicenter, open-label study of DKN-01 in combination with tislelizumab and chemotherapy as 1L therapy in patients with unresectable, locally advanced or metastatic gastric or gastroesophageal junction adenocarcinoma (G/GEJ; DisTinGuish). J Clin Oncol 2023;41(4_suppl):TPS484. https://doi.org/10.1200/JCO.2023.41.4_suppl.TPS484.

66. Klempner SJ, Chao J, Uronis HE, et al. DKN-01 and tislelizumab ± chemotherapy as a first-line (1L) and second-line (2L) investigational therapy in advanced gastroesophageal adenocarcinoma (GEA): DisTinGuish Trial. J Clin Oncol 2022;40(4_suppl):292. https://doi.org/10.1200/JCO.2022.40.4_suppl.292.

67. Nagatsuma AK, Aizawa M, Kuwata T, et al. Expression profiles of HER2, EGFR, MET and FGFR2 in a large cohort of patients with gastric adenocarcinoma. Gastric Cancer 2015;18(2):227–38. https://doi.org/10.1007/s10120-014-0360-4.

68. Maron SB, Alpert L, Kwak HA, et al. Targeted therapies for targeted populations: anti-EGFR treatment for EGFR-amplified gastroesophageal adenocarcinoma. Cancer Discov 2018;8(6):696–713. https://doi.org/10.1158/2159-8290.Cd-17-1260.

69. Wang KL, Wu TT, Choi IS, et al. Expression of epidermal growth factor receptor in esophageal and esophagogastric junction adenocarcinomas: association with poor outcome. Cancer 2007;109(4):658–67. https://doi.org/10.1002/cncr.22445.

70. Galizia G, Lieto E, Orditura M, et al. Epidermal growth factor receptor (EGFR) expression is associated with a worse prognosis in gastric cancer patients undergoing curative surgery. World J Surg 2007;31(7):1458–68. https://doi.org/10.1007/s00268-007-9016-4.

71. Waddell T, Chau I, Cunningham D, et al. Epirubicin, oxaliplatin, and capecitabine with or without panitumumab for patients with previously untreated advanced oesophagogastric cancer (REAL3): a randomised, open-label phase 3 trial. Lancet Oncol 2013;14(6):481–9. https://doi.org/10.1016/s1470-2045(13)70096-2.

72. Lordick F, Kang YK, Chung HC, et al. Capecitabine and cisplatin with or without cetuximab for patients with previously untreated advanced gastric cancer (EXPAND): a randomised, open-label phase 3 trial. Lancet Oncol 2013;14(6):490–9. https://doi.org/10.1016/s1470-2045(13)70102-5.

73. Dutton SJ, Ferry DR, Blazeby JM, et al. Gefitinib for oesophageal cancer progressing after chemotherapy (COG): a phase 3, multicentre, double-blind, placebo-controlled randomised trial. Lancet Oncol 2014;15(8):894–904. https://doi.org/10.1016/s1470-2045(14)70024-5.

74. Lordick F, Kang Y-K, Salman P, et al. Clinical outcome according to tumor HER2 status and EGFR expression in advanced gastric cancer patients from the EXPAND study. J Clin Oncol 2013;31(15_suppl):4021.

75. Smyth EC, Vlachogiannis G, Hedayat S, et al. EGFR amplification and outcome in a randomised phase III trial of chemotherapy alone or chemotherapy plus panitumumab for advanced gastro-oesophageal cancers. Gut 2021;70(9):1632–41. https://doi.org/10.1136/gutjnl-2020-322658.

76. Maron SB, Moya S, Morano F, et al. Epidermal growth factor receptor inhibition in epidermal growth factor receptor-amplified gastroesophageal cancer: retrospective global experience. J Clin Oncol 2022;40(22):2458–67. https://doi.org/10.1200/jco.21.02453.

77. Lam LL, Pavlakis N, Shitara K, et al. INTEGRATE II: randomised phase III controlled trials of regorafenib containing regimens versus standard of care in refractory advanced gastro-oesophageal cancer (AGOC): a study by the Australasian Gastro-Intestinal Trials Group (AGITG). BMC Cancer 2023;23(1):180. https://doi.org/10.1186/s12885-023-10642-7.

78. Pavlakis N, Shitara K, Sjoquist KM, et al. INTEGRATE IIa: a randomised, double-blind, phase III study of regorafenib versus placebo in refractory advanced gastro-oesophageal cancer (AGOC)—A study led by the Australasian Gastro-intestinal Trials Group (AGITG). J Clin Oncol 2023;41(4_suppl): LBA294.

79. Kawazoe A, Fukuoka S, Nakamura Y, et al. Lenvatinib plus pembrolizumab in patients with advanced gastric cancer in the first-line or second-line setting

(EPOC1706): an open-label, single-arm, phase 2 trial. Lancet Oncol 2020;21(8): 1057–65. https://doi.org/10.1016/s1470-2045(20)30271-0.

80. Fukuoka S, Hara H, Takahashi N, et al. Regorafenib plus nivolumab in patients with advanced gastric or colorectal cancer: an open-label, dose-escalation, and dose-expansion phase Ib Trial (REGONIVO, EPOC1603). J Clin Oncol 2020;38(18):2053–61. https://doi.org/10.1200/jco.19.03296.

Upper Gastrointestinal Cancers and the Role of Genetic Testing

Emily C. Harrold, MB BCh, BAO, MRCPI[a,b], Zsofia K. Stadler, MD[a],*

KEYWORDS

- Germline pathogenic variants • Upper gastrointestinal cancer • Gastric cancer
- Pancreatic cancer • Esophageal cancer • Genetic testing

KEY POINTS

- There are currently well-defined criteria for germline genetic testing in the setting of gastric and pancreatic cancer whereas these criteria are in evolution for esophageal and esophagogastric junction tumors beyond a limited number of well-defined genetic syndromes.
- Identification of novel associations is likely with expansion of access to germline genetic testing and the use of multi-gene panel testing.
- Germline variants in the homologous recombination deficiency (HRD) genes (*BRCA1/2, ATM, PALB2*) are increasingly being identified across a broad spectrum of tumor types beyond breast and ovarian cancer with potential therapeutic implications.
- Somatic-germline integration will be critical to determine relative causality of a particular germline pathogenic variant (gPV) to upper gastrointestinal carcinogenesis.

UPPER GASTROINTESTINAL CANCERS AND THE ROLE OF GENETIC TESTING

Evaluating the contribution of germline pathogenic variants (gPV) to the risk of any cancer is critical both for the appropriate estimation of lifetime cancer risks and potential preventative interventions but also increasingly due to potential therapeutic actionability.[1] Herein the authors will address the historical model of genetic testing and reflect on the limitations of this model,[2] define the most common high-risk genetic predisposition syndromes implicated in upper gastrointestinal carcinogenesis, and describe how germline genetic testing should be considered integral to the delivery of high-quality oncological care to both patients and their at-risk relatives.

The classic models of genetic testing for cancer are historically predicated on 3 basic factors: patient age at diagnosis with early-onset cancer conventionally being

[a] Department of Medicine, Memorial Sloan Kettering Cancer Center, New York, NY, USA;
[b] Department of Medical Oncology, Mater Misericordiae University Hospital, Dublin, Ireland
* Corresponding author.
E-mail address: stadlerz@mskcc.org
Twitter: @EmilyHarrold6 (E.C.H.); @StadlerZsofia (Z.K.S.)

Hematol Oncol Clin N Am 38 (2024) 677–691
https://doi.org/10.1016/j.hoc.2024.01.006
0889-8588/24/© 2024 Elsevier Inc. All rights reserved.
hemonc.theclinics.com

defined as cancer between 18 to 49 years, rarity of tumor type, and/or family cancer history. The aim of this approach is to identify those with the highest pre-test probability of having a gPV, while reducing the likelihood of obtaining uncertain results with limited clinical utility (eg, Variant of Uncertain Significance, VUS). This approach is centered on assessment as to whether a patient meets the "clinical criteria" for genetic testing. These criteria may be established by national guidelines specific to a particular cancer type, such as the National Comprehensive Cancer Network(NCCN) for Gastric Cancer,[3] or syndrome-specific criteria, such as the Amsterdam Criteria and Bethesda Guidelines[4,5] for assessment of and tumor screening for Lynch Syndrome (LS). While these criteria typically capture those at *highest* risk for having a gPV, over the last several years, an increasing amount of data has demonstrated that a significant portion of patients with gPVs in high penetrance cancer risk genes, such as the mismatch repair (MMR) genes diagnostic of LS, are missed through such stringent criteria. In a large cohort of patients with microsatellite instability (MSI) tumors, of those patients with LS presenting with cancers other than the canonical cancers (colorectal or endometrial cancers), only half met clinical testing criteria based on personal and/or family cancer history,[6] highlighting that relying on this "classic"testing model misses nearly half of LS diagnoses. Importantly, this is not unique to LS, as multiple studies have demonstrated a significant incremental pick-up rate for gPV in cancer susceptibility genes when classic testing criteria are relaxed.[7–9]

Gastric Cancer

Approximately 1% to 3% of gastric cancers are associated with gPVs[10] and genetically driven tumors are more common amongst patients with early onset disease. The most common syndrome is Hereditary Diffuse Gastric Cancer, associated with mutations in the *CDH1* [11–13] and more recently implicated *CTNNA1*[14] genes. Histologically this type of gastric cancer is characterized by multifocal diffuse spread with signet rings in the gastric mucosa. It is also associated with invasive lobular breast cancer when it arises in the context of a *gCDH1* mutation.

Hereditary Diffuse Gastric Cancer

Hereditary diffuse gastric cancer (HDGC) accounts for approximately 1% of diffuse gastric cancer[15] and in 46% to 48% of these patients an e cadherin (*CDH1*) germline mutation is detectable.[15,16] *CDH1* is a tumor suppressor gene that encodes the for E-cadherin protein, an integral component of the adherens junctional complex in epithelial cells. This complex is implicated in cell-cell adhesion, invasion suppression, and signal transduction.[17] The description of a clear molecular basis for hereditary diffuse gastric cancer was first reported in 3 Maori kindred[13] with early onset diffuse type gastric cancer in the presence of germline inactivating e-cadherin/*CDH1* mutations. This was subsequently corroborated by a study of British and Irish familial gastric cancer kindreds[18] and in 3 European gastric cancer kindreds.[19] By 1999, 9 different germline *CDH1* mutations had been identified in European familial gastric cancer kindreds[18–20] and 14 had been described overall. A total of 80% of these carriers generate premature termination codons which ultimately result in impaired transcript loss and subsequent early onset gastric cancer.[21] These e-cadherin mutations in HDGC can occur throughout the *CDH1* gene[22] whereas in sporadic diffuse gastric cancer the mutations are observed in exons 7 to 9 of the gene.[23] In sporadic gastric cancer, truncating mutations are uncommon and sequence changes usually result in either missense mutations or exon skipping.[24] A further 13 novel mutations in *CDH1* were described in 2004[15] and a further 6 in 2007.[25]

The cumulative risk of developing gastric cancer in a patient with gPV in *CDH1* is approximately 37% to 64% in men and 24% to 47% in women.[18,26] The risk of breast cancer is approximately 39% to 55%[11,12,26,27] and the estimated combined risk of breast and gastric cancer by 75 is 78%.[12]

In 2010, recommendations for *CDH1* testing by the International Gastric Cancer Consortium[28] identified 4 criteria for *CDH1* testing: (I) Two family members with gastric carcinoma, 1 of which is confirmed diffuse gastric cancer; (II) 3 family members with gastric carcinoma in first-degree or second-degree relatives including 1 with diffuse gastric cancer; (III) One member with diffuse gastric cancer before the age of 40; (IV) Personal or family history of diffuse gastric cancer and lobular breast cancer including 1 diagnosed before 50. This was further refined in 2015[29] to recommend testing if (I) 2 gastric cancer cases in family members regardless of age, at least 1 confirmed to be diffuse gastric cancer, (II) One case of Diffuse Gastric Cancer <40, or (III) Personal or family history of Diffuse gastric cancer or Lobular breast cancer, 1 diagnosed <50. Patients and families in whom testing can be considered include those with bilateral lobular breast cancer or family history of 2 or more cases of lobular breast cancer at least 1 <50, a personal or family history of cleft palate in a patient with diffuse gastric cancer, or in situ signet ring cells and/or pagetoid spread of signet ring cells.

A confirmed gPV in *CDH1* should prompt prophylactic gastrectomy with large series demonstrating a high rate of signet ring cancers found in patients undergoing prophylactic risk-reducing surgeries.[30] Recent data, based on individuals with *CDH1* gPVs who declined surgical intervention, provocatively suggested endoscopic screening (Cambridge protocol) in dedicated centers with appropriate expertise may be an alternative to prophylactic surgery.[31] However, at the present time, this is not considered international best practice.

CTNNA1

Approximately 40% of hereditary diffuse gastric cancer was noted in families negative for CDH1 gPVs.[12] Beyond *CDH1* gPVs, hereditary diffuse gastric cancer can also be seen in the setting of truncating mutations in the *CTNNA1* (α catenin) gene inferring a genocopy of *CDH1*[12,32] although this represents a minority of diffuse gastric cancer families.[11] *CTNNA1* encodes for α catenin which partners with the e-cadherin protein in the adherens junctional complex. *CTNNA1* has only recently been classified as an HDGC predisposing gene due to the identification of loss of function variants in families fitting clinical criteria for hereditary diffuse gastric cancer.[31] Current guidelines now recommend similar surveillance (Cambridge protocol) for patients with confirmed truncating mutation in *CTNNA1* and prophylactic gastrectomy can be considered regardless of endoscopy findings. The clinical spectrum and age range of *CTNNA1* gPV carriers is less clearly characterized than CDH1 gPV carriers. Early onset diffuse gastric cancer is a frequently associated phenotype[14]; however, pathogenic *CTNNA1* variants are not associated with lobular breast cancer.

Gastric Adenocarcinoma and Proximal Polyposis of the Stomach

Additionally, an autosomal dominant syndrome has been identified characterized by gastric adenocarcinoma and proximal polyposis of the stomach (GAPPS) without duodenal or colonic involvement in most individuals reported.[33,34] GAPPS arises in the context of *APC* promoter 1B mutations (c.-191T > C, c.-192A > G, and c.-195A > C) which reduce the binding activity of the transcription factor Yin Yang 1 (YY1) and transcriptional activity of the promoter.[35] The key clinical features of GAPPS are proximal gastric polyposis with hyperplastic and adenomatous polyps with antral sparing; the malignant transformation potential of these polyps is also noted to be higher than in familial adenomatous polyposis (FAP). GAPPS is typically associated with intestinal type adenocarcinoma. In one of the most comprehensive overviews of 3 families[33] with this syndrome, the gastric phenotype was apparent from the age of 10 and the first gastric cancer occurred at age 38. It is not yet clear whether prophylactic gastrectomy should be considered in patients with GAPPS.

Lynch Syndrome

Lynch syndrome, caused by gPVs in *MLH1, MSH2, MSH6, PMS2*, and terminal deletions in *EPCAM*[36] is one of the most common cancer predisposition syndromes with a prevalence of approximately 1 in 279 people. It is characterized by a high proportion of tumors with MSI or deficient MMR on immunohistochemistry with protein loss reflective of the underlying germline variant. Furthermore, MSI-associated Lynch syndrome cancers should prompt reflexive germline genetic testing. A 2019 publication reported that among over 15,000 patients representing a pan-cancer cohort of MSI tumors (>50 cancer types), LS was identified in approximately 16% of the cases.[37] Early onset gastric cancer (non-diffuse type) may occur in the setting of Lynch syndrome. Cumulative incidences at 75 years (risks) for upper gastrointestinal (gastric, duodenal, bile duct, or pancreatic) cancers were 10%, 17%, and 13% in path_MLH1, path_MSH2, and path_MSH6 carriers, respectively, per the Prospective Lynch syndrome registry.[38] The identification of MSI gastric cancer may have important implication for treatment with immune checkpoint blockade in both the locally advanced and the metastatic disease settings,[39,40] as well as the need for on-going high-risk surveillance even in immunotherapy-treated Lynch syndrome patients.[41]

Li Fraumeni

Li Fraumeni is an autosomal dominant syndrome caused by pathogenic variants in *TP53*. LFS confers an 80% to 90% lifetime risk of cancer with up to 21% of cancers occurring before age 15[42] Classical Li Fraumeni-associated cancers include sarcoma, brain tumors, leukemia, breast cancer, and adrenocortical tumors; however, increasingly early onset gastric cancer has been recognized as a component of the syndrome[43] and endoscopic surveillance is considered an important component of comprehensive Li Fraumeni surveillance.[44]

Familial Adenomatous Polyposis Syndrome

Familial adenomatous polyposis (FAP) is caused by gPVs in *APC*.[36,45,46] Whilst the risk of colorectal cancer is very clearly defined and underpins the recommendation for prophylactic colectomy when *gAPC* is confirmed,[47] the risk of gastric cancer appears more modest[48] particularly amongst Western carriers of *gAPC* variants.

Peutz Jeghers

Peutz–Jeghers is an autosomal dominant condition distinguished by hamartomatous polyps in the gastrointestinal tract and pigmented mucocutaneous lesions. It is by caused by gPVs in *STK11*[49,50] and confers an increased risk of gastrointestinal, pancreatic, lung, breast, uterine, and testicular cancers.

Juvenile Polyposis Syndrome

Juvenile polyposis syndrome is caused by gPVs in *SMAD4* or *BMPR1A*.[51,52] It is also an autosomal dominant syndrome characterized by distinct polyps throughout the gastrointestinal tract both upper and lower. Gastric cancer risk appears to be greatest with gPV in *SMAD4*[53] with a rare but important phenotypic variant presenting with massive gastric polyposis and often very early onset gastric cancer.[54]

Importantly, many of the aforementioned syndromes have classic, well-described phenotypic presentations, allowing for better estimations of pre-test probability of a true-positive result in such cases.

Homologous Recombination DNA Repair Pathway

Mutations in the homologous recombination DNA (HRD) pathway are thought to account for a significant proportion of families with diffuse gastric cancer in the absence of *CDH1* or *CTNNA1* gPVs. Fewings and colleagues[55] performed whole exome sequencing in 22 families who had previously tested negative for *CDH1*. *PALB2* loss of function variants were significantly more common than in the general population. However, *PALB2* germline variants have also been identified amongst patients [56] with non-diffuse histology suggesting potential association with heterogenous histologic subtypes.[57]

Deleterious mutations in *ATM* have been found at a significantly higher frequency amongst patients with gastric cancer from diverse ethnic backgrounds [58]; this is further corroborated by genome-wide association studies.[58,59] Gastric cancers arising in patients with *gATM* may potentially be susceptible to targeted approaches.[60]

The association with *BRCA1/2* with gastric cancer risk has been considered an issue of debate for some time. In a large cohort of over 5000 *BRCA* families, the relative risk of gastric cancer was increased in both *BRCA1* and *BRCA2* carriers, 2.17 (95% CI 1.25–3.77)-fold and 3.69 (95% CI 2.4–5.67)-fold, respectively.[61] This association appears to be stronger with *BRCA2* than with *BRCA1*.[62–65] Additionally, risk appears to potentially be modified by the presence of *Helicobacter pylori*.[66] At the present time, these data are not robust enough to recommend routine surveillance gastroscopy in all carriers of gPVs in *BRCA* but it would not be unreasonable in the setting of both gPVs and a family history of gastric cancer.[67] Arguably these current data would suggest that screening patients with gPV in *BRCA* at baseline for the presence of *Helicobacter pylori* should be considered.

Similar to data from other cancer types with increasing access to multigene panel testing (MGPT), gPVs potentially implicated in gastric cancer will be identified even in patients without a family history.[68]

Esophageal Cancer

Per the most recent NCCN guidelines (Version 3, 2023), specific referral guidelines for esophageal and esophagogastric junction (EGJ) cancers from the perspective of genetic risk assessment are not yet possible at this time. In contrast to gastric cancer, there are a relatively limited number of defined genetic syndromes recognized to be associated with an increased risk of esophageal cancer.

Esophageal Cancer, Tylosis with Non-epidermolytic Palmoplantar Keratoderma (PPK), and Howel–Evans Syndrome

Tylosis with esophageal cancer (TEC) is a very rare condition with an autosomal dominant pattern of inheritance and is caused by germline mutations in the *RHBDF2* gene. Individuals with germline RHBDF2 mutations have an increased risk for squamous cell carcinoma (SCC) of the middle and distal esophagus. Palmoplantar keratoderma (PPK) is divided into diffuse, punctate, or focal patterns of skin thickening on palms and soles. The risk of esophageal carcinoma has been calculated to be 95% by 65 years of age in 1 large family but the frequency of the disorder in the general population is unknown.[69]

Bloom Syndrome

Bloom syndrome (BS) is a rare autosomal recessive disorder characterized by mutations of the *BLM* gene at 15q26.1[70] and is associated with strikingly elevated sister chromatid exchange rates in all cells. Patients with BS are affected by acute myeloid leukemia, acute lymphoblastic leukemia, or lymphoid neoplasms at an early age and one-third of patients with BS have multiple independent malignancies.[71] Patients with BS appear to have 150 to 300 times greater risk of cancer development than those without this disorder[72] including SCC of the esophagus after 20 years of age.

Fanconi Anemias

The genes involved in Fanconi anemia (FA) include FA complementation groups A–E, with FA-A (FANCA) located at 16q24.3; FA-B (FANCB), unknown; FA-C (FANCC) at 9q22.3; FA-D (FANCD) at 3p26–p22; and FA-E (FANCE), unknown. Patients with germline variants *FANCA* and *FANCC* are affected by pancytopenia and chromosome breakage and hematologic abnormalities, including anemia, bleeding, and easy bruising. An increased frequency of SCC of the esophagus has been described in these patients.[73]

Familial Barrett esophagus

Familial Barrett esophagus[74] (FBE) includes adenocarcinoma of the esophagus and EGJ. Inheritance appears to be autosomal dominant and several potential candidate genes have been identified but causality has not been clearly validated.

Two more contemporary studies[75,76] have raised the question of the contribution of gPVs in ATM to esophageal adenocarcinoma risk, a potential association that will require further evaluation.

Gastroesophageal Junction Cancer

Gastroesophageal Junction (GEJ) cancers are unique in that these tumors are thought to reflect a mix of true GEJ tumors as well as proximal gastric and distal esophageal cancers, which may be clinically indistinguishable. Indeed, The Tumor Genome Atlas analysis of esophageal cancers found a gradual transition of molecular subtypes from the distal esophagus to the GEJ and then to the proximal stomach.[77] In line with this observation, in studies utilizing MGPT, the prevalence of gPV in GEJ cancers was higher than in esophageal but lower than in gastric cancers.[78] Given the difficulty in accurately classifying the origin of any GEJ cancer, following guidelines for gastric cancer genetic testing recommendation are probably a reasonable recommendation.

Pancreatic Cancer

The contribution of pPVs, particularly those in the HRD pathway, is increasingly being recognized in pancreatic cancer. In a pan cancer analysis of approximately 12,000 patients, 19.6% of the patients with pancreatic ductal adenocarcinoma (PDAC) were found to harbor pathogenic germline variants.[1] The likelihood of a positive genetic test appears higher amongst patients with early onset disease; in a cohort of 450 early onset pancreatic cancer patients diagnosed between 2008 to 2018 at a large academic institution,[79] approximately 32% were found to harbor at least 1 gPV, with 27.5% of gPVs identified in high and moderate penetrance genes.[79] This is corroborated by a large study from another US tertiary center which demonstrated that patients with early onset (EO) pancreatic cancer had a significantly higher odds of testing positive than older patients for germline mutations (OR 1.93; 95% CI 1.03–3.7), although the definition of early onset pancreatic cancer for the purposes of this study was defined as aged <60.[80] Of particular concern is that, the incidence in patients <50 years of age appears to be rising.[81–83] Understanding the contribution of gPV to this rising incidence is important particularly as the efficacy of pancreatic cancer screening amongst carriers of implicated gPVs is increasingly being corroborated.[84]

The HRD genes most commonly implicated in pancreatic cancer are *BRCA2* (5%–10%),[85,86] PALB2 (2%–3%),[87,88] ATM(3%–4%),[89,90] and BRCA1 (1%).[91] The initial studies from the Breast Cancer Linkage Consortium valuating contribution of BRCA1/2 to breast cancer risk[92,93] also suggested an association between *BRCA1* and *BRCA2* mutations and prostate and pancreatic adenocarcinomas as well (particularly for *BRCA2*), and subsequent research has further confirmed these associations. The potential actionability of these germline findings was underscored by the efficacy of polyp ADP ribose polymerase inhibitor (PARPi) in the POLO study of maintenance Olaparib among g*BRCA*-carriers with metastatic pancreatic cancer.[94]

Table 1
High and moderate penetrance gPVs in upper gastrointestinal cancer and therapeutic actionability

Pathogenic Germline Variant	Cancer Subtype	Gene Penetrance	Targetable	Therapeutic Agent
ATM	Gastric Esophageal Pancreas Biliary	Moderate	No	-
APC	Gastric	High	No	-
BRCA1/2	Pancreas Gastric[a] Biliary	High	Yes	PARPi
PALB2	Gastric Pancreas Biliary	Moderate	Yes	PARPi
CDH1	Gastric	High	No	-
CDKN2A	Pancreas	High	Not at present	Negative trial of CDK4/6i
CTNNA1	Gastric	High	No	-
MLH1	Gastric Pancreas	High	Yes[a]	ICB
MSH2	Gastric Pancreas	High	Yes[a]	ICB
MSH6	Gastric Pancreas	High	Yes[a]	ICB
PMS2	Gastric Biliary	High	Yes[a]	ICB
PRSS1	Pancreas	High or low dependent on variant	No	-
STK11	Gastric Pancreas	High	No	-
SMAD4	Gastric	High	No	-
BMPR1A	Gastric	High	No	-
TP53	Gastric Esophageal	High	No	-

Abbreviations: CDK4/6i, cyclin-dependent kinase inhibitor; ICB, immune checkpoint blockade; PARPI, polyp ADP ribose polymerase inhibitor.
[a] Actionable in the setting of tumors with Microsatellite Instability (MSI).

The association of *ATM* with pancreatic cancer was identified through genome-wide sequencing in 2012[89] and has been further corroborated in a number of studies.[90] More recent data characterizing somatic and germline *ATM* variants arising in association with pancreatic ductal adenocarcinoma demonstrated an improved OS in this cohort[95,96]; interestingly *ATM* was not found to confer an HRD signature suggesting limited benefit from strategies exploiting this pathway.

Germline variants in *CDKN2A* have been reported to confer a 12.3-fold increased risk of pancreatic cancer[91,96,97] while additionally, although rare, *gSTK11* mutations have been reported to confer a 130-fold increased risk.[49] Pancreatic cancer has also been described in association with the LS-associated genes; this risk of pancreatic cancer may vary by germline MMR variant[98] and the risk is approximately 8.6-fold greater than the general population.[99] Recognition of LS-associated pancreas cancer is potentially actionable given recent data regarding the utility of immune checkpoint blockade in this cohort in the setting of MSI disease.[40,100]

NCCN guidelines[101] now recommend germline genetic testing for all patients diagnosed with pancreatic cancer with results guiding need for cascade testing within families and potentially enrollment into pancreatic surveillance protocols for unaffected familial carriers of gPVs. Notably, despite extensive gene discovery research efforts, a large proportion of familial pancreatic cancer, defined as a kindred with at least a pair of first-degree relatives with pancreas cancer,[102] remains genetically unexplained.[96] As in patients with gPV in pancreas-associated cancer susceptibility genes and a family history of the disease, pancreatic surveillance should also be considered in the context of individualized decision-making in first-degree relatives of individuals with familial pancreatic cancer.[103]

Biliary Tract Cancer

The data for the contribution of gPVs to biliary tract cancers inclusive of cholangiocarcinoma and gallbladder cancer are much more limited. One study in a predominantly Caucasian population reported gPVs in 16% of the patients[104] with 9.9% of these in high and moderate penetrance cancer predisposition genes. This is comparable to a reported gPV rate of 11% in a Japanese cohort of patients with biliary cancer[105] although the variants identified differed. These rates are comparable to other solid tumors, however, and support integration of germline genetic testing in the management of these patients.

SUMMARY

With increasing availability of commercial multigene panel testing (MGPT) and expansion of the cancer types in which MGPT is recommended, particularly in patients with early onset cancer, we will undoubtedly detect more gPVs which are of clinical relevance for the cancer-affected patient as well as at-risk relatives. While criteria for germline genetic testing are more clearly defined for gastric cancer[3] and pancreatic cancer,[101,106] guidelines in relation to the role of genetic testing for more novel genes[75] in the setting of esophageal cancer beyond a limited number of cancer predisposition syndromes, and in biliary cancer, is in evolution.[105,107] Increased access to commercial panels and more widespread integration of genetic testing into cancer care will enhance appreciation of novel associations and our understanding of the contribution of these variants to gastrointestinal carcinogenesis will become more clearly defined (**Table 1**).

It is important to caution that the relative contribution of a gPV detected on MGPT to causation of the index cancer particularly in the setting of genes not classically associated with that cancer subtype is challenging to deduce. Integration of germline and somatic analysis is critical to elucidate the role of germline variants in upper gastrointestinal carcinogenesis by evaluating bi-allelic loss, which, when assessed, seems to be consistently higher among patients with early onset cancer than in average onset cancer.[108,109] This suggests that these gPVs are driving cancer development at least in a proportion of these cancers. Determination of causality is imperative in order to identify novel treatment approaches exploiting underlying germline drivers implicated in carcinogenesis. Potential actionability of these underlying gPvs as exemplified by the utility of PARPi and immunotherapy is particularly pertinent.

While the prevalence of gPVs is consistently higher amongst patients with early onset cancers, decisions regarding germline genetic testing should not be restricted by age alone or by an arbitrary designation of young onset. In a review of 25,035 patients with cancer,[2] an age cutoff of 50 for early onset cancer was >1 standard deviation below the mean age at diagnosis in 20 cancer types resulting in 2226 patients who would not have been classified as having early onset cancer, inclusive of 394 patients who tested positive for a germline LP/P, representing 26.1% of all germline early onset cancer positives. These findings are particularly relevant as the therapeutic implication of gPVs expands.[110,111]

CLINICS CARE POINTS: PEARLS AND PITFALLS

- Comprehensive management of upper gastrointestinal cancers should incorporate germline genetic testing.
- Stringent application of clinical criteria for genetic testing in any cancer type, including gastric, esophageal, GEJ, pancreatic, or biliary cancer, may miss a significant proportion of patients with underlying germline pathogenic variants (gPVs).
- Critically, germline genetic testing should not be restricted exclusively by definition of early onset cancer as cancer arising <50 years of age, and family history should always be integrated into clinical decision-making
- Identification of germline pathogenic variants may increasingly have implications for systemic therapy decisions

DISCLOSURE

E.C. Harrold has received funding from the Conquer Cancer, the ASCO Foundation, United States. She also served as a consultant to Pfizer Ireland on one occasion in 2021. She reports education grants from Merck and Amgen to attend GI ASCO in 2020. Z.K. Stadler's immediate family member serves as a consultant in Ophthalmology for Adverum, Genentech, Neurogene, Novartis, Optos Plc, Outlook Therapeutics, and Regeneron outside the submitted work. Z.K. Stadler serves as an Associate Editor for *JCO Precision Oncology* and as a Section Editor for UpToDate.

REFERENCES

1. Stadler ZK, Maio A, Chakravarty D, et al. Therapeutic implications of germline testing in patients with advanced cancers. J Clin Oncol 2021;39(24):2698.
2. Stadler ZK, Maio A, Khurram A, et al. Redefining early-onset cancer and risk of hereditary cancer predisposition. American Society of Clinical Oncology; 2023.

3. Ajani JA, D'Amico TA, Bentrem DJ, et al. Gastric Cancer, Version 2.2022, NCCN Clinical Practice Guidelines in Oncology. J Natl Compr Cancer Netw 2022;20(2): 167–92.

4. Hampel H, Frankel WL, Martin E, et al. Screening for the Lynch syndrome (hereditary nonpolyposis colorectal cancer). N Engl J Med 2005;352(18):1851–60.

5. Lipton LR, Johnson V, Cummings C, et al. Refining the Amsterdam Criteria and Bethesda Guidelines: testing algorithms for the prediction of mismatch repair mutation status in the familial cancer clinic. J Clin Oncol 2004;22(24):4934–43.

6. Latham A, Srinivasan P, Kemel Y, et al. Microsatellite Instability Is Associated With the Presence of Lynch Syndrome Pan-Cancer. J Clin Oncol 2019;37(4): 286–95.

7. Ceyhan-Birsoy O, Jayakumaran G, Kemel Y, et al. Diagnostic yield and clinical relevance of expanded genetic testing for cancer patients. Genome Med 2022; 14(1):92.

8. Fiala EM, Jayakumaran G, Mauguen A, et al. Prospective pan-cancer germline testing using MSK-IMPACT informs clinical translation in 751 patients with pediatric solid tumors. Nature Cancer 2021. https://doi.org/10.1038/s43018-021-00172-1.

9. Mandelker D, Zhang L, Kemel Y, et al. Mutation Detection in Patients With Advanced Cancer by Universal Sequencing of Cancer-Related Genes in Tumor and Normal DNA vs Guideline-Based Germline Testing. JAMA 2017;318(9): 825–35.

10. Oliveira C, Pinheiro H, Figueiredo J, et al. Familial gastric cancer: genetic susceptibility, pathology, and implications for management. Lancet Oncol 2015; 16(2):e60–70.

11. Blair VR, McLeod M, Carneiro F, et al. Hereditary diffuse gastric cancer: updated clinical practice guidelines. Lancet Oncol 2020;21(8):e386–97.

12. Hansford S, Kaurah P, Li-Chang H, et al. Hereditary Diffuse Gastric Cancer Syndrome: CDH1 Mutations and Beyond. JAMA Oncol 2015;1(1):23–32.

13. Guilford P, Hopkins J, Harraway J, et al. E-cadherin germline mutations in familial gastric cancer. Nature 1998;392(6674):402–5.

14. Lobo S, Benusiglio PR, Coulet F, et al. Cancer predisposition and germline CTNNA1 variants. Eur J Med Genet 2021;64(10):104316.

15. Brooks-Wilson A, Kaurah P, Suriano G, et al. Germline E-cadherin mutations in hereditary diffuse gastric cancer: assessment of 42 new families and review of genetic screening criteria. J Med Genet 2004;41(7):508–17.

16. Oliveira C, Senz J, Kaurah P, et al. Germline CDH1 deletions in hereditary diffuse gastric cancer families. Hum Mol Genet 2009;18(9):1545–55.

17. Knights AJ, Funnell AP, Crossley M, et al. Holding tight: cell junctions and cancer spread. Trends Cancer Res 2012;8:61.

18. Richards FM, McKee SA, Rajpar MH, et al. Germline E-cadherin gene (CDH1) mutations predispose to familial gastric cancer and colorectal cancer. Hum Mol Genet 1999;8(4):607–10.

19. Gayther SA, Gorringe KL, Ramus SJ, et al. Identification of germ-line E-cadherin mutations in gastric cancer families of European origin. Cancer Res 1998; 58(18):4086–9.

20. Keller G, Vogelsang H, Becker I, et al. Diffuse type gastric and lobular breast carcinoma in a familial gastric cancer patient with an E-cadherin germline mutation. Am J Pathol 1999;155(2):337–42.

21. Karam R, Carvalho J, Bruno I, et al. The NMD mRNA surveillance pathway downregulates aberrant E-cadherin transcripts in gastric cancer cells and in CDH1 mutation carriers. Oncogene 2008;27(30):4255–60.

22. Oliveira C, Pinheiro H, Figueiredo J, et al. E-cadherin alterations in hereditary disorders with emphasis on hereditary diffuse gastric cancer. Progress in Molecular Biology and Translational Science 2013;116:337–59.

23. Berx G, Becker KF, Höfler H, et al. Mutations of the human E-cadherin (CDH1) gene. Hum Mutat 1998;12(4):226–37.

24. Caldas C, Carneiro F, Lynch HT, et al. Familial gastric cancer: overview and guidelines for management. J Med Genet 1999;36(12):873–80.

25. Kaurah P, MacMillan A, Boyd N, et al. Founder and recurrent CDH1 mutations in families with hereditary diffuse gastric cancer. JAMA 2007;297(21):2360–72.

26. Xicola RM, Li S, Rodriguez N, et al. Clinical features and cancer risk in families with pathogenic CDH1 variants irrespective of clinical criteria. J Med Genet 2019;56(12):838–43.

27. Roberts ME, Ranola JMO, Marshall ML, et al. Comparison of CDH1 penetrance estimates in clinically ascertained families vs families ascertained for multiple gastric cancers. JAMA Oncol 2019;5(9):1325–31.

28. Fitzgerald RC, Hardwick R, Huntsman D, et al, International Gastric Cancer Linkage Consortium. Hereditary diffuse gastric cancer: updated consensus guidelines for clinical management and directions for future research. J Med Genet 2010;47(7):436–44.

29. van der Post RS, Vogelaar IP, Carneiro F, et al. Hereditary diffuse gastric cancer: updated clinical guidelines with an emphasis on germline CDH1 mutation carriers. J Med Genet 2015;52(6):361–74.

30. Vos EL, Salo-Mullen EE, Tang LH, et al. Indications for total gastrectomy in CDH1 mutation carriers and outcomes of risk-reducing minimally invasive and open gastrectomies. JAMA Surgery 2020;155(11):1050–7.

31. Asif B, Sarvestani AL, Gamble LA, et al. Cancer surveillance as an alternative to prophylactic total gastrectomy in hereditary diffuse gastric cancer: a prospective cohort study. Lancet Oncol 2023;24(4):383–91.

32. Majewski IJ, Kluijt I, Cats A, et al. An alpha-E-catenin (CTNNA1) mutation in hereditary diffuse gastric cancer. J Pathol 2013;229(4):621–9.

33. Worthley DL, Phillips KD, Wayte N, et al. Gastric adenocarcinoma and proximal polyposis of the stomach (GAPPS): a new autosomal dominant syndrome. Gut 2012;61(5):774–9.

34. Yen T., Stanich P.P., Axell L., et al., APC-Associated Polyposis Conditions. 1998. [Updated 2022 May 12]. In: Adam M.P., Feldman J., Mirzaa G.M., et al., editors. GeneReviews® [Internet]. Seattle (WA): University of Washington, Seattle; 1993-2024. Available at: https://www.ncbi.nlm.nih.gov/books/NBK1345/.

35. Rudloff U. Gastric adenocarcinoma and proximal polyposis of the stomach: diagnosis and clinical perspectives. Clin Exp Gastroenterol 2018;11:447–59.

36. Fornasarig M, Magris R, De Re V, et al. Molecular and Pathological Features of Gastric Cancer in Lynch Syndrome and Familial Adenomatous Polyposis. Int J Mol Sci 2018;19(6). https://doi.org/10.3390/ijms19061682.

37. Latham A, Srinivasan P, Kemel Y, et al. Microsatellite instability is associated with the presence of Lynch syndrome pan-cancer. J Clin Oncol 2019;37(4):286.

38. Møller P, Seppälä TT, Bernstein I, et al, Mallorca Group. Cancer risk and survival in path_MMR carriers by gene and gender up to 75 years of age: a report from the Prospective Lynch Syndrome Database. Gut 2018;67(7):1306–16.

39. André T, Tougeron D, Piessen G, et al. Neoadjuvant nivolumab plus ipilimumab and adjuvant nivolumab in localized deficient mismatch repair/microsatellite instability–high gastric or esophagogastric junction adenocarcinoma: The GERCOR NEONIPIGA phase II study. J Clin Oncol 2023;41(2):255.

40. Marabelle A, Le DT, Ascierto PA, et al. Efficacy of pembrolizumab in patients with noncolorectal high microsatellite instability/mismatch repair–deficient cancer: results from the phase II KEYNOTE-158 study. J Clin Oncol 2020;38(1):1.

41. Harrold EC, Foote MB, Rousseau B, et al. Neoplasia risk in patients with Lynch syndrome treated with immune checkpoint blockade. Nat Med 2023;29(10):2458–63.

42. Amadou A, Waddington Achatz MI, Hainaut P. Revisiting tumor patterns and penetrance in germline TP53 mutation carriers: temporal phases of Li–Fraumeni syndrome. Curr Opin Oncol 2018;30(1):23–9.

43. Masciari S, Dewanwala A, Stoffel EM, et al. Gastric cancer in individuals with Li-Fraumeni syndrome. Genet Med 2011;13(7):651–7.

44. Katona BW, Powers J, McKenna DB, et al. Upper gastrointestinal cancer risk and surveillance outcomes in Li-Fraumeni syndrome. Am J Gastroenterol 2020;115(12):2095.

45. Leone PJ, Mankaney G, Sarvapelli S, et al. Endoscopic and histologic features associated with gastric cancer in familial adenomatous polyposis. Gastrointest Endosc 2019;89(5):961–8.

46. Mankaney G, Leone P, Cruise M, et al. Gastric cancer in FAP: a concerning rise in incidence. Fam Cancer 2017;16(3):371–6.

47. Bisgaard ML, Fenger K, Bülow S, et al. Familial adenomatous polyposis (FAP): frequency, penetrance, and mutation rate. Hum Mutat 1994;3(2):121–5.

48. Walton S-J, Frayling IM, Clark SK, et al. Gastric tumours in FAP. Fam Cancer 2017;16(3):363–9.

49. Giardiello FM, Brensinger JD, Tersmette AC, et al. Very high risk of cancer in familial Peutz-Jeghers syndrome. Gastroenterology 2000;119(6):1447–53.

50. Hearle N, Schumacher V, Menko FH, et al. Frequency and spectrum of cancers in the Peutz-Jeghers syndrome. Clin Cancer Res 2006;12(10):3209–15.

51. Dal Buono A, Gaiani F, Poliani L, et al. Juvenile polyposis syndrome: An overview. Best Pract Res Clin Gastroenterol 2022;58-59:101799.

52. MacFarland SP, Ebrahimzadeh JE, Zelley K, et al. Phenotypic Differences in Juvenile Polyposis Syndrome With or Without a Disease-causing SMAD4/BMPR1A Variant. Cancer Prev Res (Phila) 2021;14(2):215–22.

53. Singh AD, Gupta A, Mehta N, et al. Occurrence of gastric cancer in patients with juvenile polyposis syndrome: a systematic review and meta-analysis. Gastrointest Endosc 2023;97(3):407–14.e1.

54. Stadler ZK, Salo-Mullen E, Zhang L, et al. Juvenile polyposis syndrome presenting with familial gastric cancer and massive gastric polyposis. J Clin Oncol 2012;30(25):e229–32.

55. Fewings E, Larionov A, Redman J, et al. Germline pathogenic variants in PALB2 and other cancer-predisposing genes in families with hereditary diffuse gastric cancer without CDH1 mutation: a whole-exome sequencing study. Lancet Gastroenterol Hepatol 2018;3(7):489–98.

56. Sahasrabudhe R, Lott P, Bohorquez M, Latin American Gastric Cancer Genetics Collaborative Group. Germline mutations in PALB2, BRCA1, and RAD51C, which regulate DNA recombination repair, in patients with gastric cancer. Gastroenterology 2017;152(5):983–6.e6.

57. Carvajal-Carmona LG. PALB2 as a familial gastric cancer gene: is the wait over? Lancet Gastroenterol Hepatol 2018;3(7):451–2.

58. Huang D-S, Tao H-Q, He X-J, et al. Prevalence of deleterious ATM germline mutations in gastric cancer patients. Oncotarget 2015;6(38):40953.

59. Helgason H, Rafnar T, Olafsdottir HS, et al. Loss-of-function variants in ATM confer risk of gastric cancer. Nat Genet 2015;47(8):906–10.

60. Bang Y-J, Im S-A, Lee K-W, et al. Randomized, double-blind phase II trial with prospective classification by ATM protein level to evaluate the efficacy and tolerability of olaparib plus paclitaxel in patients with recurrent or metastatic gastric cancer. J Clin Oncol 2015;33(33):3858–65.

61. Li S, Silvestri V, Leslie G, et al. Cancer Risks Associated With BRCA1 and BRCA2 Pathogenic Variants. J Clin Oncol 2022;40(14):1529–41.

62. Lubinski J, Phelan CM, Ghadirian P, et al. Cancer variation associated with the position of the mutation in the BRCA2 gene. Fam Cancer 2004;3(1):1–10.

63. Jakubowska A, Nej K, Huzarski T, et al. BRCA2 gene mutations in families with aggregations of breast and stomach cancers. Br J Cancer 2002;87(8):888–91.

64. Risch HA, McLaughlin JR, Cole DE, et al. Population BRCA1 and BRCA2 mutation frequencies and cancer penetrances: a kin-cohort study in Ontario, Canada. J Natl Cancer Inst 2006;98(23):1694–706.

65. Moran A, O'Hara C, Khan S, et al. Risk of cancer other than breast or ovarian in individuals with BRCA1 and BRCA2 mutations. Fam Cancer 2012;11(2):235–42.

66. Usui Y, Taniyama Y, Endo M, et al. Helicobacter pylori, homologous-recombination genes, and gastric cancer. N Engl J Med 2023;388(13):1181–90.

67. Buckley KH, Niccum BA, Maxwell KN, et al. Gastric Cancer Risk and Pathogenesis in BRCA1 and BRCA2 Carriers. Cancers (Basel) 2022;14(23). https://doi.org/10.3390/cancers14235953.

68. Slavin T, Neuhausen SL, Rybak C, et al. Genetic gastric cancer susceptibility in the international clinical cancer genomics community research network. Cancer genetics 2017;216:111–9.

69. Ellis A, Risk JM, Maruthappu T, et al. Tylosis with oesophageal cancer: Diagnosis, management and molecular mechanisms. Orphanet J Rare Dis 2015; 10:1–6.

70. Arora H, Chacon AH, Choudhary S, et al. Bloom syndrome. Int J Dermatol 2014; 53(7):798–802.

71. German J. Bloom's syndrome. XX. The first 100 cancers. Cancer Genet Cytogenet 1997;93(1):100–6.

72. Ababou M. Bloom syndrome and the underlying causes of genetic instability. Mol Genet Metabol 2021;133(1):35–48.

73. Akbari MR, Malekzadeh R, Lepage P, et al. Mutations in Fanconi anemia genes and the risk of esophageal cancer. Hum Genet 2011;129:573–82.

74. Sun X, Elston R, Barnholtz-Sloan J, et al. A segregation analysis of Barrett's esophagus and associated adenocarcinomas. Cancer Epidemiol Biomark Prev 2010;19(3):666–74.

75. El Jabbour T, Misyura M, Cowzer D, et al. ATM germline-mutated gastroesophageal junction adenocarcinomas: Clinical descriptors, molecular characteristics, and potential therapeutic implications. J Natl Cancer Inst 2022;114(5): 761–70.

76. Lee M, Eng G, Handte-Reinecker A, et al. Germline Determinants of Esophageal Adenocarcinoma. Gastroenterology 2023;165(5):1276–9.e7.

77. Network CGAR, Analysis Working Group: Asan University, BC Cancer Agency, et al. Integrated genomic characterization of oesophageal carcinoma. Nature 2017;541(7636):169.

78. Ku GY, Kemel Y, Maron SB, et al. Prevalence of germline alterations on targeted tumor-normal sequencing of esophagogastric cancer. JAMA Netw Open 2021; 4(7):e2114753–.

79. Varghese AM, Singh I, Singh R, et al. Early-Onset Pancreas Cancer: Clinical Descriptors, Genomics, and Outcomes. J Natl Cancer Inst 2021;113(9):1194–202.

80. Bannon SA, Montiel MF, Goldstein JB, et al. High Prevalence of Hereditary Cancer Syndromes and Outcomes in Adults with Early-Onset Pancreatic Cancer. Cancer Prev Res (Phila) 2018;11(11):679–86.

81. Sung H, Siegel RL, Rosenberg PS, et al. Emerging cancer trends among young adults in the USA: analysis of a population-based cancer registry. Lancet Public Health 2019;4(3):e137–47.

82. Ben-Aharon I, van Laarhoven HWM, Fontana E, et al. Early-Onset Cancer in the Gastrointestinal Tract Is on the Rise-Evidence and Implications. Cancer Discov 2023;13(3):538–51.

83. Jayakrishnan T, Nair KG, Kamath SD, et al. Comparison of characteristics and outcomes of young-onset versus average onset pancreatico-biliary adenocarcinoma. Cancer Med 2023. https://doi.org/10.1002/cam4.5418.

84. Dbouk M, Katona BW, Brand RE, et al. The multicenter cancer of pancreas screening study: impact on stage and survival. J Clin Oncol 2022;40(28):3257.

85. Couch FJ, Johnson MR, Rabe KG, et al. The prevalence of BRCA2 mutations in familial pancreatic cancer. Cancer Epidemiol Biomark Prev 2007;16(2):342–6.

86. Hahn SA, Greenhalf B, Ellis I, et al. BRCA2 germline mutations in familial pancreatic carcinoma. J Natl Cancer Inst 2003;95(3):214–21.

87. Jones S, Hruban RH, Kamiyama M, et al. Exomic sequencing identifies PALB2 as a pancreatic cancer susceptibility gene. Science 2009;324(5924):217.

88. Yang X, Leslie G, Doroszuk A, et al. Cancer risks associated with germline PALB2 pathogenic variants: an international study of 524 families. J Clin Oncol 2020;38(7):674.

89. Roberts NJ, Jiao Y, Yu J, et al. ATM mutations in patients with hereditary pancreatic cancer. Cancer Discov 2012;2(1):41–6.

90. Shindo K, Yu J, Suenaga M, et al. Deleterious germline mutations in patients with apparently sporadic pancreatic adenocarcinoma. J Clin Oncol 2017;35(30): 3382.

91. Zhen DB, Rabe KG, Gallinger S, et al. BRCA1, BRCA2, PALB2, and CDKN2A mutations in familial pancreatic cancer: a PACGENE study. Genet Med 2015; 17(7):569–77.

92. Consortium BCL. Cancer risks in BRCA2 mutation carriers. J Natl Cancer Inst 1999;91(15):1310–6.

93. Thompson D, Easton DF, Breast Cancer Linkage Consortium. Cancer incidence in BRCA1 mutation carriers. J Natl Cancer Inst 2002;94(18):1358–65.

94. Golan T, Hammel P, Reni M, et al. Maintenance Olaparib for Germline BRCA-Mutated Metastatic Pancreatic Cancer. N Engl J Med 2019;381(4):317–27.

95. Park W, O'Connor CA, Bandlamudi C, et al. Clinico-genomic characterization of ATM and HRD in pancreas cancer: application for practice. Clin Cancer Res 2022;28(21):4782–92.

96. Roberts NJ, Norris AL, Petersen GM, et al. Whole genome sequencing defines the genetic heterogeneity of familial pancreatic cancer. Cancer Discov 2016; 6(2):166–75.

97. Hu C, Hart SN, Polley EC, et al. Association between inherited germline mutations in cancer predisposition genes and risk of pancreatic cancer. JAMA 2018;319(23):2401–9.
98. Zalevskaja K, Mecklin J-P, Seppälä TT. Clinical characteristics of pancreatic and biliary tract cancers in Lynch syndrome: A retrospective analysis from the Finnish National Lynch Syndrome Research Registry. Front Oncol 2023;13:1123901.
99. Kastrinos F, Mukherjee B, Tayob N, et al. Risk of pancreatic cancer in families with Lynch syndrome. JAMA 2009;302(16):1790–5.
100. Coston T, Desai A, Babiker H, et al. Efficacy of Immune Checkpoint Inhibition and Cytotoxic Chemotherapy in Mismatch Repair-Deficient and Microsatellite Instability-High Pancreatic Cancer: Mayo Clinic Experience. JCO Precision Oncology 2023;7:e2200706.
101. Daly MB, Pal T, Berry MP, Buys SS, Dickson P, Domchek SM, Elkhanany A, Friedman S, Goggins M, Hutton ML, CGC, Karlan BY, Khan S, Klein C, Kohlmann W, CGC, Kurian AW, Laronga C, Litton JK, Mak JS, LCGC, Menendez CS, Merajver SD, Norquist BS, Offit K, Pederson HJ, Reiser G, CGC, Senter-Jamieson L, CGC, Shannon KM, Shatsky R, Visvanathan K, Weitzel JN, Wick MJ, Wisinski KB, Yurgelun MB, Darlow SD, Dwyer MA. Genetic/familial high-risk assessment: breast, ovarian, and pancreatic, version 2.2021, NCCN clinical practice guidelines in oncology. J Natl Compr Cancer Netw 2021;19(1):77–102.
102. Petersen GM. Familial pancreatic adenocarcinoma. Hematol/Oncol Clin 2015; 29(4):641–53.
103. Goggins M, Overbeek KA, Brand R, et al, International Cancer of the Pancreas Screening CAPS consortium. Management of patients with increased risk for familial pancreatic cancer: updated recommendations from the International Cancer of the Pancreas Screening (CAPS) Consortium. Gut 2020;69(1):7–17.
104. Maynard H, Stadler ZK, Berger MF, et al. Germline alterations in patients with biliary tract cancers: A spectrum of significant and previously underappreciated findings. Cancer 2020;126(9):1995–2002.
105. Wardell CP, Fujita M, Yamada T, et al. Genomic characterization of biliary tract cancers identifies driver genes and predisposing mutations. J Hepatol 2018; 68(5):959–69.
106. Daly MB, Pal T, Maxwell KN, et al. NCCN Guidelines® Insights: Genetic/Familial High-Risk Assessment: Breast, Ovarian, and Pancreatic, Version 2.2024: Featured Updates to the NCCN Guidelines. J Natl Compr Cancer Netw 2023; 21(10):1000–10.
107. Ajani JA, D'Amico TA, Bentrem DJ, et al. Esophageal and Esophagogastric Junction Cancers, Version 2.2023, NCCN Clinical Practice Guidelines in Oncology. J Natl Compr Cancer Netw 2023;21(4):393–422.
108. Cercek A, Chatila WK, Yaeger R, et al. A Comprehensive Comparison of Early-Onset and Average-Onset Colorectal Cancers. J Natl Cancer Inst 2021;113(12): 1683–92.
109. El Jabbour T, Misyura M, Cowzer D, et al. ATM Germline-Mutated Gastroesophageal Junction Adenocarcinomas: Clinical Descriptors, Molecular Characteristics, and Potential Therapeutic Implications. J Natl Cancer Inst 2022;114(5):761–70.
110. Lord CJ, Ashworth A. PARP inhibitors: Synthetic lethality in the clinic. Science 2017;355(6330):1152–8.
111. Joris S, Denys H, Collignon J, et al. Efficacy of olaparib in advanced cancers with germline or somatic mutations in BRCA1, BRCA2, CHEK2 and ATM, a Belgian Precision tumor-agnostic phase II study. ESMO Open 2023;8(6): 102041.

The Role of Screening and Early Detection in Upper Gastrointestinal Cancers

Jin Woo Yoo, MD*, Monika Laszkowska, MD, MS,
Robin B. Mendelsohn, MD

KEYWORDS

- Upper gastrointestinal cancer • Esophageal cancer • Gastric cancer
- Small-bowel cancer • Screening • Surveillance • Early detection

KEY POINTS

- Effective strategies for early detection of upper gastrointestinal cancers in regions of modest incidence require targeted screening and surveillance of high-risk individuals.
- Risk stratification of individuals based on demographic, familial, and clinicopathologic factors is fundamental for targeted screening and surveillance.
- Assessment of precancerous lesions underlying upper gastrointestinal cancers is pivotal for risk stratification and informing surveillance strategies.
- Endoscopic surveillance of established precancerous lesions, such as Barrett esophagus, esophageal squamous dysplasia, atrophic gastritis, and gastric intestinal metaplasia and dysplasia, should be considered in high-risk patients.
- Endoscopic screening of small-bowel adenocarcinoma should be considered in individuals with hereditary gastrointestinal cancer syndromes.

INTRODUCTION

Upper gastrointestinal (GI) cancers comprise a substantial part of the global cancer burden. In 2020, worldwide, esophagogastric cancers alone represented 13% of deaths from all cancers and 36% of deaths from GI cancers.[1] Late detection is a major driver of poor outcomes for upper GI cancers,[2–4] which is largely attributable to the deficit of effective screening and surveillance programs amid a landscape of heterogeneous risk. A comprehensive understanding of the epidemiology, pathogenesis, and risk assessment is essential for overcoming these barriers.

Gastroenterology, Hepatology and Nutrition Service, Department of Medicine, Memorial Sloan Kettering Cancer Center, 1275 York Avenue, New York, NY 10065, USA
* Corresponding author.
E-mail address: yooj3@mskcc.org

Hematol Oncol Clin N Am 38 (2024) 693–710
https://doi.org/10.1016/j.hoc.2024.01.007
hemonc.theclinics.com

EPIDEMIOLOGY OF ESOPHAGEAL CANCER

Esophageal cancer (EC) is the eighth most common cancer and sixth leading cause of cancer deaths responsible for 604,100 new cases and 544,100 deaths in 2020 globally.[5] EC is highly lethal with an overall 5-year survival rate of 21%,[6] which decreases to less than 5% for distant metastatic disease, which unfortunately is the presentation in the most patients with EC at the time of diagnosis.[2,3]

Esophageal adenocarcinoma (EAC) and esophageal squamous cell carcinoma (ESCC) are the main histologic subtypes of EC. ESCC is most common globally, comprising 85% of ECs in 2020.[5] ESCC incidence is concentrated in East Asia, South Central Asia, Eastern Africa, and South Africa, where the age-standardized rates (ASRs) are 11.2, 5.2, 6.4, and 5.9 per 100,000 person-years, respectively.[5] Although comprising 14% of ECs globally, EAC is the predominant subtype in developed countries.[5] EAC incidence is concentrated in Northern Europe and North America, where the rates are 3.4 and 1.9 per 100,000 person-years, respectively.[5] Incidence and mortalities for all ECs are 2- to 3-fold higher in men compared with women globally.[5] Racial disparities exist within the United States where higher incidence rates of ESCC are seen among Asians and African Americans, whereas higher rates of EAC are seen among non-Hispanic white men.[7]

CAUSE OF ESOPHAGEAL CANCER
Esophageal Adenocarcinoma

Barrett esophagus (BE) is a precancerous lesion of EAC that develops as a response to chronic inflammatory insult, such as gastroesophageal acid reflux disease (GERD), resulting in replacement of normal esophageal squamous epithelium with metaplastic intestinal-type columnar epithelium.[8] BE progresses to EAC through a carcinogenic sequence from nondysplastic BE (NDBE) to BE with low-grade dysplasia (LGD-BE) to BE with high-grade dysplasia (HGD-BE), and finally, to carcinoma (**Fig. 1A–C**).[9] The prevalence of BE is estimated to be 1% to 2% of the general adult population and 7% to 10% in patients with chronic GERD.[3] A higher degree of dysplasia correlates with an increasing risk of EAC. The pooled annual incidence rates of EAC in patients with NDBE, LGD-BE, and HGD-BE have been reported as 0.3%, 0.5%, and 7%, respectively.[10]

GERD is a well-established risk factor for both EAC and BE (**Table 1**).[3,8,11] Chronic GERD is associated with a 5- to 7-fold higher risk of EAC.[11] Other risk factors common to EAC and BE include obesity[12] and smoking.[13] Hiatal hernia is associated with a 12.7- and 2.9-fold higher risk of long- and short-segment BE, respectively.[14] A familial risk of EAC has also been described, wherein family history of EAC in patients with BE was associated with 5.5-fold higher risk of EAC.[15]

Esophageal Squamous Cell Carcinoma

Esophageal squamous dysplasia (SD) is the BE-equivalent precancerous lesion of ESCC that progresses through a carcinogenic sequence, in which a higher degree of dysplasia correlates with an increasing risk of ESCC.[2] Incident ESCC among untreated patients in a high-risk Chinese population with mild, moderate, or severe SD was found in 5%, 27%, and 65% of patients, respectively, after 3.5 years,[16] and 24%, 50%, and 74% of patients, respectively, after 13.5 years.[17]

Various environmental and host-related risk factors have been linked to ESCC (see **Table 1**). Environmental factors include smoking,[18,19] alcohol consumption,[19] diets rich in nitrogenous compounds,[19] wood burning for heating and cooking,[20] history of esophageal caustic injury (eg, lye ingestion),[21] and human papillomavirus

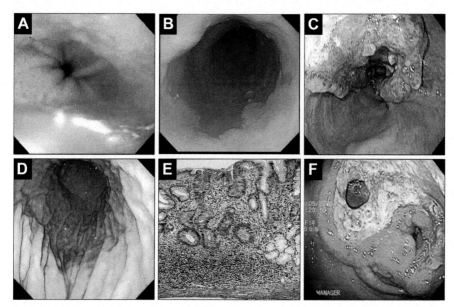

Fig. 1. Development of EAC and GAC. (*A*) Normal esophageal mucosa on endoscopic examination. (*B*) BE on endoscopic examination. (*C*) EAC on endoscopic examination. (*D*) Normal gastric mucosa on endoscopic examination. (*E*) Gastric intestinal metaplasia on histologic examination. (*F*) GAC on endoscopic examination.

infection.[22] Host-related factors include tylosis,[23] achalasia,[24] celiac sprue,[25] and a history of head and neck cancer.[26,27] Esophageal caustic injury increases risk of both ESCC and EAC, with implication in up to 4% of all ECs.[21] Tylosis is a rare autosomal dominant disorder characterized by hyperkeratosis that greatly increases lifetime risk of ESCC to as high as 95%.[23] Achalasia is associated with a 16- to 33-fold higher risk of ESCC.[24] The incidence of either synchronous or metachronous ESCC is estimated to be 3% to 14% in patients with history of head and neck cancer, which notably shares smoking and alcohol consumption as common risk factors.[26,27]

ESOPHAGEAL ADENOCARCINOMA SCREENING
Endoscopic Evaluation of Barrett Esophagus

Performance of a high-quality endoscopic examination is essential for reliable detection and prognostication of BE. Although the optimal threshold for inspection time remains unclear, European guidelines have recommended an endoscopic procedure time of $\geq$7 minutes and inspection time of $\geq$1 minute per centimeter of the circumferential length of BE to improve detection.[28] The use of virtual chromoendoscopy, an image-enhancing technique such as narrow-band imaging (NBI) that uses blue wavelengths of light to enhance fine visualization of the mucosa and microvasculature without the use of dyes as for traditional chromoendoscopy, significantly improves detection of HGD/EAC.[29] Other advanced imaging technologies, such as confocal laser endomicroscopy, may be used adjunctively to assist dysplasia detection.[30]

Informative assessment of BE requires measurement of the BE dimensions and morphologic characterization of visible lesions, which may be accomplished by using standardized reporting systems, such as the Prague and Paris classifications, respectively. Biopsies should be obtained using the Seattle biopsy protocol, which requires

Table 1
Risk factors for common esophagogastric cancers

Subtype	Risk Factors		
	Environmental	Host-Related	Demographic (U.S.)
EAC	Precancerous lesions (BE)[8–10] Obesity[12] Smoking[13]	GERD[3,8,11] Hiatal hernia[14] Family history of EAC[15]	Male gender[5] High-risk racial/ethnic background (non-Hispanic whites)[7] Immigration from high-incidence regions (Northern Europe)[5]
ESCC	Precancerous lesions (squamous dysplasia)[2,16,17] Smoking[18,19] Alcohol use[19] Diets rich in nitrogenous compounds[19] Wood burning for heating/cooking[20] Esophageal caustic injury[21] HPV infection[22]	Tylosis[23] Achalasia[24] Celiac sprue[25] History of head and neck cancer[26,27]	Male gender[5] High-risk racial/ethnic background (Asians, African American)[7] Immigration from high-incidence regions (East Asia, South Central Asia, Eastern Africa, South Africa)[5]
GAC	Precancerous lesions (AG, GIM)[47–52] Hp infection[47] Smoking[55] High-salt diets[56] Total, red, processed meat consumption[57] Heavy alcohol use[58]	AIG/PA[49,53,54] Family history of GAC[59]	High-risk racial/ethnic background (Hispanics, Asians, African Americans, Native Americans/Alaska Natives)[47] Immigration from high-incidence regions (East Asia, Central Asia, Andean Latin America)[47]

Abbreviation: HPV, human papillomavirus.

4-quadrant biopsies every 1 to 2 cm and target biopsies of visible lesions, to improve dysplasia detection.[29] Wide-area transepithelial sampling 3D is a novel method of tissue sampling that uses an abrasive brush to collect large sheets of cells maintaining their structural integrity for computer-assisted analysis, and may be used as an adjunctive technique to the Seattle biopsy protocol to further improve dysplasia detection as well as reduce interobserver variability in histopathologic interpretation.[31,32]

Nonendoscopic Evaluation of Barrett Esophagus

Although endoscopic biopsies remain the gold standard, nonendoscopic tools have emerged as minimally invasive screening tests for BE. Esophageal cell-collection devices, such as Cytosponge (Medtronic, Minneapolis, MN, USA), EsoCheck (Lucid Diagnostics, New York, NY, USA), and EsophaCap (Capnostics, Raleigh, NC, USA), use an encapsulated sponge or balloon that can be swallowed and then withdrawn orally to sample the mucosal surface of the esophagus.[33] These tests can be performed in an office setting by trained nonphysician providers without sedation and have demonstrated excellent tolerability and safety.[34] Collected specimens are submitted for cytologic evaluation combined with biomarker assays for protein or methylated DNA markers of BE.[35] This approach has been investigated in the United States and United

Kingdom, demonstrating proof-of-concept with variable performance. Studies using sponge specimens for analyses of cytology and trefoil factor 3 staining showed sensitivities of 76% to 80% and specificities of 77% to 92% for BE detection.[36,37] Other studies using sponge or balloon specimens for analyses of cytology and various panels of methylated DNA markers (eg, *AKAP12, CCNA1, FER1L4, NDRG4, NELL1, p16, TAC1, VAV3, VIM, ZNF568, ZNF682*) showed sensitivities of 92% to 94% and specificities of 62% to 94% for BE detection.[38–41]

Targeted Screening and Surveillance of Barrett Esophagus in High-Risk Individuals

Clinical practice for endoscopic management of BE is variable and continually evolving. In the United States, the American College of Gastroenterology (ACG), the American Gastroenterological Association (AGA), and the American Society for Gastrointestinal Endoscopy (ASGE) have contributed with guidelines to inform clinical practice (**Table 2**).[3,33,35,42] All guidelines suggest consideration of endoscopic screening of BE for high-risk individuals based on variable thresholds for the number and combinations of BE risk factors, including chronic GERD, male gender, age greater than 50 years, non-Hispanic white background, smoking, obesity, and family history of BE/EAC. The ACG suggests one-time screening for patients with chronic GERD and $\geq$3 additional risk factors. The AGA requires a less stringent criteria of $\geq$3 risk factors. The ASGE suggests consideration of screening for individuals of high- or moderate-risk groups, defined as those with family history of BE/EAC and those with GERD and $\geq$1 additional risk factor, respectively. For patients found to have NDBE, all guidelines recommend endoscopic surveillance at 3- to 5-year intervals. The ACG specifies that the interval length should be dictated by the length of BE, wherein a 3-year interval was recommended for segments $\geq$3 cm, and a 5-year interval was recommended for segments less than 3 cm.

When dysplastic BE is found, endoscopic eradication therapy (EET) should be considered to prevent progression to carcinoma. Both EET and continued surveillance are reasonable options for management of LGD-BE, whereas EET is preferred for treatment of HGD-BE.[35,42] For patients with LGD-BE, endoscopic surveillance at 6-month intervals for the first year and annually thereafter is universally recommended. For patients post-EET, all guidelines recommend endoscopic surveillance at intervals dictated by the degree of prior dysplasia. For prior diagnosis of HGD/EAC, surveillance at 3, 6 and 12 months and annually thereafter is recommended. For prior diagnosis of LGD, surveillance every 1 to 2 years for the first 2 to 3 years and every 2 to 3 years thereafter is recommended. Surveillance biopsies post-ETT should entail 4-quadrant random biopsies capturing the esophagogastric junction, gastric cardia, and distal 2 cm of the neosquamous epithelium in addition to targeted biopsies of visible lesions to improve capture of nonvisible recurrences.[33]

ESOPHAGEAL SQUAMOUS CELL CARCINOMA SCREENING
Population-Based Screening of Esophageal Squamous Cell Carcinoma in High-Incidence Regions

Although there are no universal screening recommendations for ESCC because of its highly variable incidence, population-based screening programs in high-incidence regions have been studied. A community assignment trial in endemic areas of China with 10-year-follow-up, in which one-time endoscopic screening with Lugol chromoendoscopy was performed with subsequent endoscopic therapy of any biopsy-proven SD, demonstrated 30% reduction in ESCC incidence and 33% reduction in cumulative ESCC-specific mortality.[43] Markov model–based analyses of strategies of mass

Table 2
US guidelines for screening and surveillance of Barrett esophagus

Source	Recommendations		
	Screening	**NDBE Surveillance**	**Dysplastic BE Surveillance**
ACG[35]	One-time endoscopic screening for patients with chronic GERD and ≥3 additional BE risk factors (male gender, non-Hispanic white background, age >50 y, smoking, obesity, family history of BE/EAC) should be considered	Endoscopic surveillance at intervals dictated by the length of BE is recommended: • 3 cm: 3 y • 3 cm: 5 y	For patients with LGD-BE, endoscopic surveillance at 6-mo intervals for the first year and annually thereafter is recommended Post-EET endoscopic surveillance is recommended at intervals dictated by prior dysplasia: • LGD: repeat exam at 1 and 3 y, then every 2 y • HGD/EAC: repeat exam at 3, 6, and 12 mo, then annually
AGA[33,42]	Endoscopic screening for individuals with ≥3 BE risk factors (male gender, non-Hispanic white background, age >50 y, smoking, chronic GERD, obesity, family history of BE/EAC) should be considered	Endoscopic surveillance every 3–5 y is recommended	For patients with LGD-BE, endoscopic surveillance at 6-mo intervals for the first year, and annually thereafter is recommended Post-EET endoscopic surveillance is recommended at intervals dictated by prior dysplasia: • LGD: repeat exam at 1 and 3 y, then every 2–3 y • HGD/EAC: repeat exam at 3, 6, and 12 mo, then annually
ASGE[3]	Endoscopic screening for individuals of high-risk group (family history of BE/EAC) and moderate-risk group (GERD and ≥1 additional BE risk factor, including male gender, age >50 y, smoking, obesity) should be considered	Endoscopic surveillance every 3–5 y is recommended	For patients with LGD-BE, endoscopic surveillance at 6-mo intervals for the first year, and annually thereafter is recommended Post-EET endoscopic surveillance is recommended at intervals dictated by prior dysplasia: • LGD: repeat exam at 1 and 2 y, then every 3 y • HGD/EAC: repeat exam at 3, 6, and 12 mo, then annually

endoscopic screening identified one-time endoscopic screening at the age of 50 years to be cost-effective in high-incidence regions of China.[44]

Targeted Screening of Esophageal Squamous Cell Carcinoma in High-Risk Individuals

Given the modest incidence of ESCC in the United States, mass screening of ESCC is unlikely to be cost-effective. However, targeted screening should be considered for certain high-risk groups, including those with tylosis, achalasia, history of esophageal caustic injury, history of head and neck cancer, or high-risk racial/ethnic background. The AGA screening recommendations for such groups are described in **Table 3**.[45]

EPIDEMIOLOGY OF GASTRIC CANCER

Gastric cancer (GC) is the sixth most common cancer and third leading cause of cancer deaths globally, responsible for 1.1 million new cases and 770,000 deaths in 2020.[1] GC carries a dismal prognosis with an overall 5-year survival rate of 33%.[6] This is largely attributable to late detection of GC with 35% of patients diagnosed with distant-stage disease.[4]

Gastric adenocarcinoma (GAC) is the predominant histologic subtype comprising 90% to 95% of GCs,[46] characterized by highly variable incidence. High-incidence regions include East Asia, Central Asia, and Andean Latin America, where the ASRs exceed 15 per 100,000 person-years.[47] Low-incidence regions include eastern sub-Saharan Africa, North America, Western Europe, and Oceania, where the rates fall to less than 6 per 100,000 person-years.[47] In the United States, incidence is disproportionately high in certain racial/ethnic groups, including Hispanics, Asians, African Americans, and Native Americans/Alaska Natives.[47]

Table 3
American Gastroenterological Association guidelines for screening of esophageal squamous cell carcinoma

Risk Factor	Recommendations[45]
Tylosis	Endoscopic screening with 4-quadrant biopsies from the proximal, middle, and distal esophagus every 1–3 y beginning at the age of 30 y should be considered
Achalasia	Endoscopic screening annually beginning 10–15 y after disease onset should be considered
History of esophageal caustic injury	Endoscopic screening every 2–3 y beginning 10–20 y after the initial injury should be considered
History of head and neck cancer	Endoscopic screening with Lugol chromoendoscopy or narrow-band imaging every 6–12 mo for 10 y beginning 10 y after the completion of cancer treatment should be considered
High-risk racial/ethnic background (eg, Asians, African Americans)	One-time endoscopic screening with Lugol chromoendoscopy beginning at the age of 40 y should be considered

CAUSE OF GASTRIC ADENOCARCINOMA

Pathogenesis of GAC has been characterized by the Correa cascade in which chronic inflammatory insult, such as *Helicobacter pylori* (Hp) infection or autoimmune gastritis (AIG), results in the development and progression of precancerous lesions from non-atrophic gastritis to atrophic gastritis (AG) to gastric intestinal metaplasia (GIM) to dysplasia and finally to carcinoma (**Fig. 1D–F**).[48] The prevalence of AG is estimated to be 15% in the United States and likely greater in racial/ethnic minorities, immigrants from high-incidence regions, and those with family history of GAC.[47] The annual risk of AG progression to GAC is estimated to be 0.1% to 0.3%.[49] The prevalence of GIM is estimated to be 4.8%[50] with an annual risk of GAC of 0.16%,[51] which increases based on the extent and severity of GIM.[52] Extensive GIM involving both the antrum and the corpus confers 2.1-fold higher risk versus limited GIM confined to the antrum, whereas incomplete GIM resembling the colonic epithelium confers 3.3-fold higher risk versus complete GIM resembling the small intestinal epithelium.[51]

The most common inciting events for the carcinogenic sequence are Hp infection and AIG, of which Hp infection is the predominant cause (see **Table 1**). Hp is the leading global carcinogen for GAC, accounting for 6.2% of all cancers and up to 90% of GACs globally.[47] AIG is a less common cause, characterized by production of autoantibodies against parietal cells and intrinsic factor and immune-mediated destruction of oxyntic mucosa.[49] The incidence of GAC in patients with AIG is estimated to be 1% to 3%.[53] Pernicious anemia (PA) is a late manifestation and an indicator of severe AIG that confers a markedly higher risk of GAC.[54] AIG is also associated with type 1 gastric neuroendocrine tumors (NETs), with an annual incidence rate of 0.4% to 0.7%[49] Various other environmental and host-related risk factors have been established for GAC, including smoking,[55] high-salt diets,[56] consumption of total, red, or processed meat,[57] and heavy alcohol consumption.[58] Familial clustering of GAC has also been observed in approximately 10% of cases.[59]

GASTRIC ADENOCARCINOMA SCREENING
Endoscopic Evaluation of Precancerous Gastric Lesions

High-quality endoscopic examination is essential for reliable detection and prognostication of AG and GIM. The entire gastric lumen should be thoroughly inspected with an endoscopic procedure time of ≥ 7 minutes and systematic photo-documentation to optimize diagnostic yield.[47] Focal abnormalities warrant targeted examination using image-enhancing techniques, such as NBI, to improve detection of precancerous lesions.[49] Gastric biopsies for Hp testing or surveillance of precancerous lesions should be obtained following the updated Sydney protocol, which provides topographic assessment of precancerous lesions for risk stratification as well as nearly 100% sensitivity for Hp colonization.[47,49] In addition to targeted biopsies of visible lesions, biopsies should be obtained from the incisura angularis and greater and lesser curvatures of both the corpus and the antrum, collected separately in a minimum of 2 jars discriminating the biopsies of the corpus and antrum/incisura.

The Operative Link for Gastritis Assessment (OLGA) and Operative Link on Gastric Intestinal Metaplasia Assessment (OLGIM) are validated staging systems for prognosticating precancerous gastric lesions based on the anatomic extent and histologic grade of mucosal changes,[49] in which advanced stages correlate with higher risk of GAC.[47] Although both OLGA and OLGIM have been endorsed by international guidelines,[60,61] their use is not broadly adopted in current clinical practice in the United States.[47]

Population-Based Screening of Gastric Adenocarcinoma in High-Incidence Regions

Japan and Korea have distinctively implemented nationwide endoscopic and radiographic screening programs for GAC with measurable success as highlighted by their impressive 5-year survival rates exceeding 60% in contrast to 33% globally.[6,62] Several observational studies in both Japan and Korea have demonstrated superior performance of endoscopic versus radiographic screening in GAC detection and survival benefit.[63–68] Currently, the Japanese national screening guidelines recommend biennial screening by either endoscopy or radiography for individuals of aged ≥50 years with no upper age limit.[69] The Korean national guidelines recommend biennial screening by endoscopy as the first-line screening modality for individuals of aged 40 to 74 years.[63]

Targeted Surveillance of Precancerous Gastric Lesions in High-Risk Individuals

Although universal screening of GAC in the United States is unlikely to be cost-effective because of its modest incidence, targeted surveillance of high-risk individuals with established precancerous gastric lesions has been an important focus for secondary prevention. Although optimal strategies for surveillance of AG and GIM remain unclear, the AGA and ASGE have developed guidelines to address this need **(Table 4)**.[49,52,70] For patients with AG, the AGA suggests consideration of surveillance at 3-year intervals in those with advanced AG corresponding to OLGA/OLGIM stages III/IV. For patients with AIG, consideration of surveillance based on individualized assessment and shared decision making is suggested without a specified interval. For patients with PA, endoscopic evaluation at the time of PA diagnosis is recommended for staging of AG and screening of prevalent gastric neoplasia, such as NETs; consideration of surveillance at 1- to 2-year intervals is suggested depending on the burden of NETs. Similarly, the ASGE suggests endoscopic evaluation of patients with PA within 6 months of PA diagnosis. For patients with GIM, all guidelines suggest consideration of surveillance in high-risk individuals. The AGA defines high-risk individuals as those with extensive or incomplete GIM or those with any GIM plus family history of GAC, high-risk racial/ethnic background, or immigration from high-incidence regions, and suggests a surveillance interval of 3 to 5 years. The ASGE defines high-risk individuals as those with family history of GAC or high-risk racial/ethnic background, and although a surveillance interval was not specified, suggests suspension of surveillance when 2 consecutive endoscopies are negative for dysplasia.

EPIDEMIOLOGY OF SMALL-BOWEL CANCER

Small-bowel cancers (SBCs) are rare, comprising 0.6% of all cancers and 3% of GI cancers in the United States.[71] SBCs were responsible for 12,070 new cases and 2070 deaths in the United States in 2023.[6] The 5-year survival rate for SBC is 65%, which decreases to 41.2% for distant-stage disease.[72] Small-bowel adenocarcinoma (SBAC) is a major histologic subtype comprising 40% of SBCs.[72] Notably, approximately 20% of SBACs occur in the context of predisposing conditions.[73]

SMALL-BOWEL ADENOCARCINOMA SCREENING IN HEREDITARY CANCER SYNDROMES

Increased risk of SBAC is well-established in patients with hereditary GI cancer syndromes, including familial adenomatous polyposis (FAP), Peutz-Jeghers syndrome (PJS), and Lynch syndrome (LS),[74] and warrants special screening considerations.

Table 4
US guidelines for surveillance of precancerous gastric lesions

Source	Recommendations	
	AG	GIM
AGA[49,52]	Endoscopic surveillance every 3 y should be considered for patients with advanced AG corresponding to OLGA/OLGIM stages III/IV For patients with AIG, endoscopic surveillance should be considered based on individualized assessment and shared decision making; optimal surveillance interval is unclear For patients with PA, endoscopic evaluation at the time of PA diagnosis is recommended to assess AG and rule out prevalent gastric neoplasia, such as NETs; surveillance every 1–2 y should be considered depending on the burden of NETs	Endoscopic surveillance every 3–5 y should be considered for patients at increased risk of GAC, if shared decision making favors surveillance Patients with GIM at increased risk of GAC include those with • Incomplete vs complete GIM • Extensive vs limited GIM • Family history of GAC Patients at overall increased risk of GAC include • Racial/ethnic minorities (eg, Hispanics, Asians, African Americans, Native Americans/Alaska Natives) • Immigrants from high-incidence regions
ASGE[70]	For patients with PA, endoscopic evaluation within 6 mo of PA diagnosis is suggested	Endoscopic surveillance should be considered for patients at increased risk of GAC due to family history of GAC or high-risk racial/ethnic background (eg, Asians) Optimal surveillance interval is unclear; surveillance may be suspended when 2 consecutive endoscopies are negative for dysplasia

The ACG has provided important insights for SBAC screening in this population (**Table 5**).[75]

FAP is an autosomal dominant disorder owing to a germline mutation in the adenomatous polyposis coli (*APC*) gene, characterized by development of innumerable adenomatous polyps throughout the colorectum as well as the small intestine typically beginning at the age of 10 years. The duodenum is the most common extracolonic site of polyposis[76] and cancer,[72] with 88% lifetime risk of duodenal polyposis and 18% cumulative risk of cancer by the age of 75 years.[77] The Spigelman classification is a validated staging system for prognosticating duodenal polyposis based on the number, size, histologic features, and degree of dysplasia, in which advanced stages correlate with higher risk of SBAC.[72] The ACG recommends SBAC screening by upper endoscopy in patients with FAP beginning at the age of 25 to 30 years, with repeat examinations at intervals dictated by the Spigelman staging. For stages 0, I, II, and III, intervals of 4 years, 2 to 3 years, 1 to 3 years, and 6 to 12 months, respectively, are recommended; for stage IV, surgical evaluation is recommended.

PJS is an autosomal dominant disorder owing to a germline mutation in the serine/threonine kinase 11 (*STK11*) gene, characterized by focal mucocutaneous pigmentation as well as hamartomatous polyposis throughout the GI tract. Polyps occur mainly in the small bowel with a prevalence of 65%,[78] of which the jejunum is the most commonly involved segment.[79] The incidence of SBAC has been estimated to be as high as 13% in patients with PJS.[72] The ACG recommends SBAC screening by video capsule endoscopy in patients with PJS beginning at the age of 8 years, with repeat examinations at 3-year intervals.

LS is an autosomal dominant disorder owing to a germline mutation in DNA mismatch repair genes (*MLH1, MSH2, MSH6, PMS2, EPCAM*) and confers greater

---

Table 5
American College of Gastroenterology guidelines for screening of small-bowel adenocarcinoma in hereditary cancer syndromes

Syndrome	Recommendations[75]
Familial adenomatous polyposis	Screening by upper endoscopy beginning at the age of 25–30 y, with repeat exams at intervals dictated by the Spigelman staging of duodenal polyposis, is recommended: • Stage 0: 4 y • Stage I: 2–3 y • Stage II: 1–3 y • Stage III: 6–12 mo • Stage IV: surgical evaluation No specific recommendations for screening of the small bowel beyond the reach of upper endoscope are provided
Peutz-Jeghers syndrome	Screening by video capsule endoscopy every 3 y beginning at the age of 8 y is recommended
Lynch syndrome	Screening by upper endoscopy beginning at the age of 30–35 y should be considered with repeat exams every 3–5 y for patients with family history of duodenal cancer No specific recommendations for screening of the small bowel beyond the reach of upper endoscope are provided

than 100-fold higher risk of SBAC compared with the general population with as high as 12% lifetime risk.[72] The duodenum is the most commonly involved segment of the small bowel, accounting for 43% of SBACs.[80] The ACG suggests consideration of SBAC screening by upper endoscopy in patients with LS beginning at the age of 30 to 35 years, with repeat examinations at 3- to 5-year intervals for those with family history of duodenal cancer.

DISCUSSION
Identifying High-Risk Individuals for Targeted Screening and Surveillance

Strategies for screening and early detection of upper GI cancers are complicated by their highly variable global footprint, rendering universal screening ineffective in most populations globally. Although some success has been demonstrated for universal endoscopic or radiographic screening programs for ESCC and GAC, it has been limited to regions of Asia with exceptionally high disease burdens.[43,63–69] In regions of modest incidence, such as the United States, a targeted approach for high-risk individuals is more optimal. However, identifying high-risk individuals who are often asymptomatic remains challenging and requires comprehensive informed risk assessment of demographic, familial, and clinicopathologic factors. Detection of precancerous lesions can be highly informative, as they represent quantifiable disease states with prognostic values that can guide clinical decisions regarding surveillance. Risk prediction models have been developed to aid risk stratification of patients with known precancerous lesions. The Progression in Barrett's Esophagus score is a validated risk prediction model for predicting BE progression to HGD/EAC that stratifies patients into low-, intermediate-, or high-risk groups based on male gender, smoking, length of BE, and the presence of baseline LGD, wherein a greater than 16-fold higher risk was seen in high- versus low-risk group.[81] Integration of risk prediction models into clinical practice requires a coordinated effort of gastroenterologists and pathologists to ensure collection of necessary clinicopathologic data in their evaluation of precancerous lesions.

Innovations in Screening and Early Detection of Upper Gastrointestinal Cancers

Numerous exciting advances in screening and early detection of upper GI cancers are on the horizon and likely to bring major shifts in clinical paradigms in the future. Notably, recent progress in artificial intelligence is promising for enhancing endoscopic detection of precancerous lesions in the luminal GI tract and reducing operator dependency.[82,83] There is also an ongoing flurry of research in high-throughput molecular diagnostics of upper GI cancers, such as liquid biopsies using blood, urine, and saliva for detection of biomarkers, which may potentially generate cost-effectiveness ratios that rationalize mass screening programs for upper GI cancers.[84,85] Furthermore, advances in deep sequencing technologies may augment risk stratification of patients at the molecular level via epigenomic, genomic, or transcriptomic profiling.[86]

SUMMARY

Early detection of upper GI cancers and improvement of patient outcomes may be achieved by targeted endoscopic screening and surveillance of high-risk individuals. Identification of such individuals who warrant screening and surveillance is fundamental to this task and requires a comprehensive risk assessment that involves evaluation of precancerous lesions for prognostication. Refinement and validation of risk prediction models should be an area of future focus.

CLINICS CARE POINTS

- Effective screening of upper gastrointestinal cancers in regions of modest incidence, such as the United States, requires a targeted approach for high-risk individuals based on demographic, familial, and clinicopathologic risk factors.
- Assessment of precancerous lesions is pivotal for risk stratification of patients and informing clinical decisions for surveillance.
- Endoscopic evaluation of precancerous lesions should follow standardized reporting systems, such as the Prague and Paris classifications for Barrett esophagus, and biopsy protocols, such as the Seattle biopsy protocol for Barrett esophagus and updated Sydney protocol for atrophic gastritis/gastric intestinal metaplasia, to optimize diagnostic yield.
- Image-enhancing techniques, such as narrow-band imaging, improve detection of precancerous lesions and should be standard-of-care in screening and surveillance endoscopies.
- Validated staging systems, such as the Operative Link for Gastritis Assessment/Operative Link on Gastric Intestinal Metaplasia Assessment for atrophic gastritis/gastric intestinal metaplasia and Spigelman classification for duodenal polyposis, should be used routinely to improve risk stratification of patients.
- Endoscopic screening of esophageal adenocarcinoma should be considered for patients with multiple Barrett esophagus risk factors, including chronic gastroesophageal acid reflux disease, male gender, age greater than 50 years, non-Hispanic white background, smoking, obesity, and family history of Barrett esophagus/esophageal adenocarcinoma; for patients with nondysplastic Barrett esophagus, endoscopic surveillance at 3- to 5-year intervals based on the length of Barrett esophagus is recommended.
- Endoscopic screening of esophageal squamous cell carcinoma should be considered for individuals with tylosis, achalasia, history of esophageal caustic injury, history of head and neck cancer, or high-risk racial/ethnic background.
- Endoscopic screening of gastric adenocarcinoma at 3-year intervals should be considered for patients with advanced atrophic gastritis corresponding to Operative Link for Gastritis Assessment/Operative Link on Gastric Intestinal Metaplasia Assessment stages III/IV; endoscopic evaluation is recommended for patients with autoimmune gastritis and Pernicious anemia at the time of Pernicious anemia diagnosis.
- Endoscopic screening of gastric adenocarcinoma at 3- to 5-year intervals should be considered for patients with gastric intestinal metaplasia at higher risk of progression to gastric adenocarcinoma based on the extent and severity of gastric intestinal metaplasia and the presence of familial or demographic risk factors.
- Endoscopic screening of small-bowel adenocarcinoma should be considered in patients with hereditary gastrointestinal cancer syndromes.

DISCLOSURE

None.

REFERENCES

1. Sung H, Ferlay J, Siegel RL, et al. Global Cancer Statistics 2020: GLOBOCAN Estimates of Incidence and Mortality Worldwide for 36 Cancers in 185 Countries. CA Cancer J Clin 2021;71(3):209–49.
2. Codipilly DC, Qin Y, Dawsey SM, et al. Screening for esophageal squamous cell carcinoma: recent advances. Gastrointest Endosc 2018;88(3):413–26.

3. Asge Standards Of Practice C, Qumseya B, Sultan S, et al. ASGE guideline on screening and surveillance of Barrett's esophagus. Gastrointest Endosc 2019; 90(3):335–359 e332.

4. Thrift AP, El-Serag HB. Burden of Gastric Cancer. Clin Gastroenterol Hepatol 2020;18(3):534–42.

5. Morgan E, Soerjomataram I, Rumgay H, et al. The Global Landscape of Esophageal Squamous Cell Carcinoma and Esophageal Adenocarcinoma Incidence and Mortality in 2020 and Projections to 2040: New Estimates From GLOBOCAN 2020. Gastroenterology 2022;163(3):649–658 e642.

6. Siegel RL, Miller KD, Wagle NS, et al. Cancer statistics, 2023. CA Cancer J Clin 2023;73(1):17–48.

7. Xie SH, Rabbani S, Petrick JL, et al. Racial and Ethnic Disparities in the Incidence of Esophageal Cancer in the United States, 1992-2013. Am J Epidemiol 2017; 186(12):1341–51.

8. Standards of Practice C, Wani S, Qumseya B, et al. Endoscopic eradication therapy for patients with Barrett's esophagus-associated dysplasia and intramucosal cancer. Gastrointest Endosc 2018;87(4):907–931 e909.

9. Qumseya BJ, Wani S, Gendy S, et al. Disease Progression in Barrett's Low-Grade Dysplasia With Radiofrequency Ablation Compared With Surveillance: Systematic Review and Meta-Analysis. Am J Gastroenterol 2017;112(6):849–65.

10. Shaheen NJ, Falk GW, Iyer PG, et al. ACG Clinical Guideline: Diagnosis and Management of Barrett's Esophagus. Am J Gastroenterol 2016;111(1):30–50 [quiz: 51].

11. Alcedo J, Ferrandez A, Arenas J, et al. Trends in Barrett's esophagus diagnosis in Southern Europe: implications for surveillance. Dis Esophagus 2009;22(3): 239–48.

12. Kubo A, Corley DA. Body mass index and adenocarcinomas of the esophagus or gastric cardia: a systematic review and meta-analysis. Cancer Epidemiol Biomarkers Prev 2006;15(5):872–8.

13. Oze I, Matsuo K, Ito H, et al. Cigarette smoking and esophageal cancer risk: an evaluation based on a systematic review of epidemiologic evidence among the Japanese population. Jpn J Clin Oncol 2012;42(1):63–73.

14. Andrici J, Tio M, Cox MR, et al. Hiatal hernia and the risk of Barrett's esophagus. J Gastroenterol Hepatol 2013;28(3):415–31.

15. Tofani CJ, Gandhi K, Spataro J, et al. Esophageal adenocarcinoma in a first-degree relative increases risk for esophageal adenocarcinoma in patients with Barrett's esophagus. United European Gastroenterol J 2019;7(2):225–9.

16. Dawsey SM, Lewin KJ, Wang GQ, et al. Squamous esophageal histology and subsequent risk of squamous cell carcinoma of the esophagus. A prospective follow-up study from Linxian, China. Cancer 1994;74(6):1686–92.

17. Wang GQ, Abnet CC, Shen Q, et al. Histological precursors of oesophageal squamous cell carcinoma: results from a 13 year prospective follow up study in a high risk population. Gut 2005;54(2):187–92.

18. Lee CH, Lee JM, Wu DC, et al. Independent and combined effects of alcohol intake, tobacco smoking and betel quid chewing on the risk of esophageal cancer in Taiwan. Int J Cancer 2005;113(3):475–82.

19. Wheeler JB, Reed CE. Epidemiology of esophageal cancer. Surg Clin North Am 2012;92(5):1077–87.

20. Mlombe YB, Rosenberg NE, Wolf LL, et al. Environmental risk factors for oesophageal cancer in Malawi: A case-control study. Malawi Med J 2015;27(3):88–92.

21. Kochhar R, Sethy PK, Kochhar S, et al. Corrosive induced carcinoma of esophagus: report of three patients and review of literature. J Gastroenterol Hepatol 2006;21(4):777–80.

22. Sur M, Cooper K. The role of the human papilloma virus in esophageal cancer. Pathology 1998;30(4):348–54.

23. Harper PS, Harper RM, Howel-Evans AW. Carcinoma of the oesophagus with tylosis. Q J Med 1970;39(155):317–33.

24. ASoP Committee, Evans JA, Early DS, et al. The role of endoscopy in Barrett's esophagus and other premalignant conditions of the esophagus. Gastrointest Endosc 2012;76(6):1087–94.

25. Ferguson A, Kingstone K. Coeliac disease and malignancies. Acta Paediatr Suppl 1996;412:78–81.

26. Abemayor E, Moore DM, Hanson DG. Identification of synchronous esophageal tumors in patients with head and neck cancer. J Surg Oncol 1988;38(2):94–6.

27. Kim JA, Shah PM. Screening and prevention strategies and endoscopic management of early esophageal cancer. Chin Clin Oncol 2017;6(5):50.

28. Bisschops R, Areia M, Coron E, et al. Performance measures for upper gastrointestinal endoscopy: a European Society of Gastrointestinal Endoscopy (ESGE) Quality Improvement Initiative. Endoscopy 2016;48(9):843–64.

29. Wani S, Yadlapati R, Singh S, et al. Post-Endoscopy Esophageal Neoplasia Expert Consensus P. Post-endoscopy Esophageal Neoplasia in Barrett's Esophagus: Consensus Statements From an International Expert Panel. Gastroenterology 2022;162(2):366–72.

30. Xiong YQ, Ma SJ, Hu HY, et al. Comparison of narrow-band imaging and confocal laser endomicroscopy for the detection of neoplasia in Barrett's esophagus: A meta-analysis. Clin Res Hepatol Gastroenterol 2018;42(1):31–9.

31. Codipilly DC, Krishna Chandar A, Wang KK, et al. Wide-area transepithelial sampling for dysplasia detection in Barrett's esophagus: a systematic review and meta-analysis. Gastrointest Endosc 2022;95(1):51–59 e57.

32. Vennalaganti P, Kanakadandi V, Goldblum JR, et al. Discordance Among Pathologists in the United States and Europe in Diagnosis of Low-Grade Dysplasia for Patients With Barrett's Esophagus. Gastroenterology 2017;152(3):564–570 e564.

33. Muthusamy VR, Wani S, Gyawali CP, et al. AGA Clinical Practice Update on New Technology and Innovation for Surveillance and Screening in Barrett's Esophagus: Expert Review. Clin Gastroenterol Hepatol 2022;20(12):2696–2706 e2691.

34. Januszewicz W, Tan WK, Lehovsky K, et al. Safety and Acceptability of Esophageal Cytosponge Cell Collection Device in a Pooled Analysis of Data From Individual Patients. Clin Gastroenterol Hepatol 2019;17(4):647–656 e641.

35. Shaheen NJ, Falk GW, Iyer PG, et al. Diagnosis and Management of Barrett's Esophagus: An Updated ACG Guideline. Am J Gastroenterol 2022;117(4):559–87.

36. Ross-Innes CS, Debiram-Beecham I, O'Donovan M, et al. Evaluation of a minimally invasive cell sampling device coupled with assessment of trefoil factor 3 expression for diagnosing Barrett's esophagus: a multi-center case-control study. PLoS Med 2015;12(1):e1001780.

37. Shaheen NJ, Komanduri S, Muthusamy VR, et al. Acceptability and Adequacy of a Non-endoscopic Cell Collection Device for Diagnosis of Barrett's Esophagus: Lessons Learned. Dig Dis Sci 2022;67(1):177–86.

38. Iyer PG, Taylor WR, Johnson ML, et al. Accurate Nonendoscopic Detection of Barrett's Esophagus by Methylated DNA Markers: A Multisite Case Control Study. Am J Gastroenterol 2020;115(8):1201–9.

39. Iyer PG, Taylor WR, Slettedahl SW, et al. Validation of a methylated DNA marker panel for the nonendoscopic detection of Barrett's esophagus in a multisite case-control study. Gastrointest Endosc 2021;94(3):498–505.

40. Moinova HR, LaFramboise T, Lutterbaugh JD, et al. Identifying DNA methylation biomarkers for non-endoscopic detection of Barrett's esophagus. Sci Transl Med 2018;10(424).

41. Wang Z, Kambhampati S, Cheng Y, et al. Methylation Biomarker Panel Performance in EsophaCap Cytology Samples for Diagnosing Barrett's Esophagus: A Prospective Validation Study. Clin Cancer Res 2019;25(7):2127–35.

42. Sharma P, Shaheen NJ, Katzka D, et al. AGA Clinical Practice Update on Endoscopic Treatment of Barrett's Esophagus With Dysplasia and/or Early Cancer: Expert Review. Gastroenterology 2020;158(3):760–9.

43. Wei WQ, Chen ZF, He YT, et al. Long-Term Follow-Up of a Community Assignment, One-Time Endoscopic Screening Study of Esophageal Cancer in China. J Clin Oncol 2015;33(17):1951–7.

44. Yang J, Wei WQ, Niu J, et al. Cost-benefit analysis of esophageal cancer endoscopic screening in high-risk areas of China. World J Gastroenterol 2012;18(20): 2493–501.

45. Wang KK, Wongkeesong M, Buttar NS, et al. American Gastroenterological Association medical position statement: Role of the gastroenterologist in the management of esophageal carcinoma. Gastroenterology 2005;128(5):1468–70.

46. Richman DM, Tirumani SH, Hornick JL, et al. Beyond gastric adenocarcinoma: Multimodality assessment of common and uncommon gastric neoplasms. Abdom Radiol (NY) 2017;42(1):124–40.

47. Huang RJ, Laszkowska M, In H, et al. Controlling Gastric Cancer in a World of Heterogeneous Risk. Gastroenterology 2023;164(5):736–51.

48. Correa P. A human model of gastric carcinogenesis. Cancer Res 1988;48(13): 3554–60.

49. Shah SC, Piazuelo MB, Kuipers EJ, et al. AGA Clinical Practice Update on the Diagnosis and Management of Atrophic Gastritis: Expert Review. Gastroenterology 2021;161(4):1325–1332 e1327.

50. Altayar O, Davitkov P, Shah SC, et al. AGA Technical Review on Gastric Intestinal Metaplasia-Epidemiology and Risk Factors. Gastroenterology 2020;158(3): 732–744 e716.

51. Gawron AJ, Shah SC, Altayar O, et al. AGA Technical Review on Gastric Intestinal Metaplasia-Natural History and Clinical Outcomes. Gastroenterology 2020; 158(3):705–731 e705.

52. Gupta S, Li D, El Serag HB, et al. AGA Clinical Practice Guidelines on Management of Gastric Intestinal Metaplasia. Gastroenterology 2020;158(3):693–702.

53. Yoon H, Kim N. Diagnosis and management of high risk group for gastric cancer. Gut Liver 2015;9(1):5–17.

54. Vannella L, Lahner E, Osborn J, et al. Systematic review: gastric cancer incidence in pernicious anaemia. Aliment Pharmacol Ther 2013;37(4):375–82.

55. Ladeiras-Lopes R, Pereira AK, Nogueira A, et al. Smoking and gastric cancer: systematic review and meta-analysis of cohort studies. Cancer Causes Control 2008;19(7):689–701.

56. Tsugane S, Sasazuki S. Diet and the risk of gastric cancer: review of epidemiological evidence. Gastric Cancer 2007;10(2):75–83.

57. Gonzalez CA, Jakszyn P, Pera G, et al. Meat intake and risk of stomach and esophageal adenocarcinoma within the European Prospective Investigation Into Cancer and Nutrition (EPIC). J Natl Cancer Inst 2006;98(5):345–54.

58. Wang PL, Xiao FT, Gong BC, et al. Alcohol drinking and gastric cancer risk: a meta-analysis of observational studies. Oncotarget 2017;8(58):99013–23.
59. Oliveira C, Pinheiro H, Figueiredo J, et al. Familial gastric cancer: genetic susceptibility, pathology, and implications for management. Lancet Oncol 2015;16(2):e60–70.
60. Banks M, Graham D, Jansen M, et al. British Society of Gastroenterology guidelines on the diagnosis and management of patients at risk of gastric adenocarcinoma. Gut 2019;68(9):1545–75.
61. Pimentel-Nunes P, Libanio D, Marcos-Pinto R, et al. Management of epithelial precancerous conditions and lesions in the stomach (MAPS II): European Society of Gastrointestinal Endoscopy (ESGE), European Helicobacter and Microbiota Study Group (EHMSG), European Society of Pathology (ESP), and Sociedade Portuguesa de Endoscopia Digestiva (SPED) guideline update 2019. Endoscopy 2019;51(4):365–88.
62. Allemani C, Matsuda T, Di Carlo V, et al. Global surveillance of trends in cancer survival 2000-14 (CONCORD-3): analysis of individual records for 37 513 025 patients diagnosed with one of 18 cancers from 322 population-based registries in 71 countries. Lancet 2018;391(10125):1023–75.
63. Jun JK, Choi KS, Lee HY, et al. Effectiveness of the Korean National Cancer Screening Program in Reducing Gastric Cancer Mortality. Gastroenterology 2017;152(6):1319–1328 e1317.
64. Kim H, Hwang Y, Sung H, et al. Effectiveness of Gastric Cancer Screening on Gastric Cancer Incidence and Mortality in a Community-Based Prospective Cohort. Cancer Res Treat 2018;50(2):582–9.
65. Choi KS, Jun JK, Park EC, et al. Performance of different gastric cancer screening methods in Korea: a population-based study. PLoS One 2012;7(11):e50041.
66. Hamashima C, Ogoshi K, Okamoto M, et al. A community-based, case-control study evaluating mortality reduction from gastric cancer by endoscopic screening in Japan. PLoS One 2013;8(11):e79088.
67. Hamashima C, Shabana M, Okada K, et al. Mortality reduction from gastric cancer by endoscopic and radiographic screening. Cancer Sci 2015;106(12):1744–9.
68. Hamashima C, Okamoto M, Shabana M, et al. Sensitivity of endoscopic screening for gastric cancer by the incidence method. Int J Cancer 2013;133(3):653–9.
69. Hamashima C. Systematic Review G, Guideline Development Group for Gastric Cancer Screening G. Update version of the Japanese Guidelines for Gastric Cancer Screening. Jpn J Clin Oncol 2018;48(7):673–83.
70. Committee ASoP, Evans JA, Chandrasekhara V, et al. The role of endoscopy in the management of premalignant and malignant conditions of the stomach. Gastrointest Endosc 2015;82(1):1–8.
71. Vlachou E, Koffas A, Toumpanakis C, et al. Updates in the diagnosis and management of small-bowel tumors. Best Pract Res Clin Gastroenterol 2023;64-65:101860.
72. Sanchez-Mete L, Stigliano V. Update on small bowel surveillance in hereditary colorectal cancer syndromes. Tumori 2019;105(1):12–21.
73. Aparicio T, Zaanan A, Mary F, et al. Small Bowel Adenocarcinoma. Gastroenterol Clin North Am 2016;45(3):447–57.
74. Aparicio T, Zaanan A, Svrcek M, et al. Small bowel adenocarcinoma: epidemiology, risk factors, diagnosis and treatment. Dig Liver Dis 2014;46(2):97–104.

75. Syngal S, Brand RE, Church JM, et al. ACG clinical guideline: Genetic testing and management of hereditary gastrointestinal cancer syndromes. Am J Gastroenterol 2015;110(2):223–62 [quiz: 263].

76. Bulow S, Bjork J, Christensen IJ, et al. Duodenal adenomatosis in familial adenomatous polyposis. Gut 2004;53(3):381–6.

77. Bulow S, Christensen IJ, Hojen H, et al. Duodenal surveillance improves the prognosis after duodenal cancer in familial adenomatous polyposis. Colorectal Dis 2012;14(8):947–52.

78. Utsunomiya J, Gocho H, Miyanaga T, et al. Peutz-Jeghers syndrome: its natural course and management. Johns Hopkins Med J 1975;136(2):71–82.

79. Giardiello FM, Brensinger JD, Tersmette AC, et al. Very high risk of cancer in familial Peutz-Jeghers syndrome. Gastroenterology 2000;119(6):1447–53.

80. Cheung DY, Kim JS, Shim KN, et al. Korean Gut Image Study G. The Usefulness of Capsule Endoscopy for Small Bowel Tumors. Clin Endosc 2016;49(1):21–5.

81. Parasa S, Vennalaganti S, Gaddam S, et al. Development and Validation of a Model to Determine Risk of Progression of Barrett's Esophagus to Neoplasia. Gastroenterology 2018;154(5):1282–1289 e1282.

82. Dilaghi E, Lahner E, Annibale B, et al. Systematic review and meta-analysis: Artificial intelligence for the diagnosis of gastric precancerous lesions and Helicobacter pylori infection. Dig Liver Dis 2022;54(12):1630–8.

83. Meinikheim M, Messmann H, Ebigbo A. Role of artificial intelligence in diagnosing Barrett's esophagus-related neoplasia. Clin Endosc 2023;56(1):14–22.

84. Ma S, Zhou M, Xu Y, et al. Clinical application and detection techniques of liquid biopsy in gastric cancer. Mol Cancer 2023;22(1):7.

85. Rai V, Abdo J, Agrawal DK. Biomarkers for Early Detection, Prognosis, and Therapeutics of Esophageal Cancers. Int J Mol Sci 2023;24(4).

86. Huang KK, Ramnarayanan K, Zhu F, et al. Genomic and Epigenomic Profiling of High-Risk Intestinal Metaplasia Reveals Molecular Determinants of Progression to Gastric Cancer. Cancer Cell 2018;33(1):137–150 e135.

Advances in the Imaging of Esophageal and Gastroesophageal Junction Malignancies

Lisa Ruby, MD, Vetri Sudar Jayaprakasam, MBBS, FRCR,
Maria Clara Fernandes, MD, MSc, Viktoriya Paroder, MD, PhD*

KEYWORDS

- Staging • Esophageal cancer • Computed tomography
- Positron emission tomography • MRI • Radiomics • HER2

KEY POINTS

- Accurate imaging is key for the diagnosis and treatment of esophageal and gastroesophageal junction malignances because of their complex anatomic location and variable presentation.
- Standard-of-care imaging modalities (computed tomography [CT] and ^{18}F-FDG [2-deoxy-2-[18F]fluoro-D-glucose] positron emission tomography [PET]/CT) for esophageal and gastroesophageal junction malignances are limited in tumor (T) and lymph node (N) staging.
- Advances in MRI technology offer promising solutions for T and N staging, especially in detecting residual disease and assessing treatment response.
- Novel PET tracers targeting biomarkers like HER2 and FAP are being explored to enhance diagnostic accuracy and treatment planning.
- Emerging methods like radiomics and artificial intelligence and theranostics have the potential to revolutionize esophageal cancer imaging, enabling personalized treatment approaches.

INTRODUCTION

Accurate imaging is key for the diagnosis and treatment of esophageal and gastroesophageal junction malignancies, particularly because of their complex anatomic location, often asymptomatic early stages, and the inherent challenges of surgical options. Currently, of the available imaging modalities, contrast-enhanced computed

Department of Radiology, Memorial Sloan Kettering Cancer Center, 1275 York Avenue, New York, NY 10065, USA
* Corresponding author.
E-mail address: paroderv@mskcc.org

Hematol Oncol Clin N Am 38 (2024) 711–730
https://doi.org/10.1016/j.hoc.2024.02.003
0889-8588/24/© 2024 Elsevier Inc. All rights reserved.

tomography (CT), endoscopic ultrasound (EUS), and 2-deoxy-2-[18F]fluoro-D-glucose positron emission tomography (PET)-CT (^{18}F-FDG PET/CT) are crucial for prognostication and treatment planning for these malignancies. In the current clinical practice, endoscopic resection is used to treat early stage disease; trimodality therapy (chemotherapy and radiotherapy followed by surgical resection) is used to treat resectable, locally advanced disease, and chemotherapy and radiotherapy are used to treat unresectable locally advanced or metastatic disease.[1]

Contrast-enhanced CT and ^{18}F-FDG PET/CT are the current standard-of-care imaging modalities for the staging of esophageal cancer, with ^{18}F-FDG PET/CT findings leading to changes in the therapeutic protocol in up to one-third of patients.[2] However, there are well-known limitations pertaining to the diagnostic accuracy of both CT and ^{18}F-FDG PET/CT for tumor (T) staging, and of ^{18}F-FDG PET/CT for regional nodal (N) staging. In terms of T staging, CT cannot distinguish between the different esophageal wall layers, making it unreliable for distinguishing between T1, T2, and T3 tumors; and in terms of N staging, CT-based assessment relies on unreliable size criterion.[3,4] Meanwhile, on ^{18}F-FDG PET/CT, peritumoral para-esophageal lymph nodes can be masked by ^{18}F-FDG uptake in the primary tumor.[5,6] Apart from CT and ^{18}F-FDG PET/CT, EUS is commonly used for T and N staging, but its applicability is limited by interoperator variability and nonfeasibility in up to one-third of patients presenting with high-grade strictures.[7]

In recent years, cutting-edge research and technological breakthroughs have offered increasing valuable insights into tumor morphology, vascularity, and molecular characteristics, enabling personalized treatment strategies. In this context, newer imaging techniques have also been explored to improve the staging and treatment response assessment of esophageal cancer. MRI with high soft tissue resolution can distinguish between the different gastrointestinal wall layers and appears to be a promising tool for T staging and the assessment of residual disease after treatment.[8] Meanwhile, advances in CT, including dynamic multiphase and dual-energy CT, have led to improved visualization of esophageal tumors.[9,10] Additionally, novel PET tracers have been investigated with the goal of improving staging and treatment response assessment.[11] Innovative radiolabeled probes targeting biomarkers such as human epidermal growth factor receptor 2 (HER2), epidermal growth factor receptor (EGFR), and fibroblast activating protein inhibitor (FAPI) are being explored to enhance diagnostic accuracy and improve treatment planning in patients with esophageal cancer.[12–16] Finally, recent strides in artificial intelligence have led to improvements and streamlining of image segmentation, feature extraction, and pattern recognition, with various applications such as the identification and characterization of lesions, the prediction of patient outcomes, and the optimization of treatment planning.

This article aims to describe current limitations in the imaging of esophageal and gastroesophageal junction malignancies for staging and treatment planning, and to explore the latest advances in imaging, with a focus on their implications for early detection, accurate staging, and improved therapeutic outcomes.

ANATOMY OF ESOPHAGEAL AND GASTROESOPHAGEAL JUNCTION MALIGNANCIES

Primary esophageal cancers are divided into cervical (between the hypopharynx to the sternal notch), thoracic (between the sternal notch to the gastroesophageal junction), and abdominal esophagus (between the gastroesophageal junction to 2 cm below the gastroesophageal junction) esophageal cancers. Thoracic esophageal cancers are further divided into upper (between the sternal notch to the azygos vein), middle (lower border of the azygos vein to the inferior pulmonary vein), and lower (lower border of the inferior pulmonary vein to the gastroesophageal junction) thoracic esophageal cancers. Of note, in the eighth version of the American Joint Committee of Cancer (AJCC) cancer staging manual, the anatomic boundary between the esophagus and the stomach was changed to include tumors involving the gastroesophageal junction with an epicenter of no more than 2 cm in the proximal stomach; meanwhile, esophageal tumors with an epicenter of more than 2 cm into the proximal stomach are considered gastric cancers even if the gastroesophageal junction is involved.[17]

STAGING USING COMPUTED TOMOGRAPHY AND ENDOSCOPIC ULTRASOUND

Table 1 presents the main stages for esophageal and gastroesophageal malignancies according to the eighth edition of the AJCC cancer staging manual. The T stage of the primary tumor is determined based on the depth of invasion of the esophageal wall layers (mucosa, submucosa, and the muscularis propria). Taking into consideration the difference in prognosis, pathologic T1 (pT1) is now subcategorized into pT1a and pT1b; additionally, there are unique stage groupings for clinical tumor node metastasis (cTNM) and post-neoadjuvant pathologic TNM (ypTNM).[18]

On CT, the primary esophageal tumor can present as an ill-defined mass or circumferential or eccentric mural thickening, or it can be visually occult (**Fig. 1**). Esophageal wall thickening is a nonspecific finding and is often seen as a result of inflammatory changes in the esophagus or in the setting of underdistension.[19] It is widely accepted that the thickness of the normal esophageal wall thickness on CT should be no more than 5 mm (3 mm in the distended esophagus), but this is rarely consistently achieved.[20] Differences in attenuation between the preoperative esophageal cancer and the background normal esophageal wall on contrast-enhanced CT can potentially differentiate the tumor from normal esophagus.[21] However, multiple studies have shown a wide range in sensitivity (60%–90%) and specificity (70%–95%) for tumor identification and significant interobserver variability in the localization of primary tumor on CT.[22] Crucially, because of its limited soft tissue contrast, CT cannot distinguish the different esophageal wall layers and thereby cannot distinguish between

Table 1 Esophageal cancer staging, American Joint Committee on Cancer Staging Manual, eighth edition[4]	
Stage	**Description**
Tis	High-grade dysplasia
T1	T1a: invasion of lamina propria or muscularis mucosa T1b: invasion of submucosa
T2	Invasion of muscularis propria
T3	Invasion of the adventitia
T4	T4a: invasion of adjacent structures, such as pleura, pericardium, azygos vein, diaphragm, and peritoneum T4b: invasion of major adjacent structures, such as the aorta, vertebral body, or trachea
N	Based on the number of regional lymph nodes involved
M	
M0	No distant metastases
M1	Presence of distant metastases

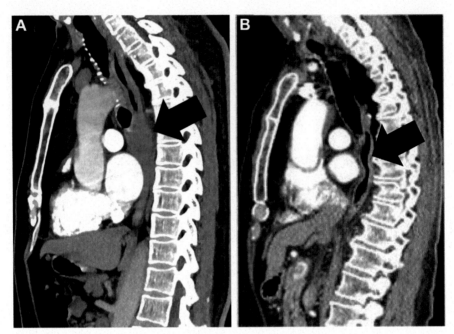

Fig. 1. Localization of esophageal tumors on CT. *(A)* Example of a midesophageal mass. *(B)* Example of a patient with a visually occult esophageal cancer on CT.

T1, T2 and T3 tumors.[3] On the other hand, CT can demonstrate the loss of the fat plane between the tumor and adjacent structures and the displacement of adjacent mediastinal structures with moderate to high accuracy.[23–25]

On EUS, it is possible to distinguish the different esophageal wall layers, including superficial mucosa (hyperechoic), muscularis mucosa (hypoechoic), submucosa (hyperechoic), muscularis propria (hypoechoic), and adventitia (hyperechoic). Thus, EUS has an accuracy of 71% to 92% for T staging.[7] For the discrimination of mucosal (T1a) and submucosal (T1b) tumors, which is important for identifying patients who can benefit from endoluminal treatment, EUS has a sensitivity of 72% to 85% and specificity of 49% to 87%; thereby, its value for distinguishing between T1a and T1b tumors continues to be a topic of debate.[26–28]

Lymph node involvement in esophageal cancer is a significant prognostic factor and an independent risk factor for long-term survival.[29] Once the submucosa is invaded (T1b), the risk of lymph node metastases is increased, with a 5-year cumulative incidence of over 30%.[30] The regional lymph nodes for esophageal cancer extend from the periesophageal lymph nodes to the celiac nodes, irrespective of tumor location (see **Table 1**). On CT, the evaluation of the lymph nodes is limited, as it is based mainly on size criteria, with a short axis of greater than 1 cm previously considered to indicate that a lymph node is likely metastatic. However, in a study of 1196 lymph nodes from 40 patients with esophageal cancer, the average size of positive lymph nodes was shown to be just under 0.7 cm, and fewer than 10% of all the resected lymph nodes were 1.0 cm or more.[4] Furthermore, lymph nodes that are in direct contact with the tumor and therefore indistinguishable can lead to false-negative results. All nodes visualized on CT should be noted on the imaging report, as AJCC recommends endoscopically guided fine needle aspiration for the confirmation of diagnosis with the intent of delineating the radiation therapy field accordingly.[18] Meanwhile, on EUS, features of suspicious lymph nodes include a size greater than 10 mm, round morphology, hypoechogenicity, and location in the vicinity of the primary tumor.[31] Drawbacks of EUS include interobserver variability and nonfeasibility in patients presenting with a high-grade strictures, which comprise 20% to 36% of patients with esophageal cancer.[7]

EVALUATION USING 2-DEOXY-2-[18F]FLUORO-D-GLUCOSE] POSITRON EMISSION TOMOGRAPHY/COMPUTED TOMOGRAPHY

^{18}F-FDG PET/CT has been used in evaluation of esophageal cancers for over 2 decades and has become a standard-of-care tool for staging, treatment response assessment, radiotherapy and surgical planning, post-treatment evaluation, follow-up, and surveillance.[2] Esophageal squamous cell carcinomas typically show high tracer uptake on ^{18}F-FDG PET/CT compared with adenocarcinomas, which exhibit low tracer uptake.[32] High tracer uptake on ^{18}F-FDG PET/CT can be helpful for the identification and localization of the primary tumors when they are not clearly demarcated on CT. However, false-positive results can be seen in esophagitis because of conditions such as gastroesophageal reflux disease, postinstrumentation inflammation, medication, or infection, and false-negative results may be seen in patients with small or early stage tumors.

^{18}F-FDG PET/CT has limited utility in the T staging of esophageal cancers and for regional lymph node staging. Of relevance to regional lymph node staging, squamous cell cancers typically advance locally first and subsequently involve the lymph nodes, whereas nodal metastases are seen early on with adenocarcinoma. For regional lymph node staging, ^{18}F-FDG PET/CT has low-to-moderate sensitivity (55%–66%) and moderate-to-high specificity (76%–96%).[33,34] However, ^{18}F-FDG PET/CT outperforms contrast-enhanced CT in terms of the positive predictive value for determining regional lymph nodal metastases (93.8% versus 62.5%).[35] False-negative nodal uptake can occur because of the limited spatial resolution of PET, leading to obscuration of the periesophageal lymph nodes by tracer uptake in the primary tumor and insufficient tracer uptake in the smaller lymph nodes.[5,6] False-positive nodal uptake can also occur in benign conditions, such as granulomatous diseases or other forms of inflammation.[36]

The greatest advantage of ^{18}F-FDG PET/CT is in the detection of metastases that may not be seen on conventional imaging modalities (**Fig. 2**). Indeed, ^{18}F-FDG PET/ CT findings can result in clinically significant changes to the initial staging of the malignancy and concurrently the treatment strategy in up to one-third of the patients.[37].[18]F-FDG PET/CT has also been shown to be of value for detecting metastases at restaging after treatment with curative intent.[38] Of note, for treatment planning, Toya and colleagues also observed reduced interobserver variability in the determination of gross tumor volume when using baseline ^{18}F-FDG PET/CT for tumor delineation and treatment planning.[39]

Regarding the value of ^{18}F-FDG PET/CT for treatment response assessment, following induction chemotherapy, a decrease in the maximum standardized uptake value (SUVmax) of over 35% on ^{18}F-FDG PET/CT has been significantly associated with improved disease-free survival and overall survival.[40] Meanwhile, following chemoradiotherapy, albeit locoregional assessment can be difficult because of radiation-induced inflammatory changes, ^{18}F-FDG PET/CT has been shown to be helpful in the detection of development of interval metastases that occur in approximately 8% of patients precluding potentially high-risk surgery.[41] Exemplary cases depicting the utility of ^{18}F-PET/CT for treatment response assessment are shown in **Fig. 3** and **4**.

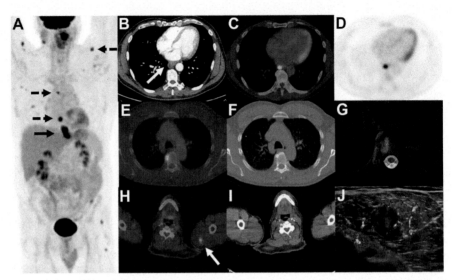

Fig. 2. Utility of PET/CT for the identification of metastatic disease in a 64-year-old patient with esophageal cancer. Coronal maximum intensity projection (MIP) (*A*) shows the primary gastroesophageal junction mass (*black arrow*) and sites of metastatic disease (dashed *lines*). CT (*B*), fused PET/CT (*C*), and PET (*D*) images of an FDG-avid periesophageal node are shown. Fused PET/CT (*E*), CT (*F*), and T2-weighted images (*G*) of a vertebral bone metastasis are depicted. A proximal left upper extremity soft tissue nodular lesion, which is not visible on contrast-enhanced CT (*I*), is FDG avid on PET/CT (*H*) and appears solid on ultrasound (*J*).

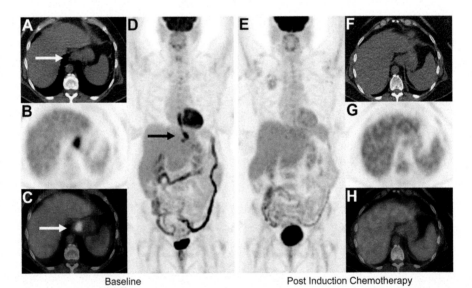

Baseline   Post Induction Chemotherapy

Fig. 3. Utility of PET/CT for treatment response assessment in a 56-year-old patient with esophageal cancer who responded to induction chemotherapy. Baseline axial CT (*A*), PET (*B*), fused PET/CT (*C*) and coronal PET maximum intensity projection (MIP) (*D*) depict hypermetabolic wall thickening at the gastroesophageal junction (*arrows*). Postinduction chemotherapy axial CT (*F*), PET (*G*), fused PET/CT (*H*), and coronal PET MIP (*E*) depict metabolic complete response.

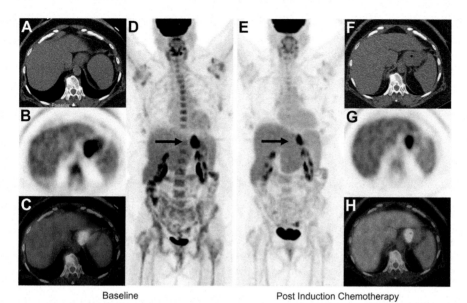

Baseline   Post Induction Chemotherapy

Fig. 4. Utility of FDG PET/CT for treatment response assessment in a 67-year-old patient with esophageal adenocarcinoma who did not respond to induction chemotherapy. Baseline axial CT (*A*), PET (*B*), fused PET/CT (*C*), and coronal PET MIP (*D*) show hypermetabolic wall thickening at the gastroesophageal junction (*arrow*). Postinduction chemotherapy axial CT (*F*), PET (*G*), fused PET/CT (*H*), and coronal PET MIP (*E*) depict persistent hypermetabolic wall thickening (*arrow*), consistent with nonresponse.

Although SUVmax is the most used parameter to assess the intensity of tracer uptake and to determine the metabolic activity of the tumor, this parameter is not representative of the entire tumor. In recent years, there is increasing interest in other quantitative PET parameters such as metabolic tumor volume (MTV), total lesion glycolysis (TLG), and intratumoral metabolic heterogeneity, which may provide better assessment and understanding of the metabolic and volumetric characteristics of the primary tumor. In a study of 62 patients with esophageal cancer, MTV of the primary tumor and total tumor burden were significantly associated with 1- and 5-year survival.[42] In other studies, baseline MTV and TLG have been found to be prognostic factors for overall survival and progression-free survival.[43–45] Higher intratumoral metabolic heterogeneity has also been shown to be associated with reduced progression-free survival.[46]

ADVANCES IN IMAGING
MRI

T staging
Given MRI's high soft tissue resolution and ability to distinguish between the different gastrointestinal wall layers, and further continuing advances in its technology, MRI has received increasing attention for the imaging of esophageal and gastroesophageal junction malignancies in recent years. On T2-weighted images, the esophageal wall can be divided into inner hypo-/intermediate signal mucosa, hyperintense submucosa, and outer hypointense muscularis layers.[8] Moreover, Yamada and colleagues showed that the depth of invasion can be accurately determined on T2-weighted images for 20 gastric carcinoma specimens using a 7 T scanner.[47]

Several studies have investigated the utility of MRI for T staging. A meta-analysis showed that MRI has a sensitivity of 92% for differentiating T0 (noninvasive) disease from T1 or higher disease, and a sensitivity of 86% for differentiating T2 or lower disease from T3 or higher disease.[48] A study by Chen and colleagues showed that dynamic contrast-enhanced (DCE) MRI aided in the diagnosis of early stage disease.[49] Given these results demonstrating the utility of MRI for detecting early stage disease, MRI might be of value to identify high-risk patients for invasive carcinoma, such as those with Barrett esophagus or dysplastic lesions.[48]

For those patients with locally advanced disease who undergo neoadjuvant therapy, in particular chemoradiotherapy, 29% to 43% will achieve complete pathologic response.[50] In contrast to currently utilized imaging methods, which show an insufficient diagnostic accuracy for detecting residual invasive disease after neoadjuvant therapy,[51,52] MRI might offer the opportunity to detect residual disease noninvasively.[48,53]

Comparing MRI with EUS, Qu and colleagues found MRI to be superior to EUS for the staging of T3/T4 lesions, whereas MRI and EUS were comparable for the staging of T1/T2 lesions.[54] In a small study by Giganti and colleagues comparing the use of MRI with diffusion-weighted imaging (DWI), multidetector CT, EUS, and ^{18}F-FDG PET/CT for the staging of esophageal cancer in 18 patients, MRI with DWI showed the highest specificity (92%) and accuracy (83%), whereas EUS showed the highest sensitivity (100%) for T staging.[55] In another small study by Harino and colleagues, the diagnostic performance of MRI (whereby MRI diagnostic criteria included the loss of the fat plane between the tumor and adjacent organs, displacement or indentation of adjacent mediastinal structures, disruption of the layer structure of adjacent organs and fibrosis of the tumor margins) was shown to be superior to CT for T4b esophageal cancer.[56] An exemplary case depicting the utility of MRI for local staging is shown in **Fig. 5**.

N staging
Wu and colleagues showed in their study involving 60 patients that DWI with a b value of 500 s/mm^2 can determine lymph node metastasis with a sensitivity of 94% and a

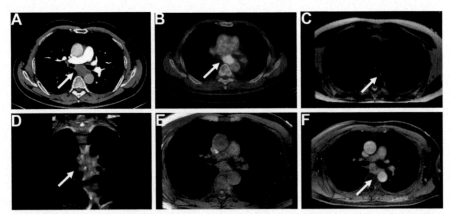

Fig. 5. Utility of MRI for local staging in a 58-year-old man with biphasic carcinoma (favoring salivary gland type) at the gastroesophageal junction. CT (A) and FDG PET/CT (B) show possible mediastinal invasion. Axial (C) and coronal (D) T2-weighted imaging depict an intermediate signal mass with adjacent mediastinal fat. Axial precontrast (E) and postcontrast (F) T1-weighted imaging show aortic abutment of less than 90° without invasion, compatible with T4a disease.

specificity of 73%.[57] Pultrum and colleagues showed in a small study involving 9 patients with esophageal cancer that MRI with ultrasmall superparamagnetic iron oxide identified most mediastinal and celiac lymph nodes suspicious for metastatic disease, suggesting that this technique may have additional value in locoregional staging in the future.[58] In a study involving 49 patients by Malik and colleagues, whole-body MRI was shown to have similar accuracy to PET/CT, not only for the detection of the primary tumor, but also for the detection of nodal deposits and the exclusion of systemic metastatic disease.[59]

Regarding nodal response assessment, Liu and colleagues were able to predict the effect of concurrent chemoradiotherapy using the combination of DCE-MRI and DWI 3 weeks after treatment, with a sensitivity of 98.6% and specificity of 73.8%.[60] **Figs. 6** and **7** show the potential of DCE-MRI and DWI in assessing treatment response.

Several factors, such as the fact that the esophagus is relatively narrow and is located deep within the thorax, cardiac motion and respiratory motion, and long imaging acquisition time are challenges in the efforts to obtain high quality MR images.[61] Using an external surface coil and cardiac gating with T2-weighted fast spin-echo sequences can aid in the improvement of MR image quality.[62]

Computed Tomography

Using a triple-phase dynamic contrast-enhanced CT protocol, Umeoka and colleagues found that the arterial phase acquired 35 seconds after the attenuation of 200 HU at the descending aorta to be the optimal phase for the visualization of esophageal cancer.[9]

Dual-energy spectral CT (DECT) imaging is an evolving field with more and more gastrointestinal applications. Although relatively few studies have been published on the use of DECT for the staging of esophageal cancer, Cheng and colleagues demonstrated an improvement of esophageal cancer lesion conspicuity with DECT and a high diagnostic accuracy for the differentiation of T1/2 from T3/4 disease (AUC 0.84).[10] Another study by Xi and colleagues investigated the potential of DECT for

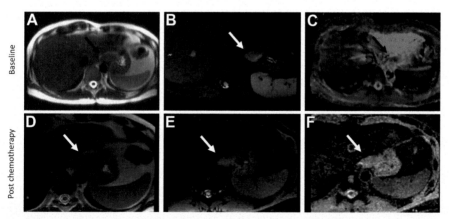

Fig. 6. Utility of MRI for treatment response assessment in a 59-year-old man with gastroesophageal junction adenocarcinoma. The mass shows intermediate signal on T2-weighted imaging (*A*) and diffusion restriction on DWI (*B*) and apparent diffusion coefficient (ADC) mapping (*C*). Post-treatment imaging show persistent intermediate signal on T2-weighted imaging (*D*) and reduced diffusion restriction (*E, F*), which corresponded to a 80% regression of tumor on pathology.

Baseline

Post neoadjuvant
chemotherapy

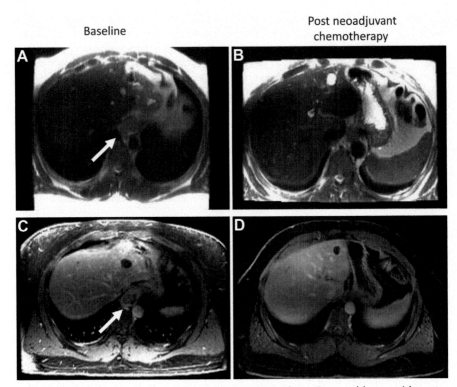

Fig. 7. Utility of MRI for treatment response assessment in a 49-year-old man with gastro-esophageal junction adenocarcinoma. T2-weighted imaging (*A*) intermediate gastroesophageal mass with hypoenhancement on postcontrast T1-weighted imaging (*C*) is shown. Post-neoadjuvant chemotherapy imaging shows resolution of the mass on T2-weighted imaging (*B*) and postcontrast imaging (*D*), consistent with radiologic complete response.

assessing treatment response to chemoradiotherapy and showed that normalized arterial and venous iodine concentrations were significantly lower in responsive patients compared with nonresponsive patients.[63]

2-Deoxy-2-[18F]Fluoro-ᴅ-Glucose][18] Positron Emission Tomography/MRI

Technological advances in the recent years have made ^{18}F-FDG PET/MRI a clinically feasible and practical investigative tool, although its use in esophageal cancers is still in the early stages. With the potential to provide a more comprehensive assessment of metabolic and anatomic characteristics, its role in disease evaluation continues to expand (**Fig. 8**). In a preliminary study comparing ^{18}F-FDG PET/MRI with ^{18}F-FDG PET/CT for the staging of primary esophageal/gastroesophageal cancer, ^{18}F-FDG PET/MRI showed nonsignificant higher concordance for T staging.[64] A year later, Wang and colleagues showed that ^{18}F-FDG PET/MRI achieved the highest accuracy of 85.7% for T staging in comparison with MRI and contrast-enhanced CT, and ^{18}F-FDG PET/MRI also achieved the highest accuracy of 96.2% for N staging in comparison with ^{18}F-FDG PET/CT, MRI, and contrast-enhanced CT.[65] Elsewhere, Yu and colleagues showed that the ratio of metabolic tumor volume and minimal apparent diffusion coefficient were inversely correlated with progression-free and overall survival in patients with esophageal squamous cell carcinoma.[66]

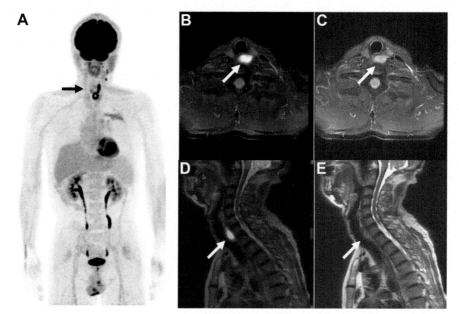

Fig. 8. Utility of ^{18}F-FDG PET/MRI for the assessment of locoregional disease extent in a 66-year-old patient with esophageal squamous cell carcinoma. MIP coronal ^{18}F-FDG PET (*A*), axial fused ^{18}F-FDG PET/MRI (*B*), axial postcontrast T1-weighted imaging (*C*), sagittal fused ^{18}F-FDG PET/MRI (*D*), and sagittal T2-weighted imaging (*E*) show an FDG-avid proximal esophageal mass-like wall thickening, extending to the left piriform recess.

Novel positron emission tomography tracers

[89]Zr-HER2. Approximately one-fourth of esophageal cancers exhibit HER2 overexpression.[67–69] Two phase III trials have shown an increased response rate and survival when trastuzumab, a HER2 antibody, was added to chemotherapy or chemotherapy in combination with PD1 blockade.[70,71] 89-Zirconium ([89]Zr)-labeled HER2 PET offers a noninvasive method to assess HER2 status, reflecting intratumoral heterogeneity that

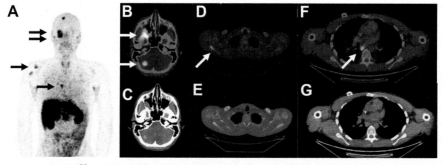

Fig. 9. Utility of [89]Zr-HER2 PET to demonstrate HER2 expression in a 38-year-old patient with esophageal cancer. [89]Zr-HER2 PET coronal MIP (*A*) shows several sites of metastatic disease (*black arrows*). Fused PET/CT and nonenhanced CT show a radiotracer avid right cerebellar and right orbital metastasis (*B, C, white arrows*). Chest images depict a radiotracer avid right scapula (*D, E*) and mediastinal node (*F, G*) metastasis (*white arrows*).

cannot be not evaluated on conventional imaging or using single biopsy[12] (**Fig. 9**). The radiopharmaceutical is assembled by conjugating trastuzumab with a deferoxamine chelator followed by radiolabeling with the positron emitter ^{89}Zr, which has a half-life of 78.4 h.[13] Two to five mCi of the radiolabeled trastuzumab or pertuzumab, containing approximately 2 mg of the antibody, is combined with non-radiolabeled antibody to make up a total mass of 50 mg. PET is performed 5 days after tracer injection, based on optimal tumor visualization from days 5 to 8 as described by O'Donoghue and colleagues.[13] Preliminary results by Lumish and colleagues in a small patient cohort indicate that at least 1 lesion with an SUV of at least 10 on ^{89}Zr-HER2 PET may be associated with response to HER2-directed therapy.[12] In addition, there was a trend showing a slightly higher progression-free survival in patients with at least 1 intense or very intense lesion on baseline ^{89}Zr-HER2 PET in patients receiving first-line HER2-directed therapy. Further studies are needed to validate these hypotheses. A limitation of ^{89}Zr-HER2 PET is its high background tracer uptake in organs, such as the liver, which may hinder the assessment of metastases.[12]

^{68}Ga-fibroblast activation protein inhibitor. Fibroblast activation protein (FAP) is highly expressed in the major cell population in tumor stroma and is associated with invasion, metastasis, and prognosis.[72,73] In a preliminary study, Giesel and colleagues studied the biodistribution and dosimetry estimates of 2 ^{68}Ga-FAP inhibitor (FAPI) agents for PET/CT, indicating the potential of ^{68}Ga-FAPI PET/CT as a new diagnostic method for cancer imaging.[74] They found an equal or even better tumor-to-background contrast ratio for ^{68}Ga-FAPI PET/CT compared with ^{18}F-FDG PET/CT. Recently, Liu and colleagues demonstrated that ^{68}Ga-DOTA-FAPI-04 PET was superior to standard ^{18}F-FDG PET/CT for detecting primary and metastatic esophageal lesions.[14] Elsewhere, good diagnostic performance has been shown for ^{68}Ga-FAPI PET/CT for the detection of lymph node metastases of esophageal cancer, which is limited with ^{18}F-FDG PET/CT.[15,34] ^{68}Ga-FAPI PET/CT has further demonstrated favorable tumor-to-background contrast in esophageal cancer, which might provide additional information in outlining the target volume for radiotherapy planning.[75] In contrast to ^{18}F-FDG PET/CT, no diet or fasting is necessary in preparation for ^{68}Ga-FAPI PET/CT.[74] Further research and clinical studies are warranted to establish the full clinical utility of ^{68}Ga-FAPI PET/CT in the management of esophageal cancer.

[18F]-3-fluoro-3-deoxy-L-thymidine. [18F]-3-fluoro-3-deoxy-L-thymidine (FLT) is a marker of proliferation, whose uptake is related to the thymidine salvage enzyme thymidine kinase 1 (TK-1), and was first applied for PET imaging in 1998 by Shields and colleagues.[76] Several years later, in the search of a more specific tracer compared with ^{18}F-FDG, Dittmann and colleagues showed that it was possible to monitor the early effects of anticancer chemotherapy using FLT uptake as a marker of tumor proliferation in an ex vivo model of human esophageal squamous cell carcinoma.[77] The utility of FLT PET has been studied in several types of cancer, including nonsmall cell lung cancer and non-Hodgkin lymphoma, showing its potential for treatment response assessment.[78,79] Compared with ^{18}F-FDG PET, ^{18}F-FLT-PET has been shown to be suitable and more specific in a preclinical esophageal cancer model for depicting early reductions in tumor proliferation, which precede tumor size changes after chemoradiotherapy, indicating a potential role in chemoradiotherapy response assessment.[80] Furthermore, ^{18}F-FLT PET has been found to result in fewer false-positive findings and higher specificity compared with ^{18}F-FDG PET/CT in the assessment of the regional lymph nodes in thoracic esophageal squamous cell carcinoma, indicating its potential for accurate locoregional staging.[81,82]

Hypoxia markers (¹⁸F- fluoroerythronitroimidazole, ¹⁸F-flouroazomycin arabinoside). Hypoxia is a critical factor in esophageal cancer, and the use of hypoxia tracers has garnered significant attention. Higher hypoxia rates have been observed in adenocarcinomas compared witho squamous cell carcinomas, which might partly explain the lower therapy response rate in adenocarcinomas.[83,84] Tumor tissue hypoxia can be identified using nitroimidazole derivatives, such as ¹⁸F- fluoroerythronitroimidazole (FETNIM) or ¹⁸F-flouroazomycin arabinoside (FAZA).[85] Hypoxia tracers have been shown to be associated with poorer response to treatment in patients following chemoradiotherapy[86] and in a mouse model following radiotherapy.[87] In a cohort with squamous cell esophageal carcinoma patients, FETNIM SUVmax values correlated with a poorer clinical response to treatment.[86] Klaassen and colleagues showed the feasibility and good repeatability of the hypoxia tracer ¹⁸F-HX4, a potentially promising tool for radiation therapy planning and treatment response monitoring in patients with esophageal cancer.[88]

⁶⁸Ga-Pentixafor. ⁶⁸Ga-Pentixafor is a radiotracer for imaging the receptor CXCR4, which has been shown to play a role in tumor growth and in the metastatic processes of esophageal cancer.[89] Linde and colleagues demonstrated the feasibility of ⁶⁸Ga-Pentixafor PET/CT in newly diagnosed and pretreated recurrent esophageal cancer.[90] Future potential applications of ⁶⁸Ga-Pentixafor include its use as a marker for metastatic development or radiation field expansion, complementary to currently utilized staging modalities.[90]

FUTURE DIRECTIONS
Radiomics and Artificial Intelligence

Radiomics is emerging as a valuable tool for the early detection and prognostication of esophageal malignancies, offering insights into the imaging characteristics of these malignancies and its potential for early diagnosis.[91] Several studies investigating the potential of radiomics in assessing response to neoadjuvant therapy have been published; although most studies lack external validation and are not used in clinical practice, several radiomic models have been developed for the assessment and prediction of treatment response and survival.[92–94] A promising recent radiomics study by Li and colleagues showed a high diagnostic performance in the training set and 2 validation sets for predicting pathologic complete response using tumor and lymph nodes contrast-enhanced CT features.[94] Meanwhile, Lu and colleagues identified the dual-region radiomic signature from the primary tumor and regional lymph nodes as an independent prognostic marker, which outperformed the single-region signature in the prediction of overall survival in patients with esophageal squamous cell cancer.[93] The potential of radiomics in esophageal cancer imaging also extends beyond diagnosis to treatment planning and assessment. For instance, radiomics has been utilized to analyze errors in margin delineation during treatment planning for esophageal radiation therapy, emphasizing its role in treatment precision and efficacy.[95]

Meanwhile, deep learning algorithms based on convolutional neural network architecture have been employed to perform semantic segmentation and diagnosis of esophageal cancer on CT.[96,97] Moreover, hyperspectral imaging combined with deep learning has shown promise for the early detection of esophageal cancer, highlighting the diverse technological approaches in this field.[98]

Theranostic nanoparticles have shown potential in drug delivery and cancer therapy, offering personalized medicine approaches.[99] Several nanoparticle platforms have been developed in esophageal cancer, providing a platform for radiosensitization and synergistic chemoradiotherapy.[100–103] Biomarkers such as VEGF are increasingly recognized as potential targets in esophageal cancer, with several studies highlighting their significance in predicting drug response and prognosis.[104,105] Moreover, specific DNA methylation markers have shown promise in the diagnosis and prognosis of esophageal cancer, offering additional avenues for precision medicine approaches.[106]

SUMMARY

In conclusion, rapid advancements in technology and a deeper understanding of tumor biology are transforming the landscape of imaging for esophageal and gastroesophageal junction malignancies. Although traditional modalities like CT, EUS, and PET/CT remain crucial, emerging techniques such as high-resolution MRI, innovative PET tracers, and the integration of artificial intelligence and radiomics are pushing the boundaries of diagnostic accuracy and treatment planning. These developments hold the promise of not only improving detection and staging capabilities but also paving the way for more personalized and effective treatment strategies. Moving forward, it is crucial to continue research and clinical validation to fully harness these innovations, ultimately enhancing patient outcomes in the complex management of esophageal cancers.

CLINICS CARE POINTS

- Multimodal imaging integrating multiple imaging modalities such as CT, ^{18}F-PET/CT, EUS, and MRI can improve the accuracy of staging and treatment planning.
- It is important not to over-rely on size criteria alone for lymph node assessment, as metastatic lymph nodes can be smaller than the traditional 1 cm size criteria for malignancy on CT.
- It is important to be aware of potential false-positive results on ^{18}F-FDG PET/CT, such as those caused by inflammation or infection.
- HER2 overexpression can guide treatment decisions and potentially improve outcomes.
- Radiomics, artificial intelligence methods and novel PET tracers hold promise but require further validation before widespread clinical use.

ACKNOWLEDGMENTS

The authors thank Joanne Chin, MFA, ELS, for her help in editing this article.

DISCLOSURE

The authors have nothing to disclose.

REFERENCES

1. Ajani JA, D'Amico TA, Bentrem DJ, et al. Esophageal and esophagogastric junction cancers, version 2.2023, NCCN Clinical Practice Guidelines in Oncology. J Natl Compr Canc Netw 2023;21(4):393–422.
2. Barber TW, Duong CP, Leong T, et al. 18F-FDG PET/CT has a high impact on patient management and provides powerful prognostic stratification in the primary staging of esophageal cancer: a prospective study with mature survival data. J Nucl Med 2012;53(6):864–71.
3. Schmidlin EJ, Gill RR. New frontiers in esophageal radiology. Ann Transl Med 2021;9(10):904.

4. Schroder W, Baldus SE, Monig SP, et al. Lymph node staging of esophageal squamous cell carcinoma in patients with and without neoadjuvant radiochemotherapy: histomorphologic analysis. World J Surg 2002;26(5):584–7.

5. van Westreenen HL, Westerterp M, Bossuyt PM, et al. Systematic review of the staging performance of 18F-fluorodeoxyglucose positron emission tomography in esophageal cancer. J Clin Oncol 2004;22(18):3805–12.

6. Luketich JD, Schauer PR, Meltzer CC, et al. Role of positron emission tomography in staging esophageal cancer. Ann Thorac Surg 1997;64(3):765–9.

7. Krill T, Baliss M, Roark R, et al. Accuracy of endoscopic ultrasound in esophageal cancer staging. J Thorac Dis 2019;11(Suppl 12):S1602–9.

8. De Cobelli F, Palumbo D, Albarello L, et al. Esophagus and Stomach: Is There a Role for MR Imaging? Magn Reson Imaging Clin N Am 2020;28(1):1–15.

9. Umeoka S, Koyama T, Togashi K, et al. Esophageal cancer: evaluation with triple-phase dynamic CT–initial experience. Radiology 2006;239(3):777–83.

10. Cheng F, Liu Y, Du L, et al. Evaluation of optimal monoenergetic images acquired by dual-energy CT in the diagnosis of T staging of thoracic esophageal cancer. Insights Imaging 2023;14(1):33.

11. van Dongen G, Beaino W, Windhorst AD, et al. The role of (89)Zr-immuno-PET in navigating and derisking the development of biopharmaceuticals. J Nucl Med 2021;62(4):438–45.

12. Lumish MA, Maron SB, Paroder V, et al. Noninvasive assessment of human epidermal growth factor receptor 2 (HER2) in esophagogastric cancer using (89)Zr-trastuzumab PET: a pilot study. J Nucl Med 2023;64(5):724–30.

13. O'Donoghue JA, Lewis JS, Pandit-Taskar N, et al. Pharmacokinetics, biodistribution, and radiation dosimetry for (89)zr-trastuzumab in patients with esophagogastric cancer. J Nucl Med 2018;59(1):161–6.

14. Liu H, Hu Z, Yang X, et al. Comparison of [(68)Ga]Ga-DOTA-FAPI-04 and [(18)F] FDG uptake in esophageal cancer. Front Oncol 2022;12:875081.

15. Liu H, Yang X, You Z, et al. Role of 68Ga-FAPI-04 PET/CT in the initial staging of esophageal cancer. Nuklearmedizin 2023;62(1):38–44. Rolle von 68Ga-FAPI-04 PET/CT in der Erstinszenierung von Speiserohrenkrebs.

16. Ayyappan S, Prabhakar D, Sharma N. Epidermal growth factor receptor (EGFR)-targeted therapies in esophagogastric cancer. Anticancer Res 2013; 33(10):4139–55.

17. D'Journo XB. Clinical implication of the innovations of the 8(th) edition of the TNM classification for esophageal and esophago-gastric cancer. J Thorac Dis 2018;10(Suppl 22):S2671–81.

18. Amin MB, Edge SB, Greene FL, et al. AJCC cancer staging manual, 1024. Springer; 2017.

19. Reinig JW, Stanley JH, Schabel SI. CT evaluation of thickened esophageal walls. AJR Am J Roentgenol 1983;140(5):931–4.

20. Xia F, Mao J, Ding J, et al. Observation of normal appearance and wall thickness of esophagus on CT images. Eur J Radiol 2009;72(3):406–11.

21. Li R, Chen TW, Wang LY, et al. Quantitative measurement of contrast enhancement of esophageal squamous cell carcinoma on clinical MDCT. World J Radiol 2012;4(4):179–85.

22. Vesprini D, Ung Y, Dinniwell R, et al. Improving observer variability in target delineation for gastro-oesophageal cancer–the role of (18F)fluoro-2-deoxy-D-glucose positron emission tomography/computed tomography. Clin Oncol 2008;20(8):631–8.

23. Picus D, Balfe DM, Koehler RE, et al. Computed tomography in the staging of esophageal carcinoma. Radiology 1983;146(2):433–8.

24. Daffner RH, Halber MD, Postlethwait RW, et al. CT of the esophagus. II. Carcinoma. AJR Am J Roentgenol 1979;133(6):1051–5.

25. Pongpornsup S, Posri S, Totanarungroj K. Diagnostic accuracy of multidetector computed tomography (MDCT) in evaluation for mediastinal invasion of esophageal cancer. J Med Assoc Thai 2012;95(5):704–11.

26. Thosani N, Singh H, Kapadia A, et al. Diagnostic accuracy of EUS in differentiating mucosal versus submucosal invasion of superficial esophageal cancers: a systematic review and meta-analysis. Gastrointest Endosc 2012;75(2):242–53.

27. Bergeron EJ, Lin J, Chang AC, et al. Endoscopic ultrasound is inadequate to determine which T1/T2 esophageal tumors are candidates for endoluminal therapies. J Thorac Cardiovasc Surg 2014;147(2):765–71. Discussion 771-3.

28. He LJ, Shan HB, Luo GY, et al. Endoscopic ultrasonography for staging of T1a and T1b esophageal squamous cell carcinoma. World J Gastroenterol 2014; 20(5):1340–7.

29. Cense HA, van Eijck CH, Tilanus HW. New insights in the lymphatic spread of oesophageal cancer and its implications for the extent of surgical resection. Best Pract Res Clin Gastroenterol 2006;20(5):893–906.

30. Gotink AW, van de Ven SEM, Ten Kate FJC, et al. Individual risk calculator to predict lymph node metastases in patients with submucosal (T1b) esophageal adenocarcinoma: a multicenter cohort study. Endoscopy 2022;54(2):109–17.

31. Committee ASoP, Evans JA, Early DS, et al. The role of endoscopy in the assessment and treatment of esophageal cancer. Gastrointest Endosc 2013;77(3): 328–34.

32. Yang GY, Wagner TD, Jobe BA, et al. The role of positron emission tomography in esophageal cancer. Gastrointest Cancer Res 2008;2(1):3–9.

33. Shi W, Wang W, Wang J, et al. Meta-analysis of 18FDG PET-CT for nodal staging in patients with esophageal cancer. Surg Oncol 2013;22(2):112–6.

34. Jiang C, Chen Y, Zhu Y, et al. Systematic review and meta-analysis of the accuracy of 18F-FDG PET/CT for detection of regional lymph node metastasis in esophageal squamous cell carcinoma. J Thorac Dis 2018;10(11):6066–76.

35. Okada M, Murakami T, Kumano S, et al. Integrated FDG-PET/CT compared with intravenous contrast-enhanced CT for evaluation of metastatic regional lymph nodes in patients with resectable early stage esophageal cancer. Ann Nucl Med 2009;23(1):73–80.

36. Asad S, Aquino SL, Piyavisetpat N, et al. False-positive FDG positron emission tomography uptake in nonmalignant chest abnormalities. AJR Am J Roentgenol 2004;182(4):983–9.

37. You JJ, Wong RK, Darling G, et al. Clinical utility of 18F-fluorodeoxyglucose positron emission tomography/computed tomography in the staging of patients with potentially resectable esophageal cancer. J Thorac Oncol 2013;8(12): 1563–9.

38. Goense L, van Rossum PS, Reitsma JB, et al. Diagnostic Performance of (1)(8) F-FDG PET and PET/CT for the detection of recurrent esophageal cancer after treatment with curative intent: a systematic review and meta-analysis. J Nucl Med 2015;56(7):995–1002.

39. Toya R, Matsuyama T, Saito T, et al. Impact of hybrid FDG-PET/CT on gross tumor volume definition of cervical esophageal cancer: reducing interobserver variation. J Radiat Res 2019;60(3):348–52.

40. Chhabra A, Ong LT, Kuk D, et al. Prognostic significance of PET assessment of metabolic response to therapy in oesophageal squamous cell carcinoma. Br J Cancer 2015;113(12):1658–65.
41. Goense L, Ruurda JP, Carter BW, et al. Prediction and diagnosis of interval metastasis after neoadjuvant chemoradiotherapy for oesophageal cancer using (18)F-FDG PET/CT. Eur J Nucl Med Mol Imag 2018;45(10):1742–51.
42. Karahan Sen NP, Aksu A, Capa Kaya G. Volumetric evaluation of staging (18)F-FDG PET/CT images in patients with esophageal Cancer. Mol Imaging Radionucl Ther 2022;31(3):216–22.
43. Hofheinz F, Li Y, Steffen IG, et al. Confirmation of the prognostic value of pretherapeutic tumor SUR and MTV in patients with esophageal squamous cell carcinoma. Eur J Nucl Med Mol Imag 2019;46(7):1485–94.
44. Krengli M, Ferrara E, Guaschino R, et al. 18F-FDG PET/CT as predictive and prognostic factor in esophageal cancer treated with combined modality treatment. Ann Nucl Med 2022;36(5):450–9.
45. Martinez A, Infante JR, Quiros J, et al. Baseline (18)F-FDG PET/CT quantitative parameters as prognostic factors in esophageal squamous cell cancer. Rev Esp Med Nucl Imagen Mol (Engl Ed). May-Jun 2022;41(3):164–70.
46. Gopal A, Xi Y, Subramaniam RM, et al. Intratumoral metabolic heterogeneity and other quantitative (18)F-FDG PET/CT parameters for prognosis prediction in esophageal cancer. Radiol Imaging Cancer 2021;3(1):e200022.
47. Yamada I, Miyasaka N, Hikishima K, et al. Gastric carcinoma: ex vivo MR imaging at 7.0 T-correlation with histopathologic findings. Radiology 2015;275(3):841–8.
48. Lee SL, Yadav P, Starekova J, et al. Diagnostic performance of MRI for esophageal carcinoma: a systematic review and meta-analysis. Radiology 2021;299(3):583–94.
49. Chen YL, Jiang Y, Chen TW, et al. Assessing microcirculation in resectable oesophageal squamous cell carcinoma with dynamic contrast-enhanced MRI for identifying primary tumour and lymphatic metastasis. Sci Rep 2019;9(1):124.
50. Li Q, Liu T, Ding Z. Neoadjuvant immunotherapy for resectable esophageal cancer: a review. Front Immunol 2022;13:1051841.
51. van Rossum PSN, Goense L, Meziani J, et al. Endoscopic biopsy and EUS for the detection of pathologic complete response after neoadjuvant chemoradiotherapy in esophageal cancer: a systematic review and meta-analysis. Gastrointest Endosc 2016;83(5):866–79.
52. Heneghan HM, Donohoe C, Elliot J, et al. Can CT-PET and endoscopic assessment post-neoadjuvant chemoradiotherapy predict residual disease in esophageal cancer? Ann Surg 2016;264(5):831–8.
53. Gollub MJ, Costello JR, Ernst RD, et al. A primer on rectal MRI in patients on watch-and-wait treatment for rectal cancer. Abdom Radiol (NY) 2023;48(9):2836–73.
54. Qu J, Zhang H, Wang Z, et al. Comparison between free-breathing radial VIBE on 3-T MRI and endoscopic ultrasound for preoperative T staging of resectable oesophageal cancer, with histopathological correlation. Eur Radiol 2018;28(2):780–7.
55. Giganti F, Ambrosi A, Petrone MC, et al. Prospective comparison of MR with diffusion-weighted imaging, endoscopic ultrasound, MDCT and positron emission tomography-CT in the pre-operative staging of oesophageal cancer: results from a pilot study. Br J Radiol 2016;89(1068):20160087.

56. Harino T, Yamasaki M, Murai S, et al. Impact of MRI on the post-therapeutic diagnosis of T4 esophageal cancer. Esophagus 2023;20(4):740–8.

57. Wu L, Ou J, Chen TW, et al. Tumour volume of resectable oesophageal squamous cell carcinoma measured with MRI correlates well with T category and lymphatic metastasis. Eur Radiol 2018;28(11):4757–65.

58. Pultrum BB, van der Jagt EJ, van Westreenen HL, et al. Detection of lymph node metastases with ultrasmall superparamagnetic iron oxide (USPIO)-enhanced magnetic resonance imaging in oesophageal cancer: a feasibility study. Cancer Imag 2009;9(1):19–28.

59. Malik V, Harmon M, Johnston C, et al. Whole body MRI in the staging of esophageal cancer–a prospective comparison with whole body 18F-FDG PET-CT. Dig Surg 2015;32(5):397–408.

60. Liu C, Sun R, Wang J, et al. Combination of DCE-MRI and DWI in predicting the treatment effect of concurrent chemoradiotherapy in esophageal carcinoma. BioMed Res Int 2020;2020:2576563.

61. Riddell AM, Hillier J, Brown G, et al. Potential of surface-coil MRI for staging of esophageal cancer. AJR Am J Roentgenol 2006;187(5):1280–7.

62. Riddell AM, Richardson C, Scurr E, et al. The development and optimization of high spatial resolution MRI for imaging the oesophagus using an external surface coil. Br J Radiol 2006;79(947):873–9.

63. Ge X, Yu J, Wang Z, et al. Comparative study of dual energy CT iodine imaging and standardized concentrations before and after chemoradiotherapy for esophageal cancer. BMC Cancer 2018;18(1):1120.

64. Sharkey AR, Sah BR, Withey SJ, et al. Initial experience in staging primary oesophageal/gastro-oesophageal cancer with 18F-FDG PET/MRI. Eur J Hybrid Imaging 2021;5(1):23.

65. Wang F, Guo R, Zhang Y, et al. Value of (18)F-FDG PET/MRI in the preoperative assessment of resectable esophageal squamous cell carcinoma: a comparison with (18)F-FDG PET/CT, MRI, and contrast-enhanced CT. Front Oncol 2022;12: 844702.

66. Yu CW, Chen XJ, Lin YH, et al. Prognostic value of (18)F-FDG PET/MR imaging biomarkers in oesophageal squamous cell carcinoma. Eur J Radiol 2019;120: 108671.

67. Janjigian YY, Sanchez-Vega F, Jonsson P, et al. Genetic predictors of response to systemic therapy in esophagogastric cancer. Cancer Discov 2018;8(1): 49–58.

68. Chua TC, Merrett ND. Clinicopathologic factors associated with HER2-positive gastric cancer and its impact on survival outcomes–a systematic review. Int J Cancer 2012;130(12):2845–56.

69. Schoppmann SF, Jesch B, Friedrich J, et al. Expression of Her-2 in carcinomas of the esophagus. Am J Surg Pathol 2010;34(12):1868–73.

70. Bang YJ, Van Cutsem E, Feyereislova A, et al. Trastuzumab in combination with chemotherapy versus chemotherapy alone for treatment of HER2-positive advanced gastric or gastro-oesophageal junction cancer (ToGA): a phase 3, open-label, randomised controlled trial. Lancet 2010;376(9742):687–97.

71. Janjigian YY, Kawazoe A, Yanez P, et al. The KEYNOTE-811 trial of dual PD-1 and HER2 blockade in HER2-positive gastric cancer. Nature 2021;600(7890): 727–30.

72. Huang R, Pu Y, Huang S, et al. FAPI-PET/CT in cancer imaging: a potential novel molecule of the century. Front Oncol 2022;12:854658.

73. Mori Y, Dendl K, Cardinale J, et al. FAPI PET: fibroblast activation protein inhibitor use in oncologic and nononcologic disease. Radiology 2023;306(2): e220749.

74. Giesel FL, Kratochwil C, Lindner T, et al. 68)Ga-FAPI PET/CT: biodistribution and preliminary dosimetry estimate of 2 DOTA-containing FAP-targeting agents in patients with various cancers. J Nucl Med 2019;60(3):386–92.

75. Zhao L, Chen S, Chen S, et al. 68)Ga-fibroblast activation protein inhibitor PET/CT on gross tumour volume delineation for radiotherapy planning of oesophageal cancer. Radiother Oncol 2021;158:55–61.

76. Shields AF, Grierson JR, Dohmen BM, et al. Imaging proliferation in vivo with [F-18]FLT and positron emission tomography. Nat Med 1998;4(11):1334–6.

77. Dittmann H, Dohmen BM, Kehlbach R, et al. Early changes in [18F]FLT uptake after chemotherapy: an experimental study. Eur J Nucl Med Mol Imag 2002; 29(11):1462–9.

78. Herrmann K, Buck AK, Schuster T, et al. Predictive value of initial 18F-FLT uptake in patients with aggressive non-Hodgkin lymphoma receiving R-CHOP treatment. J Nucl Med 2011;52(5):690–6.

79. Everitt SJ, Ball DL, Hicks RJ, et al. Differential (18)F-FDG and (18)F-FLT uptake on serial PET/CT imaging before and during definitive chemoradiation for non-small cell lung cancer. J Nucl Med 2014;55(7):1069–74.

80. Apisarnthanarax S, Alauddin MM, Mourtada F, et al. Early detection of chemoradioresponse in esophageal carcinoma by 3'-deoxy-3'-3H-fluorothymidine using preclinical tumor models. Clin Cancer Res 2006;12(15):4590–7.

81. Han D, Yu J, Zhong X, et al. Comparison of the diagnostic value of 3-deoxy-3-18F-fluorothymidine and 18F-fluorodeoxyglucose positron emission tomography/computed tomography in the assessment of regional lymph node in thoracic esophageal squamous cell carcinoma: a pilot study. Dis Esophagus 2012;25(5):416–26.

82. van Westreenen HL, Cobben DC, Jager PL, et al. Comparison of 18F-FLT PET and 18F-FDG PET in esophageal cancer. J Nucl Med 2005;46(3):400–4.

83. Brink I, Baier P, Jüttner E, et al. Assessment of hypoxia in esophageal carcinomas using 18F-MISO PET. J Nucl Med 2008;49(supplement 1):113P.

84. Brink I, Imdahl A, Juettner E, et al. Metabolic differences between esophageal adeno- and squamous cell carcinomas measured with 18F-MISO and 18F-FDG PET. J Nucl Med 2006;47(suppl 1):229P.

85. Tao R, Ager B, Lloyd S, et al. Hypoxia imaging in upper gastrointestinal tumors and application to radiation therapy. J Gastrointest Oncol 2018;9(6):1044–53.

86. Yue J, Yang Y, Cabrera AR, et al. Measuring tumor hypoxia with (1)(8)F-FETNIM PET in esophageal squamous cell carcinoma: a pilot clinical study. Dis Esophagus 2012;25(1):54–61.

87. Melsens E, De Vlieghere E, Descamps B, et al. Hypoxia imaging with (18)F-FAZA PET/CT predicts radiotherapy response in esophageal adenocarcinoma xenografts. Radiat Oncol 2018;13(1):39.

88. Klaassen R, Bennink RJ, van Tienhoven G, et al. Feasibility and repeatability of PET with the hypoxia tracer [(18)F]HX4 in oesophageal and pancreatic cancer. Radiother Oncol 2015;116(1):94–9.

89. Domanska UM, Kruizinga RC, Nagengast WB, et al. A review on CXCR4/CXCL12 axis in oncology: no place to hide. Eur J Cancer 2013;49(1):219–30.

90. Linde P, Baues C, Wegen S, et al. Pentixafor PET/CT for imaging of chemokine receptor 4 expression in esophageal cancer - a first clinical approach. Cancer Imag 2021;21(1):22.

91. Wang J, Tang L, Lin L, et al. Imaging characteristics of esophageal cancer in multi-slice spiral CT and barium meal radiography and their early diagnostic value. J Gastrointest Oncol 2022;13(1):49–55.

92. Beukinga RJ, Poelmann FB, Kats-Ugurlu G, et al. Prediction of non-response to neoadjuvant chemoradiotherapy in esophageal cancer patients with (18)F-FDG PET radiomics based machine learning classification. Diagnostics 2022;12(5). https://doi.org/10.3390/diagnostics12051070.

93. Lu N, Zhang WJ, Dong L, et al. Dual-region radiomics signature: Integrating primary tumor and lymph node computed tomography features improves survival prediction in esophageal squamous cell cancer. Comput Methods Progr Biomed 2021;208:106287.

94. Li K, Zhang S, Hu Y, et al. Radiomics nomogram with added nodal features improves treatment response prediction in locally advanced esophageal squamous cell carcinoma: a multicenter study. Ann Surg Oncol 2023;30(13): 8231–43.

95. Yong S, Ying C, Fen Z, et al. Analysis of upper and middle segment esophageal setup errors and planning of target margins based on cone beam computed tomography for esophageal radiation with immobilized thermoplastic film. Precision Radiation Oncology 2019;3(1):4–7.

96. Chen S, Yang H, Fu J, et al. U-Net plus: deep semantic segmentation for esophagus and esophageal cancer in computed tomography images. IEEE Access 2019;7:82867–77.

97. Islam MM, Poly TN, Walther BA, et al. Deep learning for the diagnosis of esophageal cancer in endoscopic images: a systematic review and meta-analysis. Cancers 2022;14(23):5996.

98. Tsai CL, Mukundan A, Chung CS, et al. Hyperspectral imaging combined with artificial intelligence in the early detection of esophageal cancer. Cancers 2021;13(18):4593.

99. Kang H, Mintri S, Menon AV, et al. Pharmacokinetics, pharmacodynamics and toxicology of theranostic nanoparticles. 10.1039/C5NR05264E. Nanoscale 2015;7(45):18848–62.

100. Li X, Chen L, Luan S, et al. The development and progress of nanomedicine for esophageal cancer diagnosis and treatment. Semin Cancer Biol 2022;86(Pt 2): 873–85.

101. Luan S, Xie R, Yang Y, et al. Acid-responsive aggregated gold nanoparticles for radiosensitization and synergistic chemoradiotherapy in the treatment of esophageal cancer. Small 2022;18(19):e2200115.

102. Zhang X, Wang M, Feng J, et al. Multifunctional nanoparticles co-loaded with adriamycin and MDR-targeting siRNAs for treatment of chemotherapy-resistant esophageal cancer. J Nanobiotechnol 2022;20(1):166.

103. Zhou W, Liu Z, Wang N, et al. Hafnium-based metal-organic framework nanoparticles as a radiosensitizer to improve radiotherapy efficacy in esophageal cancer. ACS Omega 2022;7(14):12021–9.

104. Wang L, Yang HY, Zheng YQ. Personalized medicine of esophageal cancer. J Cancer Res Therapeut 2012;8(3):343–7.

105. Chen M, Cai E, Huang J, et al. Prognostic value of vascular endothelial growth factor expression in patients with esophageal cancer: a systematic review and meta-analysis. Cancer Epidemiol Biomarkers Prev 2012;21(7):1126–34.

106. Li D, Zhang L, Liu Y, et al. Specific DNA methylation markers in the diagnosis and prognosis of esophageal cancer. Aging (Albany NY) 2019;11(23): 11640–58.